Textbook of
NURSING
FOUNDATION

for Post Basic BSc Nursing Students

(As per the Syllabus of Indian Nursing Council)

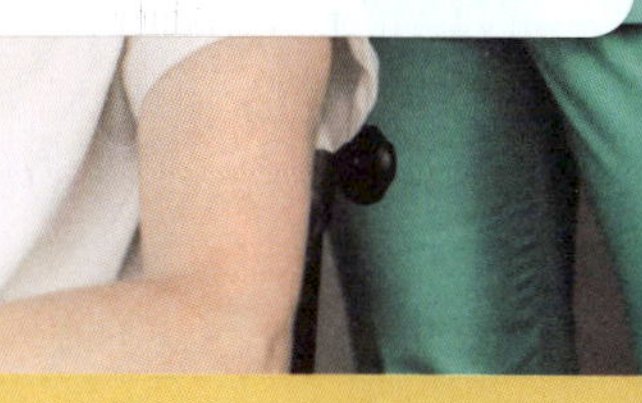

Textbook of

NURSING

FOUNDATION

for Post Basic BSc Nursing Students

(As per the Syllabus of Indian Nursing Council)

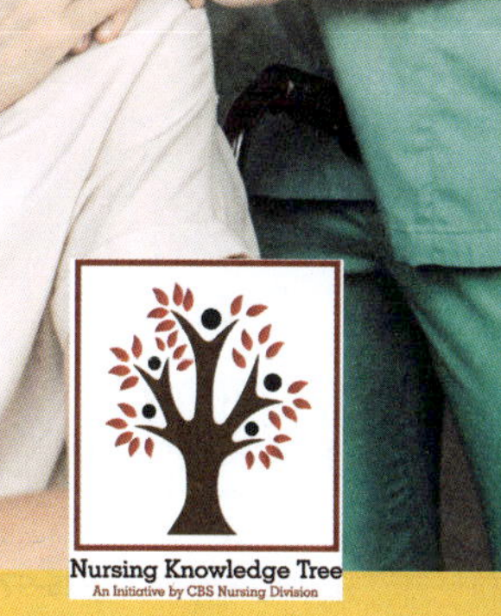

Samta Soni PhD, MSc (N), BSc (N)

Lecturer
Government College of Nursing
Jaipur, Rajasthan

CBS Publishers & Distributors Pvt Ltd

• New Delhi • Bengaluru • Chennai • Kochi • Kolkata • Lucknow • Mumbai
• Hyderabad • Jharkhand • Nagpur • Patna • Pune • Uttarakhand

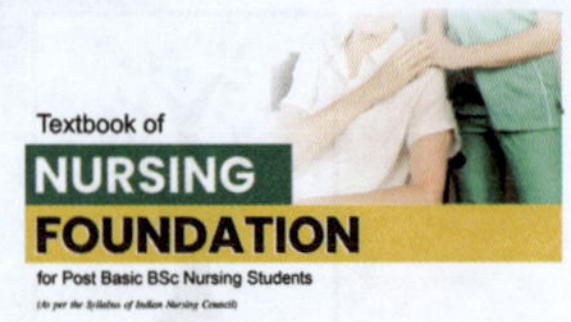

ISBN: 978-93-94525-97-9

First Edition: 2025

Published by **Satish Kumar Jain** and produced by **Varun Jain** for

CBS Publishers and Distributors Pvt Ltd

4819/XI Prahlad Street, 24 Ansari Road, Daryaganj, New Delhi 110 002, India.

Ph: +91-11-23289259, 23266861, 23266867   Website: www.cbspd.com

Fax: 011-23243014

e-mail: delhi@cbspd.com; cbspubs@airtelmail.in.

Corporate Office: 204 FIE, Industrial Area, Patparganj, Delhi 110 092

Ph: +91-11-4934 4934   Fax: 4934 4935

e-mail: feedback@cbspd.com; bhupesharora@cbspd.com

Branches

- **Bengaluru:** Seema House 2975, 17th Cross, K.R. Road, Banasankari 2nd Stage, Bengaluru-560 070, Karnataka
  Ph: +91-80-26771678/79   Fax: +91-80-26771680   e-mail: bangalore@cbspd.com

- **Chennai:** 7, Subbaraya Street, Shenoy Nagar, Chennai-600 030, Tamil Nadu
  Ph: +91-44-26680620, 26681266   Fax: +91-44-42032115   e-mail: chennai@cbspd.com

- **Kochi:** 68/1534, 35, 36-Power House Road, Opp. KSEB, Cochin-682018, Kochi, Kerala
  Ph: +91-484-4059061-65   Fax: +91-484-4059065   e-mail: kochi@cbspd.com

- **Kolkata:** Hind Ceramics Compound, 1st Floor, 147, Nilganj Road, Belghoria, Kolkata-700056, West Bengal
  Ph: +033-2563-3055/56   e-mail: kolkata@cbspd.com

- **Lucknow:** Basement, Khushnuma Complex, 7-Meerabai Marg (Behind Jawahar Bhawan), Lucknow-226001, Uttar Pradesh
  Ph: +0522-4000032   e-mail: tiwari.lucknow@cbspd.com

- **Mumbai:** PWD Shed, Gala No. 25/26, Ramchandra Bhatt Marg, Next to J.J. Hospital Gate No. 2, Opp. Union Bank of India, Noor Baug, Mumbai-400009, Maharashtra
  Ph: +91-22-66661880/89   Fax: +91-22-24902342   e-mail: mumbai@cbspd.com

Representatives

- **Hyderabad**   +91-9885175004   • **Jharkhand**   +91-9811541605   • **Nagpur**   +91-9421945513
- **Patna**   +91-9334159340   • **Pune**   +91-9623451994   • **Uttarakhand**   +91-9716462459

Printed at : Goyal Offset Works Pvt. Ltd. Haryana

Extends its Tribute to

Florence Nightingale

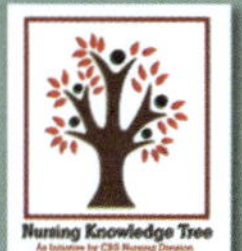

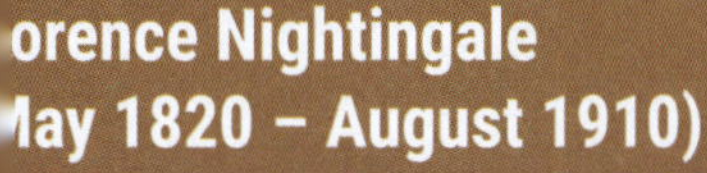

Preface

In the ever evolving landscape of healthcare, the role of nurses remains foundational to the delivery of quality patient care. The *Textbook of Nursing Foundation for Post Basic BSc Nursing*, has been meticulously crafted to align with the Indian Nursing Council (INC) and Rajasthan University of Health Sciences (RUHS) syllabus, providing nursing students with a comprehensive foundation in the art and science of nursing.

The book comprises 14 chapters which create a logical progression through the fundamental concepts of nursing, moving from theoretical foundations to practical applications. The content is structured to build your understanding systematically:

Foundation and Professional Context (Chapters 1–3)

Beginning with "Introduction of Nursing in India", the book establishes historical context before exploring contemporary "Trends and Issues in Nursing Education". The chapters on "Code of Ethics and Professional Conduct of Nurses" then set the moral framework for nursing practice.

Core Concepts and Theoretical Framework (Chapters 4–7)

The text progresses through essential theoretical understanding with chapters on "Concepts of Health and Illness", "Stress and Adaptation", "Legal and Ethical Aspects of Nursing", and the "Metaparadigm of Nursing", and provides students with a robust conceptual foundation.

Professional Practice and Quality (Chapters 8–11)

The middle part of the book focuses on practical application through chapters covering the "Nursing Process", "Quality Assurance in Nursing", "Professional Bodies in Nursing", and "Nursing Care Systems", bridging theory with real-world practice.

Clinical Skills and Patient Care (Chapters 12–14)

The final part addresses crucial practical skills through chapters on "Communication", "Patient Care During Admission, Discharge, and Surgery", and "Asepsis", ensuring students master essential clinical competencies.

Special features integrated throughout the text include:

- Step-by-step procedural instructions
- Cultural competency considerations
- Critical thinking exercises
- Quality improvement frameworks
- Professional development guidance

This textbook emphasizes both the scientific principles and the humanitarian essence of nursing. Each chapter includes carefully constructed learning objectives, practical examples, and assessment tools designed to develop clinical competence alongside critical thinking skills.

I have paid particular attention to making complex concepts accessible while maintaining the depth necessary for professional practice. The language is clear and precise, supplemented by illustrations, diagrams, and tables to enhance understanding.

As healthcare continues to evolve, I remain committed to updating this content to reflect the latest developments in nursing practice. I sincerely welcome the feedback from students, educators, and practitioners to help maintain the relevance and effectiveness of this educational resource.

May this textbook serve as your trusted companion in your journey to becoming a skilled and compassionate nursing professional.

Samta Soni

Acknowledgments

This book would never have been a reality without the belief and support of two most important people, **Mr Satish Kumar Jain** (Chairman) and **Mr Varun Jain** (Managing Director), M/s CBS Publishers and Distributors Pvt Ltd. I am thankful to them for their immense encouragement and guidance in the publication of this book. One more person who has acted like the backbone to this book is **Mr Bhupesh Aarora** [Sr. Vice President – Publishing and Marketing (Health Sciences Division)], without him this book wouldn't have been what it is today.

I sincerely thank the entire CBS team for bringing out the book with utmost care and attractive presentation. I would like to thank Ms Nitasha Arora (Assistant General Manager Publishing – Medical and Nursing), Ms Daljeet Kaur (Assistant Publishing Manager) and Dr Anju Dhir (Sr. Product Manager and Medical Development Editor) for their publishing support. I would also extend my thanks to Mr Shivendu Bhushan Pandey (Sr. Manager and Team Lead), Ms Surbhi Gupta (Sr. English Editor), Mr Ashutosh Pathak (Sr. Proofreader cum Team Coordinator) and all the production team members for devoting laborious hours in designing and typesetting the book.

Reviewers

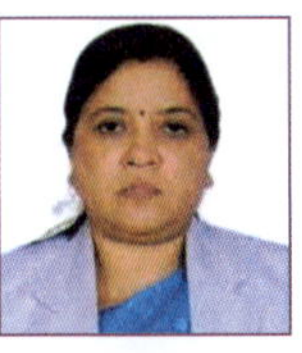

Alka Devanand Tajne
PhD (N), MSc (N), GNM, PBBSc (N)
Professor cum Principal
Vibrant Nursing College
Surat, Gujarat

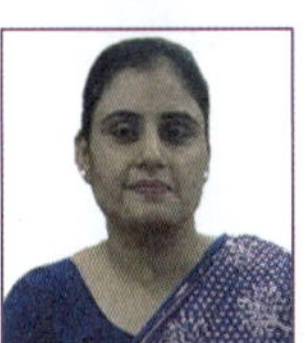

Amritpal Kaur
Community Health Nursing
PhD (N), MSc (N)
Professor cum Vice Principal
SGL Nursing College
Jalandhar, Punjab

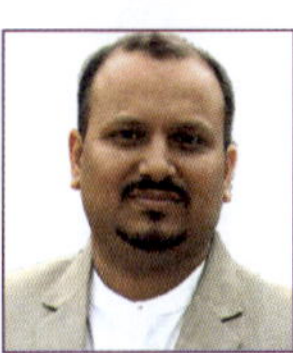

Ankit Sharma
Community Health Nursing
MSc (N)
Principal
Avadh Institute of Medical
Technology and Hospital
Lucknow, Uttar Pradesh

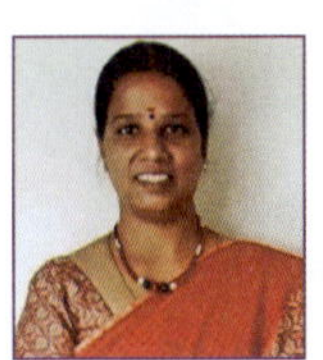

Arulmozhi Baskaran P M
Community Health Nursing
PhD (N), MSc (N)
Principal
PESU Institute of Nursing
PES University
Bengaluru, Karnataka

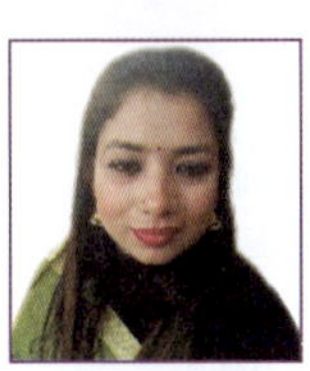

Farheen Shah
Obstetrics and Gynecological Nursing
MSc (N)
Principal
Vatsalya Nursing College
Gomti Nagar
Lucknow, Uttar Pradesh

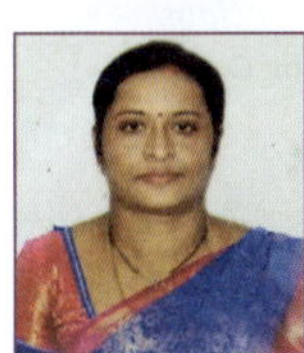

Hemamalini J
Obstetrics and Gynecological Nursing
PhD (N)
Principal
Vel Nursing College
Thiruvallur, Tamil Nadu

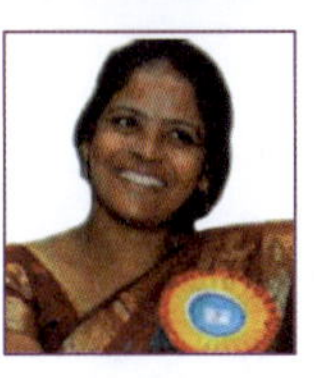

Kalpana Boddu
Community Health Nursing
PhD (N) Scholar, MSc (N)
Professor
Sree Narayana Nursing College
Nellore, Andhra Pradesh

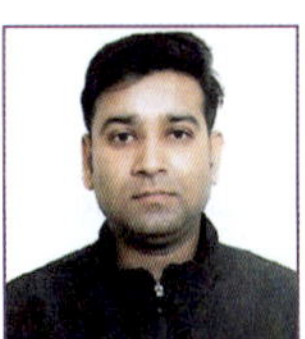

Lovelesh Singh
Medical Surgical Nursing
PhD (N) Scholar, MSc (N)
Associate Professor
Bombay Hospital College of Nursing
Indore, Madhya Pradesh

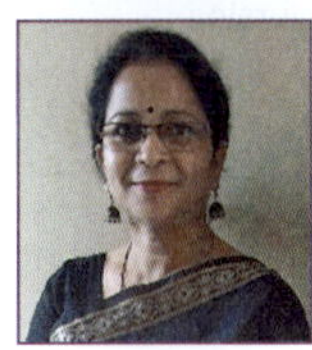

Manju Rajput
Obstetrics and Gynecological Nursing
PhD (N), MSc (N)
Principal
GNIOT Institute of Medical Sciences
& Research
Greater Noida, Uttar Pradesh

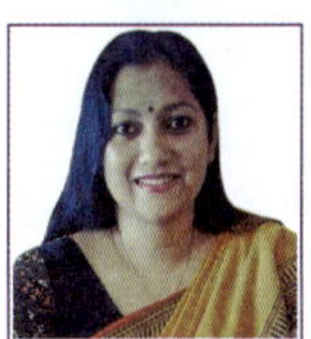

Neeta Bhide
Obstetrics and Gynecological Nursing
MSc (OBG Nursing), (Nutrition and
Dietetics), MA (Sociology),
(Psychology), (Human Rights),
MBA (Health Care Management)
Vice Principal
SAIMS College of Nursing
Indore, Madhya Pradesh

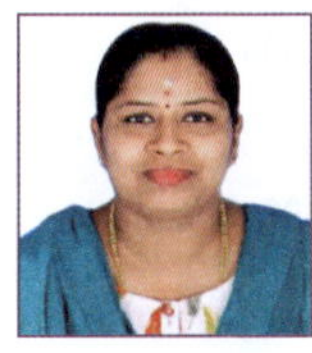

Padmavathi Kuppusamy
Medical Surgical Nursing
PhD (N), MSc (N)
Professor cum Principal
Lingayas Institute of Health Sciences
Nursing
Faridabad, Haryana

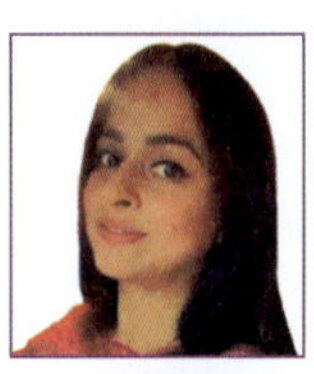

Pallavi Pathania
Medical Surgical Nursing
(Cardiac CTVS Specialty)
PhD (N) Scholar, MSc (N)
Professor
Shimla Nursing College
Shurala, Shimla, Himachal Pradesh

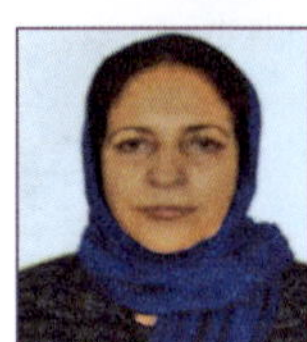

Perkash Kour
Medical Surgical Nursing
MSc (N), MA
Professor cum Principal
IBN-Sina College of Nursing and
Health Sciences, Ompura Budgam,
Jammu & Kashmir

The names of the reviewers are arranged in an alphabetical order.

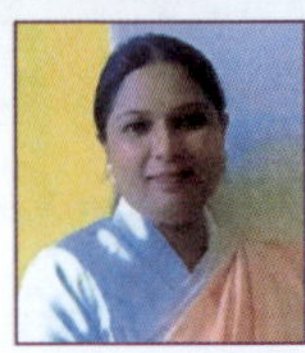

Rakhi Chandel
Child Health Nursing
PhD Pursuing, MSc (N), Master
Trainer Basic Neonatal Resuscitation
Program, Elderly and Palliative Care,
Simulation-Based Education
Professor and HOD
Choithram College of Nursing Indore,
Madhya Pradesh

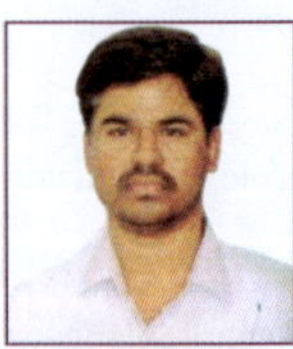

Ramakrishna Degani
Community Health Nursing
MSc (N)
Professor and HOD
Adesh University
Bathinda, Punjab

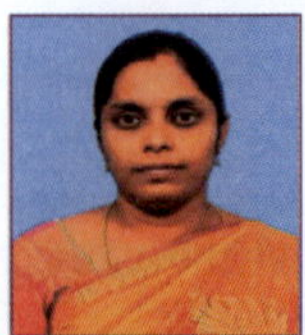

Ramya G M
Psychiatric Nursing
PhD (N) Pursuing, MSc (N)
Vice Principal
Vel Nursing College
Thiruvallur, Tamil Nadu

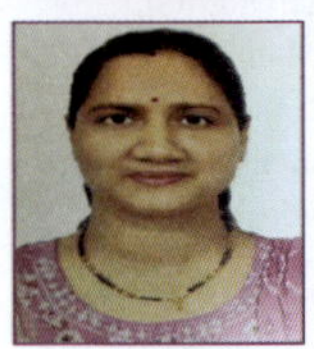

Rekha Kotnala
Medical Surgical Nursing
PhD (N), MSc (N)
Faculty
RAK College of Nursing
Lajpat Nagar, New Delhi

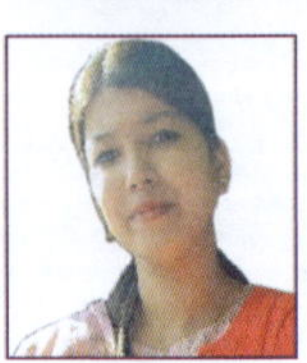

Ritika Soni
Mental Health Nursing
MSc (N), MA (Clinical Psychology)
Associate Processor
Shimla Nursing College
Shurala, Shimla
Himachal Pradesh

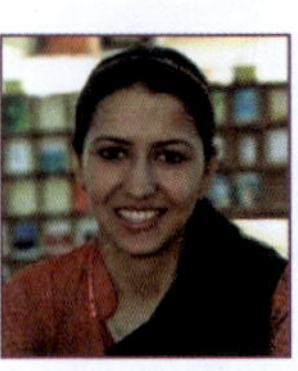

Ritu Rilta
Mental Health Nursing
MSc (N)
Associate Processor
Modern Nursing College
Shimla, Himachal Pradesh

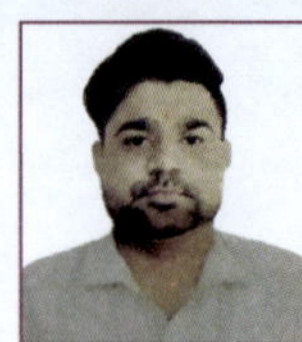

Sheeshpal Chauhan
Psychiatry Nursing
MSC (N)
Principal
Florence College of Nursing
Faridabad, Haryana

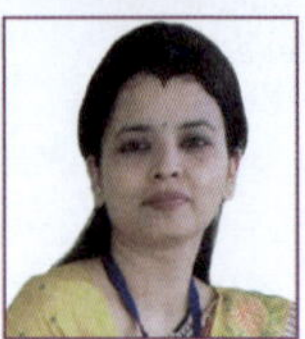

Sonam Dubey
Medical Surgical Nursing
PhD (N), MSc (N)
Professor
Smt Rukmaniben Deepchandbhai
Gardi Nurses Training Centre
Indore, Madhya Pradesh

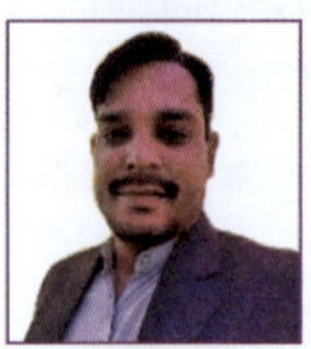

Sushil Kumar Rundle
Community Health Nursing
MSc (N)
Associate Professor
Symbiosis Institute of Nursing
Jaipur, Rajasthan

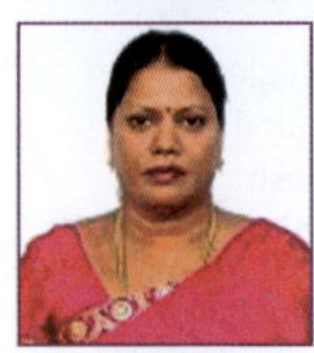

V Hemavathy
Medical Surgical Nursing
PhD (N), MSc (N), M Phil, MA
Principal
Shree Balaji College of Nursing
Chromepet, Chennai

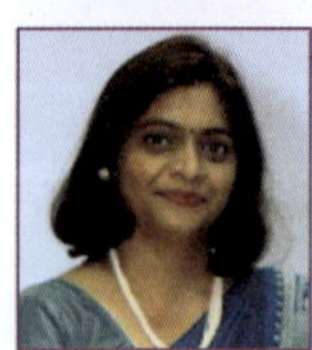

Vaishali Santosh Jadhav
Medical Surgical Nursing
PhD (N), MSc (N)
Professor cum Principal
College of Nursing
Bharati Vidyapeeth
Deemed University
Navi Mumbai, Maharashtra

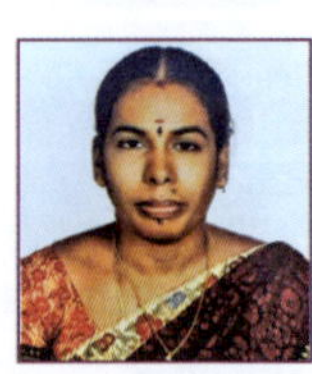

Viruthasarani K
Community Health Nursing
PhD (N) Scholar, MSc (N)
Professor cum Vice Principal
Vivekanandha Nursing College
Puducherry

The names of the reviewers are arranged in an alphabetical order.

From the Publisher's Desk

Nursing Education has a rich history, often characterized by traditional teaching techniques that have evolved over time. Primarily, teaching took place within classroom settings. Lectures, textbooks, and clinical rotations were the core teaching tools; and students majorly relied on textbooks by local or foreign publishers for quality education. However, today, technology has completely transformed the field of nursing education, making it an integral part of the curriculum. It has evolved to include a range of technological tools that enhance the learning experience and better prepare students for clinical practice.

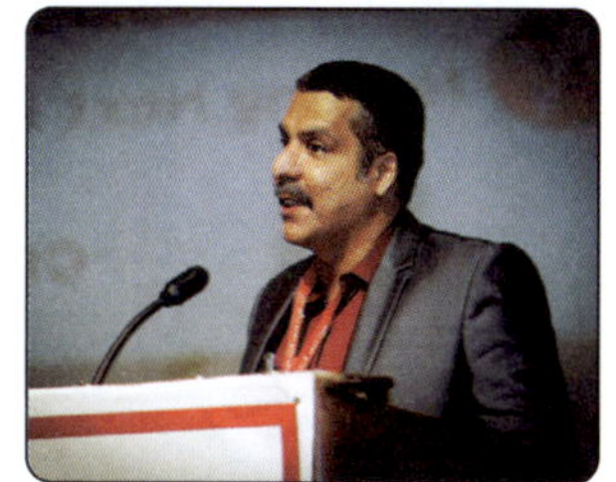

As publishers, we've been contributing to the field of Medical Science, Nursing and Allied Sciences and earned the trust of many. By supporting **Indian authors**, coupled with **nursing webinars and conferences**, we have paved an easier path for aspiring nurses, empowering them to excel in national and state level exams. With this, we're not only enhancing the quality of patient care but also enabling future nurses to adapt to new challenges and innovations in the rapidly evolving world of healthcare. Following the ideology of **Bringing learning to people instead of people going for learning**, so far, we've been doing our part by:

- Developing quality content by qualified and well-versed authors
- Building a strong community of faculty and students
- Introducing a smart approach with Digital/Hybrid Books, and
- Offering simulation Nursing Procedures, etc.

Innovative teaching methodologies, such as modern-age Phygital Books, have sparked the interest of the Next-Gen students in pursuing advanced education. The enhancement of educational standards through **Omnipresent Knowledge Sharing Platforms** has further facilitated learning, bridging the gap between doctors and nurses.

At Nursing Next Live, a sister concern of CBS Publishers and Distributors, we have long recognized the immense potential within the nursing field. Our journey in innovating nursing education has allowed us to make substantial and meaningful contributions. With the vision of strengthening learning at every stage, we have introduced several plans that cater to the specific needs of the students, including but not limited to **Plan UG** for undergraduates, **Plan MSc** for postgraduate aspirants, **Plan FDP** for upskilling faculties, **SDL** for integrated learning and **Plan NP** for bridging the gap between theoretical and practical learning. Additionally, we have successfully completed seven series of our **Target High** Book in a very short period, setting a milestone in the education industry. We have been able to achieve all this just with the sole vision of laying the foundation of diversified knowledge for all. With the rise of a new generation of educated, tech-savvy individuals, we anticipate even more remarkable advancements in the coming years.

We take immense pride in our achievements and eagerly look forward to the future, brimming with new opportunities for innovation, growth and collaborations with experienced minds such as yourself who can contribute to our mission as Authors, Reviewers and/or Faculties. Together, let's foster a generation of nurses who are confident, competent, and prepared to succeed in a technology-driven healthcare system.

Mr Bhupesh Aarora
(Sr Vice President – Publishing and Marketing)
bhupeshaarora@cbspd.com| +91 95553 53330

Special Features of the Book

LEARNING OBJECTIVES

After the completion of the chapter, the readers will be able to:
- Understand the development of nursing as a profession.
- Discuss the development of nursing education in India and trends in nursing education.

Learning Objectives of every chapter are highlighted in the beginning to help readers understand the purpose of the chapter.

CHAPTER OUTLINE

- Introduction
- Nursing as a Profession
- Development of Nursing Education in India
- Responsibilities of a Graduate Nurse
- Various Professional Bodies

Chapter Outline is given in the beginning of every chapter to provide the reader a glimpse of entire chapter.

KEY TERMS

Dignity: The right of a person to be valued and respected for their own sake, and to be treated ethically.
Ethical: Connected with beliefs of what is right or wrong.
Motivation: Changing one's mind about doing something.
Occupation: A way to earn where the values, beliefs and ethics are not prominent features.

Important **Key Terms** used in the chapter are presented to familiarize the readers with the important terminologies.

Nursing Consideration

Nursing practice falls under both public and civil law. In all states, nurses are bound by rules and regulations stipulated by the law as determined by the legislature. Public laws are designed to protect the public, when these laws are broken. A nurse can be punished by paying a fine or losing her/his license. Civil laws deal with problems occurring between a nurse and a client.

Nursing Consideration boxes throughout the book will help nurses in implementing better clinical practices.

Mnemonics

To abide by a good nursing practice with ethics, you can remember the mnemonic **"CODE"**.
C: Courage to be moral requires
O: Obligations to honor (what is right)
D: Danger to manage
E: Expression and action

Mnemonics work wonders for students as far as memorizing important facts is concerned.

Must Know boxes prove highly beneficial in memorizing the vital facts.

Must Know

The term healthcare is not synonymous with medicine or nursing but includes many professional disciplines, each of these has its own definite characteristic and independent but overlapping functions. The fields of nursing and medicine are closely related. The relationship includes the exchange of data, the sharing of ideas and the development of a plan of care. The plan of care may be recorded on a single page or in a multiple page format.

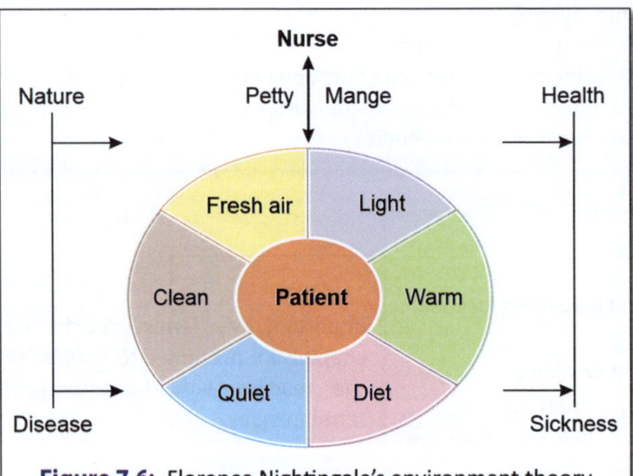

Figure 7.6: Florence Nightingale's environment theory

Studded with 100+ fully **Colored Images and Diagrams** for easy grasp of the relevant topic.

TABLE 8.1:	Types of nursing diagnoses with examples
Type of nursing diagnoses	**Examples**
Actual nursing diagnosis	Imbalanced nutrition related to nausea, disturbed sleep pattern related to cough and pain
Potential nursing diagnosis	Possible nutrition deficit leads to possible low self-esteem (related to job)
Risk nursing diagnosis	Risk for impaired skin integrity related to decreased peripheral circulation, risk for infection related to compromised immune system
Wellness diagnosis	Appropriate family coping
Syndrome (nursing) diagnosis	Rape, trauma syndrome, post trauma syndrome

Numerous informative **Tables** are used to clarify the concepts and make the reading enjoyable and interesting.

Further Readings boxes are covered to provide students with more study-related sources.

FURTHER READINGS

- Berman A, Snyder S, Frandsen G. Kozier and Erb's Fundamentals of Nursing: Concepts, Process, and Practice, 10th edition. Upper Saddle River, NJ: Pearson Prentice Hall; 2015.
- Chhugani M, James MM. Challenges faced by nurses in India—the major workforce of the healthcare system. Nurse Care Open Access J. 2017;2(4):112-4.
- Nursing Fundamentals. [online] Available from https://wtcs.pressbooks.pub/nursingfundamentals/chapter [Last accessed August, 2023].

STUDENT ASSIGNMENT

LONG ANSWER QUESTIONS

1. What do you understand by the term nursing process? What are its components? What are the benefits of applying nursing process?
2. What is data collection? Discuss the types of data along with their sources.
3. What is documentation? Explain.

SHORT ANSWER QUESTIONS

1. Define nursing diagnosis.
2. Define progress notes?
3. Write about Maslow's Hierarchy.

MULTIPLE CHOICE QUESTIONS

1. The systematic problem-solving approach toward providing individualized nursing care is known as ___________________.
   a. Nursing care plan
   b. Nursing process
   c. Nurses practice act
   d. Nursing method
2. What purpose does the nursing process serve?
   a. Assisting family members in making important healthcare decisions.
   b. Providing nurses with a framework to aid them in delivering comprehensive care.
   c. Help other healthcare professionals know what is going on with the client.
   d. Organize information so the doctor knows what is wrong with the client.

Detailed **Student Assignment** in the form of exercises in each and every chapter will facilitate structured learning and revision of the material provided in the respective chapters.

Nursing Foundation for Post Basic BSc Nursing

Placement: First Year **Time Allotted: 45 Hours**

Course Description:

This course will help students develop an understanding of the philosophy, objectives and responsibilities of nursing as a profession. The purpose of the course is to orient to the current concepts involved in the practices of nursing and developments in the nursing profession.

Objectives

At the end of the course, the student will:

- Identify professional aspects of nursing.
- Explain theories of nursing.
- Identify ethical aspects of nursing profession.
- Utilize steps of nursing process.
- Identify the role of the nurse in various levels of health services.
- Appreciate the significance of quality assurance in nursing.
- Explain current trends in health and nursing.

Course Contents

Unit I

- Development of nursing as a profession.
- Its philosophy.
- Objectives and responsibilities of a graduate nurse.
- Trends influencing nursing practices.
- Expended role of the nurse.
- Development of nursing education in India and trends in nursing education.
- Professional organization, career planning.
- Code of ethics and professional conduct for nurse.

Unit II

- Ethical, legal and other issues in nursing.
- Concept of health and illness, effects on the person.
- Stress and adaptation.
- Healthcare concept and nursing care concept.
- Development concept, needs, roles and problems of the development stages of individual newborn, infant, toddler, preadolescent, adolescent, adulthood, middle age old age.

Unit III

- Theory of nursing practices.
- Meta-paradigm of nursing—characterized by four central concepts, i.e., Nurse, person (client/patient), health and environment.

Unit IV

- Nursing process.
- Assessment: Tools for assessment, methods, recording.
- Planning: Teaching for planning care, types of care plans.
- Implementation: Different approaches to care, organizations and implementation of care, record.
- Evaluation: Tools for evaluation, process of evaluation, types of evaluation.

Unit V

- Quality assurance: Nursing standards, nursing audit, total quality management.
- Role of council and professional bodies in maintenance of standards.

Unit VI

- Primary healthcare concept.
- Community oriented nursing.
- Holistic nursing.
- Primary nursing.
- Family oriented nursing concept.
- Problem oriented nursing.
- Progressive patient care.
- Team nursing.

Contents

Chapter 1 Nursing as a Profession and Development of Nursing Education in India 1–22

Chapter 2 Trends and Issues in Nursing 23–30

Chapter 3 Code of Ethics and Professional Conduct for Nurses 31–46

Chapter 4 Concepts of Health and Illness 47–58

Chapter 5 Stress and Adaptation 59–78

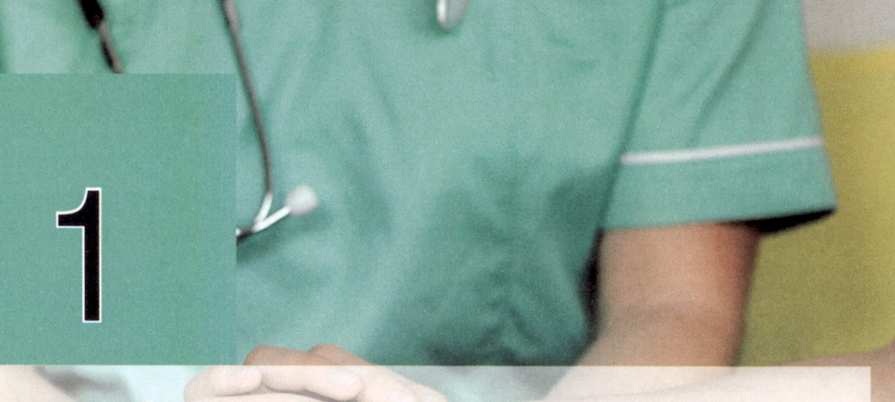

1

Nursing as a Profession and Development of Nursing Education in India

LEARNING OBJECTIVES

After the completion of the chapter, the readers will be able to:
- Understand the development of nursing as a profession.
- Discuss the development of nursing education in India and trends in nursing education.

CHAPTER OUTLINE

- Introduction
- Nursing as a Profession
- Development of Nursing Education in India
- Responsibilities of a Graduate Nurse
- Various Professional Bodies
- Recommendations of Various Committees Pertaining to Nursing Education

KEY TERMS

Dignity: The right of a person to be valued and respected for their own sake, and to be treated ethically.

Ethical: Connected with beliefs of what is right or wrong.

Motivation: Changing one's mind about doing something.

Occupation: A way to earn where the values, beliefs and ethics are not prominent features.

Profession: A vocation requiring advanced training and usually involves mental rather than manual work.

INTRODUCTION

Profession is defined as a vocation requiring advanced training. It usually involves mental rather than manual work such as teaching, engineering, medicine, law, nursing and so on. Professions are those occupations possessing a particular combination of characteristics generally considered to be the expertise, autonomy, commitment, and responsibility.

NURSING AS A PROFESSION

Nursing is a dynamic and essential profession within the healthcare system, focused on providing care to individuals, families, and communities to achieve, maintain, or recover optimal health and quality of life. Here are some key aspects of nursing as a profession.

Definition

A profession is an occupation based on specialized intellectual study and training, to supply skilled service with ethical components.

> **Must Know**
>
> **Characteristics Differences between Occupation and Profession**
> It must be noted that occupation and profession are a little different. Main characteristics differences of occupation and profession are tabulated in Table 1.1.
>
> **TABLE 1.1:** Differences between of occupation and profession
>
> | Occupation | Profession |
> | --- | --- |
> | In an occupation the values, beliefs and ethics are not prominent features. | It is basically intellectual. |
> | Training is provided during job and the duration of training may vary. | Profession is based on a body of knowledge that can be learned. |
> | In occupation people often change jobs. | Profession is practical rather than theoretical. |
> | Accountability depends on employer. | Profession can be taught through a process of professional education. |
> | | Profession has an internal organization of members. |
> | | Profession has practitioners who are motivated by altruism (desire to help others). |

Criteria

Professionalism denotes a relatively high social position. Two major criteria of profession are:

1. Autonomy
2. Controlled practice

Criteria of profession as per different educationists and reformers are as follows:

Abraham Flexner (1916)

According to Abraham Flexner, the criteria of a profession are as follows:

- **Based on knowledge:** A profession applies its body of knowledge in practical services that are vital to human welfare, and especially suited to the tradition of seasoned practitioners, shaping the skills of newcomers to the role.
- **Remain updated:** It constantly enlarges the body of knowledge it uses and subsequently, imposes a lifelong obligation on its members to remain updated in order to "do no harm".
- **Autonomous:** A profession functions autonomously (with authority) in the formulation of professional policy and in monitoring its practice and practitioners.
- **Intellectual:** It utilizes a well-defined and well-organized body of knowledge that is intellectual in nature and describes its phenomenon and practitioners.
- **Set standard:** A profession has a clear standard of educational preparation for entry into practice.
- **Follow set norms:** A profession is distinguished by the presence of specific culture, norms, and other values that are common among its members.

William Shepherd (1948)

William Shephard proposed the following criteria of a profession:

- **According to need and must be scientific:** A profession must satisfy an indispensable social need and should be based on well-established and socially accepted scientific principles. It must have developed a scientific technique which is the result of tested experience.
- **Training is must:** Profession demands adequate preprofessional and cultural training. It also demands the possession of a body of specialized and systematized training. It must give evidence of needed skills which the public does not possess, i.e., the skills which are partly inherent and partly acquired.
- **Authority to make independent choices:** Profession requires the exercise of discretion and judgment as per the time and manner of the performance of duty. This is in contrast to the kind of work which is subjected to standardization in terms of unit performance or time element.
- **Practical oriented:** It must have a group of consciousness designed to extend scientific knowledge in technical language.

Kelly (1981)

A professional is educated, caring, ethical, accountable, service-oriented, obtains knowledge through research, has the ability to practice autonomy and professional associations that encourage and support.

According to Kelly, services provided are vital to humanity and for the welfare of society. The services involve intellectual activities like:

- **Accountability:** Individual responsibility (accountability) is a strong feature.
- **Expanding knowledge:** There is a special body of knowledge that is continually enlarged through research. Practitioners are educated in institutions of higher learning.
- **Autonomous:** Practitioners are relatively independent and control their own policies and activities (autonomy).
- **Altruism:** Practitioners are motivated by service (altruism) and consider their work as an important component of their lives.
- **Guided:** There is a code of ethics to guide the decisions and conduct of practitioners.
- **Associations:** There is an organization (association) that encourages and supports high standards of practice.

Genevieve and Roy Bixler (1945)

Genevieve and Roy Bixler first wrote about the status of nursing as a profession in 1945. In nursing, the services provided are vital to humanity and for the welfare of the society. Nursing is the service that is essential to the well-being of the people and to the society. Nursing promotes, maintains and restores the health of individuals, groups and communities. Genevieve and Roy Bixler gave the seven criteria of a profession:

1. Utilizes in its practice a well-defined and well-organized body of specialized knowledge which is on the intellectual level of higher learning.
2. Constantly enlarges the body of knowledge it uses, and improves its technique of education and service by the use of scientific method.
3. Entrusts the education of its practitioners to institutions of higher education.
4. Applies its body of knowledge in practical services which are vital to human and social welfare
5. Functions autonomously in the formulation of professional policy and in the control of professional activity.
6. Attracts individuals of intellectual and personal qualities who exalts service above personal gain and who recognizes their chosen occupation as a life work.
7. Strives to compensate its practitioners by providing freedom to act on opportunity for continuous professional growth, and economic security.

Approaches to Profession

There are three approaches to a profession, discussed as follows:

1. **Process approach:** Continuum of professional development
   Position ◄————————► Profession
2. **Power approach:** Power approach uses two criteria to define a profession.
   i. Independence of profession
   ii. Amount of power the occupation controls
3. **Trait approach:** Trait approach follows high intellectual level in profession, high level of individual responsibility and accountability. Trait approach suggests need for a well-organized and strong organization, representing the members of the profession in their practice. The differences between a profession and occupation are given in Table 1.2.

TABLE 1.2:	Differences between a profession and occupation		
Sl. no.	**Basis**	**Profession**	**Occupation**
1.	Education	College or university	On the job training
2.	Length of education	Prolonged education	Length varies
3.	Activity	Mental creativity	Largely manual work
4.	Decision making	Decision based on science or theoretical constructs	Guided decision making
5.	Values, beliefs and ethics	Values, beliefs and ethics are integral part	Not part of preparation

Contd...

Sl. no.	Basis	Profession	Occupation
6.	Commitment	Strong commitment	Commitment may vary
7.	Autonomy	Autonomous	Supervised
8.	Change	No change of profession	Often change job
9.	Accountability	Individual accountability	Employer is primarily accountable

DEVELOPMENT OF NURSING EDUCATION IN INDIA

On August 15, 1947, India became independent and self-government came in action. Social changes were taking place rapidly but an alarming absence of public health and sanitary measures continued. The ratio of nurse to patient remained dangerously low.

St Stephen's hospital at Delhi was the first one to begin training the Indian women as nurses in 1867.

Basic General Nursing and Midwifery Education

Training of Dais (Birth Attendant)

Dai training continued postindependence. The goal was to train one *Dai* in each village and ultimate goal was to train all the practicing *Dais* in country. The duration of training was 30 days. No age limit was prescribed, training included theory and practice with more emphasis on 'field practice'. This training was done at subcenter and equipment was provided by United Nations International Children's Emergency Fund (UNICEF).

Auxiliary Nurse Midwife (ANM)

In 1950, INC came out with some important decisions relating to future patterns of nursing training in India. One of the important decisions was that there should be only two standards of training, nursing and midwifery, subsequently, the curriculum for these courses was prescribed. The first course was started at St. Mary Hospital Punjab, in 1951. The entrance qualification was up to seven/eight years of schooling. The period of training was 2 years which included a 9 months of midwifery and 3 months of community experience.

In 1977, as a result of the decision to prepare multipurpose health worker and vocationalize higher secondary education, curriculum was revised and designed to have 1½ years of vocational ANM program and 6 months of general education. The entrance qualification was raised from seventh passed to matriculation passed. Under multipurpose scheme, promotional venue was opened to senior ANMs for undergoing 6 months promotional training for which course was prescribed by INC.

Lady Health Visitor (LHV) Course

Training of LHV course continued postindependence. The syllabus was prepared and prescribed by INC, in 1951. The entrance qualification was matriculation. The duration was 2½ years which subsequently reduced to 2 years.

General Nursing and Midwifery (GNM) Course

The GNM course existed since early years of century. In 1951, syllabus was prescribed by INC. In 1954, a special provision was made for male nurses. Public health was integrated into basic nursing course, in 1954. The syllabus had undergone many revisions according to the changes in the health plans and policies of the government and changing trends and advancements in general education, nursing health sciences and medical technology.

Revisions of Course

- First revision of course was done in 1963. In 1964–65, psychiatric nursing was included in curriculum. The duration of course was reduced from 4 years to 3½ years. Second revision was done in 1982. The duration of the course was reduced to 3 years. The Midwifery training of 1-year duration was gradually reduced to 9 months and then 6 months. Finally a 3-year integrated program of GNM was prescribed in 1982.
- The revision of syllabus by INC, in 2004, has increased the duration of the course from 3 years to 3½ years.
- In the latest revision, in 2015, one of the major changes made in the revised curriculum is, the duration of the program. The total duration of the program has been reduced from 3½ years to 3 years, without compromising course content and objectives of the course. Internship has been integrated within the 3-year course.
- The education for basic entrance has become intermediate or class 12, instead of class 10.
- Both science and arts students are eligible for the course.
- The focus of general nursing education is, the care of sick in the hospital. Schools of nursing are generally attached to hospitals for teaching.
- The board examinations are conducted, one at the end of each year. On passing, the candidate become a registered nurse and midwife by the respective State Nursing Councils.

Philosophy

The INC believes that the basic course in nursing is a formal educational preparation which should be based on sound education principles. The council recognizes the program as the foundation on which the practice of nursing is built and on which further professional education depends. It also recognizes its responsibility toward the society, for the continued development of student as individual nurse and citizens.

Purposes

- The purpose of general nursing program is to prepare a nurse who will function as member of the health team beginning with competence for the first level position both in hospital and community.
- The program is generated due to the health needs of the society. The community and the individual assist nurses in their personal and professional development so that they can make their maximum contribution toward the society as individual citizens and nurses.

Objectives

- Demonstrate awareness and skills required in the nursing process, as mentioned in the provisions of healthcare and nursing of patients.

- Apply relevant knowledge from humanities, biological and behavioral sciences to carry out healthcare and nursing activities and functions.
- Show sensitivity and skills in human relationship and communication in his/her daily works.
- Demonstrate skills in the problem-solving methods in nursing.
- Gain knowledge of health resources in the community and the country.
- Demonstrate skills in leadership.
- Demonstrate awareness of necessity of belonging to professional organizations.
- Promotion of health, precaution against illness, restoration of health and rehabilitation.

Eligibility

- **Age:** The entrance age is 17–35 years, provided the candidate meets the minimum educational requirement, i.e., 12 years of schooling.
- **Minimum education:** All candidates should have passed 12th class or its equivalent, preferably with science subjects.
- Admission is conducted once a year.
- Candidate should be medically fit.

Selection Committee

The selection committee should comprise tutors, nurse administrators, and educationist/psychologist. The principal of the school shall be the chairperson.

Training Program

The course in general nursing is of 3½ years' duration as follows:

- 2 years practice in general nursing, 1-year community health nursing and midwifery and 6 months internship which includes nursing administration and nursing research classes.
- An alternate course is available for male students in lieu of midwifery. The ANM, who wishes to undertake general nursing course are not be given any concessions. The maximum hours per week, per student, are 36 hours, which include instructions and clinical field experiences.

Post-Basic/Post Certificate Short-Term Courses and Diploma Programs

During 1948–50, four nurses were sent to the UK by Government of India for mental health nursing diploma. During 1954, Nur Manzil Psychiatric Center, Lucknow, gave psychiatric nursing orientation course of 4–6 weeks duration. In 1951, a 1-year course in public health was started at College of Nursing, Delhi. Government of India felt urgent need for psychiatric nurses during 1953–54. This resulted in first organized course at All India Institute of Mental Health.

In 1962, Diploma in Pediatric Nursing was established at JJ Group of Hospitals, Bombay. At present, there are many other courses of 3 months duration which are monitored and recognized by INC. The ultimate aim of all the post-basic/post certificate programs, is to improve the quality of patient care and promotion of health.

Bachelor of Nursing Course (Post Certificate) for Qualified Nurses

The INC has recognized modes of programs at this level:

Regular

BSc (Post Basic) course for those who have 10+2 + and General Nursing and Midwifery (GNM) of 2 years duration.

Philosophy and Aim of the Program

Nursing is an integral part of the healthcare delivery system and shares responsibility in collaboration with other allied health professions, for the attainment of optimal health for all members of the society. Education is a lifelong learning process. It seeks to render appropriate behavioral changes in students in order to facilitate their development, which assist them to live personally satisfied and socially useful lives.

The goal of postcertificate degree program leading to bachelor of science in nursing is the preparation of the trained nurse as a specialist who accepts responsibility for enhancing the effectiveness of nursing care.

Eligibility for Admission

The candidate seeking admission must:

- Hold a certificate in general nursing.
- Be a registered nurse.
- Have minimum of 2 years of experience. Now, there is no need of experience after GNM for admission to this course.
- Have passed preuniversity exam in the arts/science/commerce or its equivalent from a recognized university.
- Be medically fit.
- Have a good personal and professional record.
- Have working knowledge of English.

Program of Study

Duration: The duration of the program is two academic years from the date of commencement of program. Terms and vacations are notified by the university from time to time.

Objectives: The goals of the postcertificate program leading to the bachelors of nursing are:

- To train nurses as a specialist who accept responsibility for enhancing the effectiveness of nursing care.
- To administer high quality nursing care to all people of all ages at homes, hospitals and other community agencies in urban and rural areas.
- To apply knowledge from the physical, social and behavioral sciences, in assessing the health status of individuals and make critical judgment in planning, directing and evaluating primary, acute and long-term care, given by themselves and others working with them.
- To investigate healthcare problems, systematically.
- To work collaboratively with members of other health disciplines.
- To teach and counsel individuals, families and other groups about health and illness.
- To understand human behavior and establish effective interpersonal relationships.
- To teach in clinical nursing situations.
- To identify underlying principles from the social and natural sciences and utilize them in adapting to or initiating changes in relation to those factors.
- To acquire professional knowledge and attitude in adapting the leadership role.

University-Level Programs

Basic BSc Nursing

First university program started just before independence in 1946, at University of Delhi and Christian Medical College (CMC), Vellore. In 1949, on recommendation of University Education Committee, Education Commission (1964–66) and conference and workshop held by TNAI, the World Health Organization (WHO) and University Grants Commission (UGC); some more colleges came up in different states, affiliated to different state universities.

The INC prescribed the syllabus which has been revised three times. The last revision was done in 2005–06. It was done on the basis of the 10+3+2 system of general education. At present, the BSc Nursing program which is recommended by the INC is of 4 years and has foundations for future study and specialization in nursing.

Graduate nursing education started in India in the year 1946 in CMC, Vellore and in the Rajkumari Amrit Kaur (RAK) College of Nursing at Delhi University. At present more than 1373 colleges have been recognized by INC to conduct the course under several universities in India.

Eligibility

A candidate seeking admission should:

- Have passed the 2 years of preuniversity exam or equivalent, by recognized university with science subjects, i.e., physics, biology and chemistry.
- Be a student of vocational course.
- Have obtained at least 45% of total marks in science subjects in the qualifying exam. If he/she belongs to a scheduled caste or tribe, should have obtained not <40% of total marks in science subjects.
- Have completed 17 years of age at the time of admission or will complete this age on or before 31st December of the year of admission.
- Be medically fit.

Objectives of the Program

The program is designed:

- To provide a balance of professional and general education.
- To enable a student to become a professional nurse practitioner who has self-direction and is a responsible citizen.

Through planned guided experiences, students are provided with opportunities to develop:

- A broad concept of the fundamental principles of nursing care based on sound knowledge and satisfactory levels of skill in providing care to people of all ages in community or institutional setting.
- Understanding of the application of principles from the physical, biological and social sciences for assessing the health status.
- Ability to investigate healthcare problems systematically.
- Ability to work collaboratively with members of allied disciplines toward attaining optimum health for all members of the society.
- Understanding of fundamental principles of administration and organization of nursing service.

- Understanding of human behavior and appreciation of effective interpersonal relationship with individuals' families and groups.
- Ability to assume responsibility for continuing learning.
- Appreciation of professional attitudes necessary for leadership roles in nursing appreciation of social and ethical obligations to society.

Course of study: The course of study leading to bachelor of nursing degree comprises four academic years having 8 semesters. INC applied "semester system" in BSc Nursing program.

Post-Basic Nursing by Distance Education Mode

Indira Gandhi National Open University (IGNOU) was established in 1985. Post-Basic BSc Nursing program was launched in 1992, which is a 3 years duration course recognized by INC.

Postgraduate Education or MSc Nursing

First 2 years course of master's in nursing was started at RAK College of Nursing in 1959 and in CMC Vellore, in 1969. At present there are many colleges imparting MSc Nursing degree course in different specialties.

- At present there are 547 colleges imparting MSc Nursing degree course in different specialties.
- INC recognized list of colleges of Nursing for MSc (N) course (updated by INC on March 31, 2021).

Philosophy

- The Master of Nursing Program is offered by institution of higher education and is built up on a recognized bachelor's curriculum in nursing (in India by INC).
- The program prepares nurses for leadership position in nursing and other healthcare fields. The nurses can function as specialists, nurse practitioners, consultants, educators, administrators and investigators in a wide variety of professional setting to meet the national priorities and the changing needs of the society.
- The program prepares nursing graduates who are professionally equipped, creative, self-directed and socially motivated to effectively meet the needs of the social change.
- The program encourages accountability and commitment to lifelong learning which fosters improvement of quality healthcare.

Objectives

Masters of MSc Nursing program demonstrates:

- Increased cognitive, affective and psychomotor competencies and the ability to utilize the potentials for effective nursing performance.
- Expertise in the utilization of concepts and theories for the assessment, planning and intervention in meeting the selfcare needs of an individual, for the attainment of fullest potentials in the field of specialty.
- Ability to practice independently as a nurse specialist.
- Ability to function effectively as nurse educators and administrators.
- Ability to interpret the health-related research.
- Ability to plan and initiate change in the healthcare system.

- Leadership qualities for the advancement of practice of professional nursing.
- Interest in lifelong learning for personal and professional learning advancement.

Eligibility

The candidate seeking admission must fulfill the following criteria:

- Candidate must have passed BSc Nursing/post certificate BSc or nursing degree from a recognized university.
- He/she must have a minimum of 1 year of experience, after obtaining BSc in hospital or nursing educational institutions or community health setting.
- For BSc nursing post certificate, no such experience is needed after graduation. The candidate shall be a registered nurse or registered midwife for admission to medical surgical nursing, community health nursing, pediatric nursing obstetric and gynecological nursing.
- Candidate must be a registered nurse for admission to psychiatric nursing.
- The candidate shall be selected on merit judged on the basis of academic performances in BSc nursing, post certificate BSc or nursing and selection tests.

Specialties

Candidate will be enrolled and get expertise in any one of the following branches:

- Medical Surgical Nursing—Cardiovascular and Thoracic Nursing
- Medical Surgical Nursing—Critical Care Nursing
- Medical Surgical Nursing—Oncology Nursing
- Medical Surgical Nursing—Neurosciences Nursing
- Medical Surgical Nursing—Nephrology Nursing
- Medical Surgical Nursing—Orthopedic Nursing
- Medical Surgical Nursing—Gastroenterology Nursing
- Obstetric and Gynecological Nursing
- Pediatric (Child Health) Nursing
- Psychiatric (Mental Health) Nursing
- Community Health Nursing

Master of Philosophy or M Phil Nursing

The INC felt need for MPhil Program as early as in 1977. For this purpose, a committee was appointed. In 1986, a 1-year duration, full time and a 2-year duration part time program was started in RAK College of Nursing, Delhi. In 1980, RAK college of nursing started MPhil program as a regular as well as a part time course. Since then, several universities started taking students for the MPhil course in nursing. Prominent among these are Dr MG Ramachandran (MGR) Medical University, Rajiv Gandhi University of Health Sciences, Shreemati Nathibai Damodar Thackersey Women's University (SNDT) University, Delhi University and Manipal Academy of Higher Education.

Philosophy

The main focus of the program is to prepare its nursing students for healthcare services and assist them to achieve a meaningful philosophy of life. The student is encouraged to develop judgment and wisdom to handle knowledge and skills and achieve mastery in problem solving and creative skills.

Commitment to lifelong learning is a mark of truly professional person. In order to maintain clinical competencies and enhance professional practice, the student must stay abreast of the new developments and contribute to the advancement of nursing knowledge.

Objectives

The objectives of MPhil degree course in nursing are:
- To strengthen the research foundations of nurses for encouraging research attitudes and problem-solving capacities.
- To provide basic training required for research in undertaking doctoral work.

Duration

Duration of the full-term MPhil course will be 1 year and part time course will be of 2 years.

Course of Study

At the time of admission, each candidate is required to indicate his/her priorities in regard to the optional courses. A candidate may opt for a course for MPhil Program, from the department of anthropology, education, sociology and physiology or any other suitable department. The MPhil studies is divided into two distinct parts, Part 1 and Part 2.

1. **Part 1:** It consists of 3 courses, i.e., research methods in nursing, major aspects of nursing and allied disciplines.
2. **Part 2:** After passing Part 1 examination, a student is required to write a dissertation. The topic and the nature of the dissertation of each candidate will be determined by the advisory committee consisting of three members. The dissertation may include results of original research, a fresh interpretation of existing facts, and date or a review article of critical nature.

Doctorate of Philosophy in Nursing or PhD in Nursing

Earlier, Indian nurses were sent abroad for PhD program. From 1992, PhD in nursing is available in India. Manipal Academy of Higher Education (MAHE) is one of the universities having PhD program. Universities where PhD programs are conducted in India, include:
- PhD Consortium by Indian Nursing Council in collaboration with Rajiv Gandhi University of Health Sciences (RUGHS) and World Health Organization (WHO)
- Rajkumari Amrit Kaur (RAK) College of Nursing
- National Institute of Mental Health and Neurosciences (NIMHANS) Bengaluru
- Manipal University

Philosophy

A candidate willing to take admission in doctorate degree of Philosophy in Medical Sciences, must have obtained an MPhil degree from a recognized university. In case the MPhil degree is not available, the candidate must have first- or second-class master's degree from a recognized Indian or foreign university in the concerned subject.

The candidate shall apply to the university for the admission stating the qualifications and the subjects he/she proposes to investigate. The candidate should enclose a statement on any work done in the concerned subject. Every application for the admission in the course, goes for analysis by the board of research studies.

Members of Board of Research Studies (Medical Sciences)

- Dean and the head of the concerned departments.
- Principals/head of institutions recognized for postgraduate medical studies.
- Two members nominated by the medical academic council.
- Three persons nominated by the medical faculty (for their special knowledge in the medical science).

Eligibility Criteria

- The candidate should be postgraduate in nursing with >55% of aggregate marks.
- The candidate should have research background.
- A candidate may or may not have published articles in journals.
- The course duration for regular PhD course is 3 years and for part time, it is 4 years.

Current Educational Patterns in Nursing

Trends in nursing education changes from basic general nursing service to doctorate education in nursing.

Non-University Programs

- Basic: ANM – GNM
- Advance: Postcertificate diploma

University Programs

- **Basic:**
    - BSc (N)
    - Post-Basic BSc (Regular)
    - Post-Basic BSc (N) (IGNOU)
- **Advance:**
    - MSc (Nursing)
    - MPhil
    - PhD

Qualities of a Professional Nurse

Professional nurse: A professional nurse is a person who has completed a basic nursing education program and is licensed in his/her country or state to practice professional nursing.

The nurse is a healthcare provider that treats the patient. A nurse should possess following qualities:

- **Honesty:** One of the qualities that makes any nurse outstanding is, honesty. He/she is taught to be truthful at all times when dealing with the patient and the family. By doing so, he/she is able to earn every one's confidence/trust.
- **Communication skills:** Communication skills are a basic foundation for any career but for nurse it is one of the most important aspects of the job. Nurse should have excellent communications skills. They should be able to follow directions without a problem and should easily be able to communicate with patients and families.
- **Caring:** A nurse should be able to give proper attention to the client. He/she must be compassionate enough to take care of the client. The comforts of the patient should be of utmost importance to him/her.
- **Empathetic:** Nurses have empathy for the pain and suffering of patient. They are able to feel compassion and provide comfort. Nurse is able to understand the feelings of the patient and

treat him the way he/she would want to be treated. Empathy is a multidimensional concept that enables the caregiver to identify, share emotions and provide care for the patient in distress. Empathy is the core of nursing.

- **Observer:** The nurse is an observant. He/she is able to monitor/observe the client closely to know when there is an improvement in the condition or when there is deterioration.
- **Intuition:** The nurse uses experience, scientific knowledge and instinct when assessing patients. Intuition in nursing is defined as the immediate understanding of a problem without the necessity of conscious thoughts. Nurses pick up the smallest cues, nuances and seemingly unrelated patient statements that may need further investigation.
- **Skillful:** Nurse is skillful in handling the problems of the patient. These skills which are enhanced by the training, enable him/her to properly deal with his client's problems.
- **Physical endurance:** Good physical health is a vital part of ensuring the stressful and high-energy demands of the nursing profession. Nurses lift heavy patients, move weighty medical equipment and may spend 12 hours or more on their feet during a shift.

RESPONSIBILITIES OF A GRADUATE NURSE

The graduate nurse practices nursing according to the code of professional conduct as laid down by the Indian Nursing Council (INC). A graduate nurse:

- Works within the scope of practice.
- Maintains a high standard of professional behavior and is accountable for practice.
- Respects and maintains the privacy, dignity and confidentiality of the patient.
- Delivers the nursing care of an assigned group of patients.
- Promotes the health, welfare and social well-being of patients.
- Assesses, plans, implements and evaluates individual person-centered care programs.
- Develops and promotes good interpersonal relationship with patient's family and significant others.
- Provides care in an empathetic and ethical manner.
- Respects the dignity and spiritual needs of the patient.
- Recognizes the social and cultural dimensions of patient care.
- Works closely and collaboratively with the patients, their families and healthcare team members.
- Provides appropriate and timely education and information to the patient and significant others.
- Maintains accurate written nursing records.
- Participates in clinical audit and review.
- Participates in community need assessment.
- Delegates and supervises the work of other nursing personnel.
- Refers patients to higher setups as required.
- Contributes to ongoing monitoring, audit and evaluation of the services.
- Participates in the development of policies/procedures and guidelines to support compliance with current legal requirements.
- Participates in the development, promotion and implementation of infection prevention programs.
- Participates in the clinical induction of all new nursing staff as required.
- Contributes to the identification of training needs related to clinical area.
- Develops teaching skill and participates in the planning and implementation training and teaching programs for nursing students and other healthcare personnel.
- Maintains professional standards including patient and data confidentiality.

- Ensures that equipment is safe to use and reports any malfunctions in a timely manner.
- Supervises the health personnel.
- Provides direct and indirect nursing care to all age group patients.
- Coordinates with nursing managers and nursing directors in managing nursing activities.
- Assists registered nurses in administering medications to patients.

VARIOUS PROFESSIONAL BODIES

Trained Nurses Association of India (TNAI)

The TNAI helps the initiation of university level education in India. Recommendations of the Bhore Committee were implemented within year. TNAI made significant achievements in the field of nursing education.

Functions of TNAI

- Passing of the INC Act.
- Deputation of Indian nurses abroad for post-basic education.
- It creates awareness among nurses through Nursing Journal of India and by organizing continuing education programs.
- TNAI also offers scholarships to deserving candidates to take up studies within the country and abroad.

Indian Nursing Council (INC)

The INC was constituted to establish a uniform standard of education for nurses, midwives, health visitors and auxiliary nurse midwives. The INC Act was passed following an ordinance on December 31, 1947. The council was constituted in 1949.

Functions of INC

- To set standards and to regulate all types of nursing education all over the country.
- To prescribe and specify minimum requirement for qualifying a particular course in nursing.
- To provide an advisory role in the state nursing council.
- To collaborate with state nursing councils, schools and colleges of nursing and examination board.

State Nursing Council (SNC)

Some of the state registration council functions are mentioned below:

Functions

- Inspect and accredit schools of nursing in their state.
- Conduct examinations.
- Prescribe rules of conduct.
- Maintain registers of nurses, midwives, ANM and health visitors in the state.

The state registration councils are autonomous except they do not have power to prescribe the syllabi for courses.

RECOMMENDATIONS OF VARIOUS COMMITTEES PERTAINING TO NURSING EDUCATION

Health Survey and Development Committee, (Bhore Committee) 1946

Appointed by the Government of India in 1943

- Sir Joseph Bhore as Chairman
  - To survey the then existing position regarding the
    - Health conditions and
    - Health organization in the country
  - To make recommendations for the future development.

Bhore committee has submitted its report in 1946.

- First time proposed a national program for improving health services in the country
- Committee observed:

  "If the nation's health is to be built, – the health program should be developed
  - On a foundation of preventive health
  - Preventive activities should proceed side by side with those concerned with the treatment of patients."

Important recommendations:

- Integration of preventive and curative services at all administrative levels
- Development of primary health centres in two stages:
  1. A short-term measure:
     - Primary health centre in the rural areas 1/40,000 population
     - Secondary health centre to serve as a supervisory, coordinating and referral institution.
  2. A long-term program (also k/a the 3 million plan)
     - Primary health units, 1/10,000 to 20,000 population with 75-bedded hospitals and
     - Secondary units with 650-bedded hospitals,
     - District hospitals with 2,500 beds;
- **Major changes in medical education:** Including 3 months' training in Preventive and Social Medicine to prepare "Social Physicians".

  It made comprehensive recommendations for remodeling of health services in India. The report, had some important recommendations like:
- Integration of preventive and curative services of all administrative levels.
  - Development of Primary Health Centres in two stages:
    - i. Short-term measure – one primary health centre as suggested for a population of 40,000. Each PHC was to be manned by 2 doctors, one nurse, four public health nurses, four midwives, four trained dais, two sanitary inspectors, two health assistants, one pharmacist and fifteen other class IV employees. Secondary health centre was also envisaged to provide support to PHC, and to coordinate and supervise their functioning.
    - ii. A long-term program (also called the 3 million plan) of setting up primary health units with 75 – bedded hospitals for each 10,000 to 20,000 population and secondary units with 650 – bedded hospital, again regionalised around district hospitals with 2500 beds.

Shetty Committee (1954)

In 1954, the government constituted Shetty Committee under the chairmanship of Attavar Balakrishna Shetty, State Health Minister of Madras, to review the condition of nursing service, emoluments, etc. of the nursing profession to standardize and for the development of nursing in India.

The committee recommendations were as follows:

- Establishment of new schools of nursing with adequate teaching and supervisory staff to trained nurses
- Provision of adequate training for nursing teachers
- Deputation to two to four nurses to undergo higher study and to take up courses in teaching, administration, and public health nursing
- Adequate facility for clinical experience and clinical supervision
- Admission criteria per Indian Nursing Council norms
- Adequate accommodation for nurse students and proper care of their health
- Improvement in nursing education standard
- Two grades of nurses: A fully trained nurse and midwives who have undergone 3.5–4 years training in nursing and midwifery and another auxiliary nurse and midwife of 2 years
- Appointment of Superintendents of Nursing in the offices of Directorates in each state
- A national minimum pay scales for nurses, midwives, and ANMs
- Improvement in working conditions of nurses
- Provision of in-service education programs
- Part-time working facilities for nurses
- Need for the training of male nurses.

Mudaliar Committee (1961)

The Government of India in 1959 appointed another committee to provide guidelines for the Five-Year Plans. This committee is known as the "Health Survey and Planning Committee." Dr AL Mudaliar, Vice Chancellor of Madras University, headed it. This committee appointed to assess the performance in the health sector based on Bhore recommendations.

This committee found the conditions in PHCs to be unsatisfactory and suggested that the PHC, already established should be strengthened before new ones are opened.

This committee suggested the following recommendations:

- Strengthening of existing PHC before the opening of new ones.
- PHC for 40,000 populations.
- PHC should provide the curative, preventive, and promotive services.
- Strengthening of subdivisional and district hospitals.
- Each district hospital should have one bed against 1,000 population; Taluk hospital should have 600-800 beds, and each PHC should have 10 beds.
- Lady health visitor (LHV) and midwife should be engaged in providing health education, personal hygiene, and nutrition.
- There should be one ANM for 5,000 population.
- There should be three grade of nurses: Basic nurses with 4 years of training, ANM with 2 years training, and degree nurses.

- The minimum qualification for General Nursing and Midwifery (GNM) should be matriculation or equivalent; and for degree nurses, the minimum qualification should be higher secondary or preuniversity.
- The medium of instruction in GNM course should be preferably in English, whereas in the degree course, it should be in English only.
- Public health nursing should be a part of the nursing curriculum. The district hospitals with bed strength with 75–100 can consider for clinical practice for nurse students; there should be provision for free accommodation, free uniform, laundry, free books, and free medical services, and stipend to student nurses.
- Each school of nursing should have an advisory committee and should have its budget.
- Train male nurses for certain jobs.
- There should be short-term special training courses such as pediatric nursing, public health nursing, theatre nursing, psychiatric nursing, nursing administration, etc.
- Dai training program, other post basic training courses such as sister tutor course, operation theater technique, public health nursing, mental disease nursing, and nursing service administration.

Chadha Committee (1963)

This committee appointed in 1963 under the chairmanship of Dr MS Chadha who was the Director General of health Services. The main aim of this committee was to give inputs regarding the maintenance phase of the NMEP.

The committee made the following suggestions:
- Basic health workers for NMEP activity.
- Basic health workers as multipurpose workers would perform malaria work and the duties of family planning and vital statistics data collection.
- They would work under the supervision of family planning health assistants.
- Integration of different nursing services.

Mukharjee Committee (1966)

The Government appointed a committee of Health Secretaries in 1966 under the chairmanship of Shri Mukherjee. He was then Union Health Secretary to work out specific health service at the block level and strengthening higher levels of administration.

The committee recommendations were as follows:
- One family planning female worker for every two subcenters
- One LHV for 40,000 populations
- One part-time worker for motivation population for acceptance of Intrauterine Devices (IUD)
- Appointment of education leaders at block and district
- Part-time availability of government doctors on an incentive basis.
- **Recommendations:**
  - Integrated approach in the entire health field - Programs of public health and medical care should be integrated to the maximum extent possible and so also the programs within each field. Health workers at the lower levels should become increasingly multipurpose workers.

In certain phases of any large national program it may be necessary to have separate staff, at the maintenance stage the activities under the program should get integrated more and more with the basic health services and to the extent possible should be taken care of through the domiciliary services.

- One basic health worker for a population of 10,000.
- At the district level there should be as much integration of the general health program with the family planning program as possible, ensuring at the same time however, that the family planning program continues to receive adequate attention and profits from such integration
- The Committee did not attempt to work out any details of the organisation that would be needed above the District level, i.e. at the Zonal , the State and the Central levels They also felt that the State Government could themselves work out better the strength and pattern and method of functioning of the health organisation at the Zonal and State levels.

Jungalwalla Committee (1964)

The Government constituted the "Committee on Integration of Health Services" in 1964 under the chairmanship of Dr N Jungalwalla. He was the Director of National Institute of Health Administration and Education. (Currently NIHFW).

Objective: The objective of the committee was to examine various problems related to the integration of health services, the abolition of private practice by doctors in government services, and the services conditions of doctors.

The committee defined "integrated health services" as:

- A service with a unified approach for all problems instead of a segmented approach for different problems.
- Medical care and public health programs should be put under charge of a single administrator at all levels of hierarchy.

Recommendations: Following steps were recommended for the integration at all levels of health organisation in the country:

- Unified cadre
- Common seniority
- Recognition of extra qualifications
- Equal pay for equal work
- Special pay for special work
- Abolition of private practice by government doctors
- Improvement in their service conditions

The recommendations given by committees and commission provided guidelines for improvement and growth of nursing education.

Kartar Singh Committee (1972–73)

- Multipurpose health worker scheme.
- Change in designation of ANM's and LHV.
- Setting up of training division at the Ministry of Health and Family Welfare.

Sarojini Varadappan Committee—A High Power Committee on Nursing and Nursing Profession (1990)

- Two levels of nursing personnel.
- Post-basic BSc nursing degree to continue.
- Masters in nursing program to be increased and strengthened.
- Doctorate in nursing program to be started in selected university.
- Continuing education and staff development for nurses.

Working Group on Nursing Education and Manpower (1991)

- By 2020 the GNM program to be phased out.
- Curriculum of BSc nursing to be modified.
- Staffing norm should be as per INC.
- There should be deliberate plan for preparation of teachers MSc/MPhil and PhD degrees
- Improvement in functioning of INC.
- Importance of continuing education for nurses.

FURTHER READINGS

- Chitty and Amp; Black, 2011, p. 66
- https://nhsrcindia.org/sites/default/files/2021-04/Mudalier%20Committee%20Report.pdf
- https://nihfw.ac.in/cms/committee--and-commission.php
- https://nihfw.ac.in/Doc/Reports/Bhore%20Committee%20Report%20-%20Vol%20II.pdf
- https://ruralindiaonline.org/hi/library/resource/report-of-the-committee-on-multipurpose-workers-under-health-and-family-planning-program/
- Preventive and social medicine, K Park, 27th edition

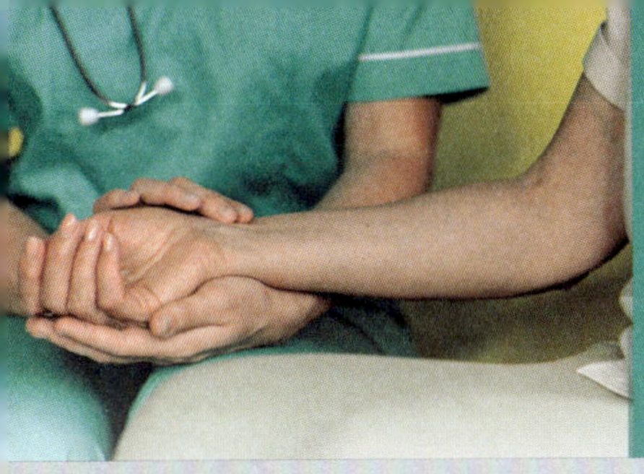

LONG ANSWER QUESTIONS

1. Discuss the development of nursing education in India in detail.
2. Describe the responsibilities of a graduate nurse.
3. Write the qualities of professional nurse.

SHORT ANSWER QUESTIONS

1. What are the differences between a profession and occupation?
2. What are the different approaches to profession?

MULTIPLE CHOICE QUESTIONS

1. **Which among the following options, of national legislation is directly related to nursing practice?**
   a. The government service conduct rules
   b. The Indian Nursing Council Act
   c. Law, based upon the English pattern
   d. The state service conduct rules

2. **What is the meaning of trends in nursing?**
   a. Professional qualification required for a nurse
   b. Job responsibilities of a professional nurse
   c. Movement in a particular direction in nursing field
   d. Code of ethics in nursing profession

3. **Current aim in nursing education includes:**
   a. All school of nursing now attached to a medical college should be upgraded to the BSc level
   b. Nursing personnel must have authority in the selection of students
   c. Nursing schools should have independent budget
   d. All of the above

4. **What is the full form of TNAI?**
   a. Training in Nursing at All India level
   b. Trained Nurses of All India
   c. Trained Nurses Association of India
   d. Training in Nurses at International level

5. **Activities of TNAI include:**
   a. Granting scholarship to nurses who wish to go for advanced study either in the country or abroad
   b. Publication of nursing journal of India
   c. Promoting the development of courses in higher education for nurses
   d. All of the above

6. **Qualities of a nurse include all; except:**
   a. Caring attitude
   c. Talkative

   b. Honesty
   d. Well balanced life
7. **Nursing is considered a profession because:**
   a. Nurse earns money
   b. It is based on science and art
   c. It provides comprehensive health services
   d. Nursing fulfills all the criteria of a profession
8. **Criteria of a profession include all; except:**
   a. A profession should be intellectual
   b. It should be self-governing
   c. In a profession, there is no place for higher education
   d. A profession should be service-oriented
9. **Characteristics of a profession include:**
   a. A profession constantly enlarges its body of knowledge
   b. A profession makes its own policies and controls its own activities
   c. A profession offers services which are related to human and social welfare
   d. All of the above

2

Trends and Issues in Nursing

LEARNING OBJECTIVES

After the completion of the chapter, the readers will be able to:
* Understand the current trends in nursing education.
* Know about the expanded roles of a nurse.

CHAPTER OUTLINE

* Introduction
* Issues in Nursing

* Expanded Roles of Nurses

KEY TERMS

Adjustment difficulties: The difficulties related to an emotional or behavioral reaction to a stressful event or change in a person's life.

Emerging: Emerging means something coming into existence.

Gerontology: The study of aging and older adults.

PAP smear: A procedure in which a small brush is used to gently remove cells from the surface of the cervix and the area around it so they can be checked under a microscope for cervical cancer or cell changes that may lead to cervical cancer.

Rehabilitation: A set of interventions designed to optimize functioning and reduce disability in individuals with health conditions in interaction with their environment.

INTRODUCTION

Trends denote general direction and tendencies, especially of events and opinions. A trend means a change or movement in a particular direction.

Trends in nursing are changes that are taking place in present days in all fields of nursing which affect the profession as a whole.

Trends in nursing refer to the direction toward which the different nursing events have moved or are moving. It also means a change currently taking place in any area of nursing and influencing the profession. These changes are:

- Social change
- Change in other nursing related professions
- Change in nursing profession in country.

Emerging Trends in Nursing

- Knowledge expansion and increasing use of technology and informatics
- Practice-based competency
- Rise of telehealth and technology in healthcare
- Self-care needs
- Evolution of workplace
- Expanding distance education
- Nurse practitioner in critical care
- Online nursing programs and education
- Nursing informatics
- Increased use of simulation
- Focus on holistic care
- Curriculum innovations
- Changing demography of nursing students
- Training of Trainees (TOT's)
- University-based education
- Innovative evaluation strategies like OSCE
- Increase in patient wearable medical devices
- Comprehensive primary healthcare

ISSUES IN NURSING

Issues at Infrastructure Level

- Lack of independent building for schools and colleges
- Separate directorate is needed
- Higher education for senior positions in nursing
- Political involvement
- Poor pay structures
- Disorganization
- Working environment

Issues in Nursing Practice

- Lack of security and safety
- Less promotional opportunities
- Harassment by other personnel
- Staff retention
- Influence of the medical fraternity
- Inadequate health supplies
- Internal conflict and influence
- Nurses' burnout

Issues at the Level of Nursing Education

- Lack of independent principal for schools and colleges
- Inadequate hostel facilities for students
- Shortage of qualified teachers in nursing
- Inadequate library facilities
- No UGC pay scales for college teachers in nursing
- Very less or no stipend for nursing students
- Less supply of AV aids
- Less promotional opportunities for teachers of both schools and colleges.

Issues with Administration

- Noninvolvement of nursing administrators in planning and decision making in hospital administration.
- Lack of knowledge in management among nursing administrators.
- Interference of non-nursing personnel in nursing administration.
- No written nursing policies or manuals.
- No separate budget.
- No proper job description for various nursing cadres.
- No organized staff development programs for nurses like orientation, in-service education, continuing education, etc.
- Inefficiency of nursing councils of state and union to maintain standards in nursing.

Legal Issues in Nursing

- Nurse Practice Act
- Standards of Professional Practice
- Licensure versus Good Samaritan Laws
- Public Health Laws

Other Issues in Nursing

- Nursing shortage
- Patient satisfaction
- National Patient Safety Initiatives

- Evidence-based practice
- Aging population
- Global burden of infectious and noninfectious diseases
- Political will

EXPANDED ROLES OF NURSES

Nurses fulfill various roles in the healthcare term. They are the most flexible of health professionals and do a number of things as well. Contemporary nursing requires possession of knowledge and skills for a variety of professional roles and responsibilities. In the past, the principal role of nurse was to provide care and comfort as they carried out specific nursing functions. Changes in nursing field have expanded the role to include increased emphasis on health promotion and illness prevention as well as concern for the client as whole.

At present nurses have different roles as depicted in Figure 2.1.

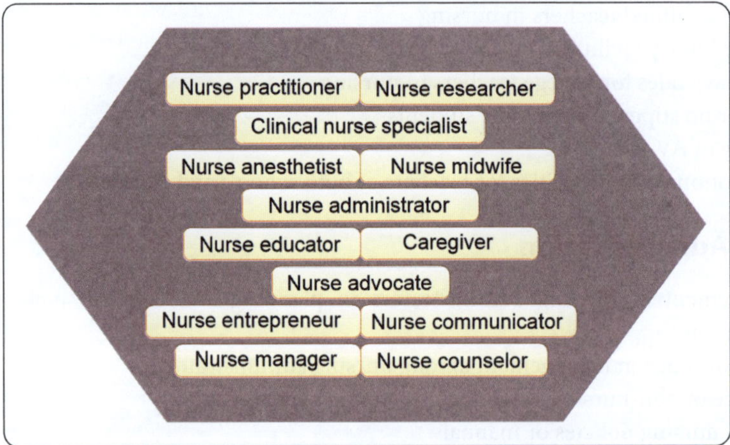

Figure 2.1: Multiple roles of a nurse in present time

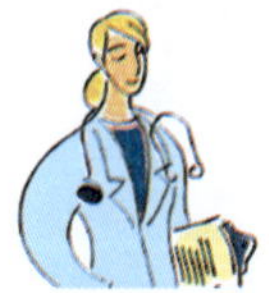

Nurse Practitioner

A nurse who has an advanced education and is a graduate, is a programmed nurse practitioner. The areas of this role are adult nurse practitioner, pediatric nurse practitioner or gerontology nurse practitioner. Nurse practitioners are employed in healthcare agencies or community-based settings. They usually deal with nonemergency, acute or chronic illness and provide primary ambulatory care.

Nurse practitioners provide healthcare to clients usually in an outpatient ambulatory care or community-based settings. They provide more holistic approach, attending to symptoms of nonpathological conditions, comfort and comprehensiveness of care.

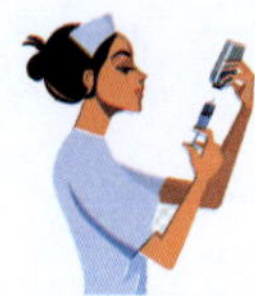

Clinical Nurse Specialist

The clinical nurse specialist is an advanced practice nurse with nursing expertise in a specialized field of practice and may work in any practice setting. Many Intensive Care

Units (ICUs) and emergency department nurses are required to have teachings in advanced cardiac life support and certification in critical care emergency nursing or trauma nursing. Hospital-based nurse may also choose to practice in specialty areas such as transportation, rehabilitation or oncology. The clinical nurse practitioners may specialize in specific disease such as diabetes mellitus, cancer or cardiac problems or in a specific field such as pediatrics or gerontology. The clinical nurse specialist functions as an expert clinician, educator, case manager, consultant and researcher to plan or improve the quality of care provided to the client and family.

Nurse Anesthetist

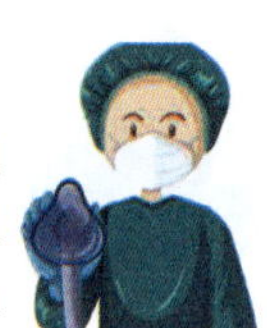

A certified registered nurse anesthetist is a registered nurse who has received advanced training in an accredited program in anesthesiology. Nurse anesthetist provides surgical anesthesia under the guidance and supervision of an anesthesiologist, who is a physician with advanced knowledge of surgical anesthesia.

Nurse Midwife

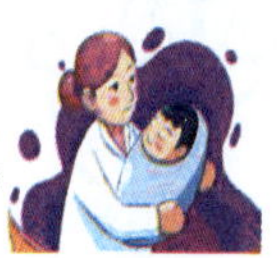

A nurse midwife is a registered nurse who is educated in midwifery. The practice enables independent care of women during normal pregnancy, labor, and delivery, as well as care of newborn. It may include some gynecological services like PAP smears, family planning and treatment for minor vaginal infections.

Nurse Researcher

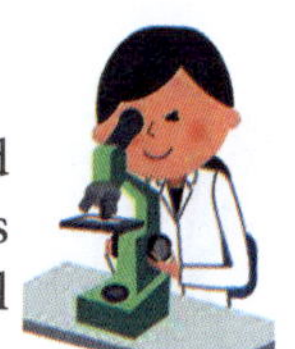

Nurse researcher investigates nursing problems to improve nursing care and to refine and expand nursing knowledge. They are employed in nursing institutions, teaching hospitals and research centers. A nurse researcher usually has advanced education at the doctoral level with at least a master's degree in nursing.

Research involves action taken to implement studies to determine the actual effect of nursing care to further the scientific base of nursing. It can include all nurses, nurse scientists, graduates and students. Research is a nurse's primary responsibility, and all nurses should be involved in research.

Nurse Administrator

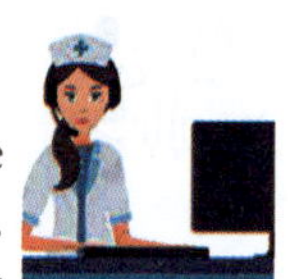

The nurse administrator manages client care including the delivery of nursing services. The administrator may have middle management position such as director of nursing services. Nurse manager's position usually requires at least bachelor's degree in nursing, and director and nurse executive positions generally require a master's degree. Chief nursing executive and vice-president positions in large healthcare organization often require preparation at the doctorate level. Nurses may have degrees such as hospital administration, public health, etc.

Nurse Educator

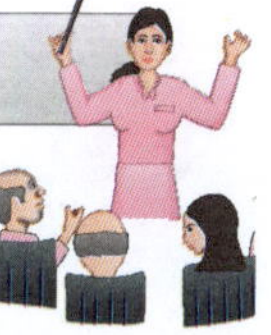

Nurse educator teaches patients and families, the community, other healthcare team members, students, business and government. In hospital setup, nurse provides information about illness, medication, treatment and rehabilitation needs. They help patients understand how to deal with the life changes necessitated by chronic illness. Nurses also teach how to adopt care to the home settings, when that is required. They also demonstrate procedures such as self-care activities.

In community settings, nurses offer classes on injury and illness prevention and health promotion. These classes are often jointly taught with other healthcare team members.

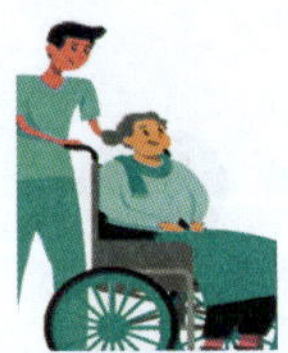

Caregiver

As a caregiver, the nurse helps the client regain health through the healing process. Healing is more than just curing specific disease. Although, treatment skills that promote physical healing are important to caregivers. A nurse addresses the holistic healthcare needs of the client, including measures to restore emotional, spiritual and social well-being. The caregiver sets goals and meets those goals with a minimal cost of time and energy.

Nurse Advocate

As a client advocate, the nurse protects the clients' human and legal rights and provides assistance in asserting those rights, if need arises. The nurse advocates for the client, keeping in mind the client's religion and culture. For example, the nurse may provide additional information for a client who is trying to decide whether or not to accept a treatment. The healthcare system is complex and needs a nurse advocate to help patient.

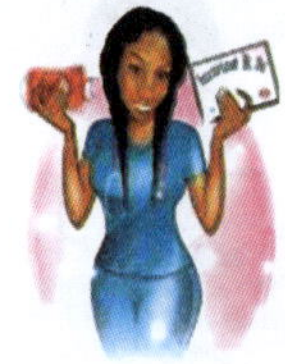

Nurse Entrepreneur

Nurse entrepreneurs are becoming more common. Nurses now have business of their own that provides direct patient services in hospitals, community setting, business, schools, homes, and many other settings. They provide services to business by conducting worksite wellness programs and by advising human resource staff on how to provide high quality health benefits to employees while reducing their cost.

The nurse should have advanced degree to manage health related business. The nurse may be involved in education, consultation and research and counseling.

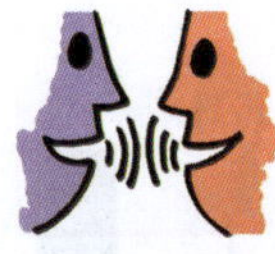

Nurse Communicator

The role of communicator is central in all nursing roles and activities. Nursing involves communication with clients and families, healthcare professionals, resource persons and the community. It is impossible to give effective care, make decisions with clients and families, protect clients in rehabilitation or offer comfort without clear communication.

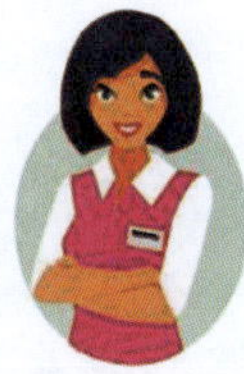

Nurse Manager

As a manager, the nurse coordinates the activities of other members of the healthcare team such as nutritionist and physical therapists, when managing care for a group of clients. To effectively manage a single client or group of clients, the nurse implements solid clinical decision-making skills. As a clinical decision and decision-maker, the nurse uses critical thinking skills throughout the nursing process to provide effective care. Before undertaking any nursing action, the nurse plans the action by deciding the best approach for each client. The nurse makes these decisions alone or in collaboration with the client and family. In each of these situations, the nurse collaborates and consults with other healthcare professionals.

The nurse managers are responsible for managing client's care and overseeing other nurses within the organization to supervise critical procedures like reporting and documentation.

Nurse Counselor

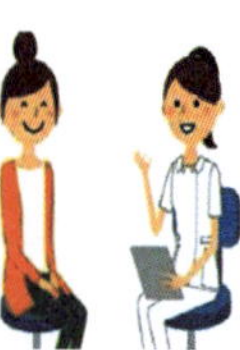

Counseling is the process of helping the client to recognize and cope with stressful psychological or social problems to develop improved interpersonal relationship and to promote personal growth. It involves providing emotional, intellectual and psychological support. The nurse counsels primarily healthy individuals with normal adjustment difficulties and focuses on helping the person to develop new attitudes, feelings and behaviors by encouraging and motivating the client.

FURTHER READINGS

- Roux G, Halstead JA. Issues and Trends in Nursing: Practice Policy and Leadership, 2nd edition. Burlington: Jones and Bartlett Publishers; 2017.
- Trained Nurses Association of India. History and Trends in Nursing in India. TNAI Publication.

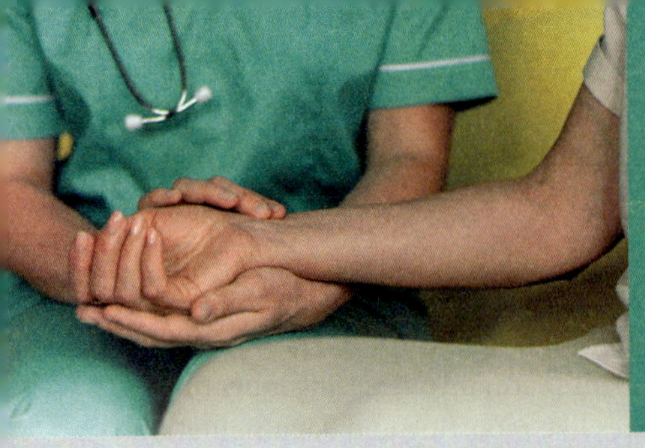

STUDENT ASSIGNMENT

LONG ANSWER QUESTIONS

1. Discuss the roles played by a nurse in the present time.
2. How is nurse practitioner different from nurse administrator?

SHORT ANSWER QUESTIONS

1. Write about trends in nursing education.
2. Write a short note on nurse managers.

MULTIPLE CHOICE QUESTIONS

1. **What is nursing education?**
   a. Educating children about nurses
   b. A specific training a nurse receives to be qualified to work with patients
   c. Training teachers to teach nurses
   d. Educating families of nurses

2. **How are nurses trained to make sure patients can take care of themselves as a preventive measure?**
   a. Educate patients
   b. Give shots
   c. Hand out good reading materials
   d. Schedule appointments

3. **What new technology allows a nurse to access patient's information immediately?**
   a. File folders
   b. Pagers
   c. Telephones
   d. Wearable technology

4. **What are the most commonly used models of care in ICUs?**
   a. Functional nursing
   b. Team nursing
   c. Primary nursing
   d. Total patient care

5. **Objectives of nursing supervision include all; except:**
   a. Promote communication
   b. Initiate disciplinary actions
   c. Promote motivation
   d. Evaluate and improve performance

ANSWER KEY

1. b   **2.** a   **3.** d   **4.** a   **5.** d

Code of Ethics and Professional Conduct for Nurses

LEARNING OBJECTIVES

After the completion of the chapter, the readers will be able to:
- Discuss the types, purposes and uses of ethics.
- Understand the INC code of professional conduct for nurses.
- Understand the ICN code of ethics.

CHAPTER OUTLINE

- Introduction
- Types of Ethics
- Ethics in Nursing
- INC Code of Ethics
- INC Code of Professional Conduct for Nurses
- International Council for Nurses (ICN) Code of Ethics

KEY TERMS

Basic nursing education: A formally recognized program of study providing a broad and sound foundation in the behavioral, life and nursing sciences for the general practice of nursing, for a leadership role, and for post-basic education for specialty or advanced nursing practice.

Code: A code may be defined as conventionalized set of rules or expectations devised for a specific purpose.

Competence: The integrated knowledge, skills, judgment and attributes required from a nurse to practice safely and ethically in a designated role and setting.

Confidentiality: Refers to the duty of the nurse to refrain from sharing patient information with third parties unrelated to the patient's care.

Conscientious objection: Refusing to participate in required action or seeking exemption from participation in classes of interventions (e.g., abortion, gender reassignment surgery, organ transplantation) that threaten a person's sense of moral integrity.

Coworkers: Nurses and other health and nonhealth related workers and professionals.

Environmental justice: It includes sustainability, representative participation, and the avoidance of environmental discrimination.

Equity: An aspect of social justice.

Ethics: The branch of philosophy that examines the difference between right and wrong.

Evidence-informed practice: A process for making informed clinical decisions. Research evidence is integrated with clinical experience, patient values, preferences and circumstances.

Family: A social unit composed of members connected through blood, kinship, emotional or legal relationships.

Fitness to practice: Having the skills, knowledge, health and character to do one's job safely and effectively.

Human rights: The rights that are fundamental in nature irrespective of race, ethnicity, sex, nationality, language, religion or any other status.

National Nurses Associations (NNAs): Any professional national nursing group that clarifies, researches, educates and promotes the continued development of nurses and nursing.

Nurse: The nurse is a person who has completed a program of basic, generalized nursing education and is authorized by the appropriate regulatory authority to practice nursing in his/her country.

Personal information: The information obtained during professional contact that is private to an individual or family, and which, when disclosed, may violate the right to privacy, cause inconvenience, embarrassment or harm to the individual or family.

Primary healthcare: A whole-of-society approach to health and well-being centered on the needs and preferences of individuals, families and communities.

Privacy: The right to freedom from intrusion into one's personal matters, information or one's body.

Professional relationship: An ongoing interaction between two people that observes a set of established boundaries or limits that is deemed appropriate under governing ethical standards.

Social determinants of health: The conditions in which people are born, grow, live, work and age.

Social media: An umbrella term to describe social interaction through technology-based tools, many of which are online like Facebook, Twitter, Instagram and LinkedIn.

Sustainable development goals: The blueprint to achieve a better and more sustainable future for all people.

Values: Sought by both the profession and in nurse-patient relationships such as dignity, respect, compassion, equity.

INTRODUCTION

The code of ethics for nurses was developed as a guide for carrying out nursing responsibilities in a manner consistent with quality in nursing care and the ethical obligations of the profession.

Code of ethics is a specific set of professional behaviors and values the professional interpreter must know and must abide by, including confidentiality, accuracy, privacy and integrity. The ethical code is adopted by an organization in an attempt to assist those in the organization called upon to make a decision, understand the difference between right and wrong; and to apply this understanding to their decisions.

TYPES OF ETHICS

There are two types of ethics: (i) Employee ethics (ii) Professional Ethics.

Employee Ethics

- A code of conduct is a document designed to influence the behavior of employees. The code of conduct sets out the procedure to be used in specific ethical situations.
- The effectiveness of such code of ethics depends on the extent to which management supports them with sanctions and rewards.
- Violations of a code of conduct may subject the violator to the organization's remedies which can, under particular circumstances, result in the termination of employment.

Professional Ethics

- A code of practice is adopted by a profession or governmental or nongovernmental organization to regulate that profession.
- A code of practice can be styled as a code of professional responsibility, which will discuss difficult issues, difficult decisions that will often need to be made and provide a clear account of what behavior is considered "ethical" or "correct" or "right" in the circumstances.
- Ethics gives the professionals various guidelines that how they should behave with each other, with public and with governments. It refers to guidelines which the professionals should follow when they are dealing with their clients.
- Ethics tells the public what they can expect from a professional; and tells the professionals what the public expects from them.

ETHICS IN NURSING

- Nursing ethics refers to ethical issues that occur in nursing practice. The code of professional conduct for nurses is critical for building professionalism and accountability.
- Ethical considerations are vital in any area dealing with human beings because they represent values, rights and relationships. A nurse must have professional competence, responsibility and accountability with moral obligations. A nurse is obliged to provide services even if they are in conflict with his/her personal beliefs and values.

Code of Ethics

Meaning

Code of ethics refers to a set of guiding principles for professional conduct and behavior. It is a guide for carrying out nursing responsibilities in a manner, consistent with quality in nursing care and the ethical obligations of the profession.

These are set of rules or guidelines that people agree to follow to be fair, honest and good in a certain area of life at work.

Definition

A code of ethics is a form of standardization at work place behavior, hence it is a more detailed general behavioral guidelines set by law (Bracknell & Cohen, 2005).

Purposes

Purposes of code of ethics are as follows:

- To inform both the nurse and the society of the minimum standards for professional conduct.
- To provide regulatory bodies a basis for decisions regarding standards of professional conduct.
- To protect the rights of individuals, families and community and also the rights of the nurse.

Uses of Codes of Ethics

Uses of codes of ethics are as follows:

- Acknowledge the rightful place of individuals in healthcare delivery system.
- Contribute toward empowerment of individuals to become responsible for their health and well-being.
- Contribute to quality care.
- Identify obligations in practice, research and relationships.
- Inform the individuals, families, community and other professionals about expectations from a nurse.

INC CODE OF ETHICS

1. **The nurse respects the uniqueness of individual in provision of care.**

   Nurse:
   1.1 Provides care for individuals without consideration of caste, creed, religion, culture, ethnicity, gender, socioeconomic and political status, personal attributes or any other grounds.
   1.2 Individualizes the care, considering the care, considering the beliefs, values and cultural sensitivities.
   1.3 Appreciates the place of the individual in family and community and facilitates participation of significant others in the care.
   1.4 Develops and promotes trustful relationship with individuals.
   1.5 Recognizes uniqueness of response of individuals to interactions and adapts accordingly.

2. **The nurse respects the rights of individuals as partners in care and helps in making informed choices.**

   Nurse:
   2.1 Appreciates individual's right to make decisions about their care and therefore, gives adequate and accurate information for enabling them to make informed choices.
   2.2 Respects the decisions made by individual(s) regarding their care.
   2.3 Protects public from misinformation and misinterpretation.
   2.4 Advocates special provisions to protect vulnerable individuals/groups.

3. **The nurse respects individual's right to privacy, maintains confidentiality and shares information judiciously.**

   Nurse:
   3.1 Respects the individual's right to privacy of their personal information.
   3.2 Maintains confidentiality of privileged information except in life-threatening situations and uses discretion in sharing information.
   3.3 Takes informed consent and maintains anonymity when information is required for quality assurance/academic/legal reasons.

3.4. Limits the access to all personal records, written and computerized, to authorized persons only.

4. **Nurse maintains competence in order to render quality nursing care.**
   4.1 Nursing care must be provided only by a registered nurse.
   4.2 Nurse strives to maintain quality nursing care and upholds the standards of core.
   4.3 Nurse values continuing education, initiates and utilizes all opportunities for self-development.
   4.4 Nurse values research as a means of development of nursing profession and participates in nursing research adhering to ethical principles.

5. **The nurse is obliged to practice within the framework of ethical, professional and legal boundaries.**
   Nurse:
   5.1 Adheres to code of ethics and code of professional conduct for nurses in India developed by Indian Nursing Council.
   5.2 Familiarizes himself/herself with relevant laws and practices in accordance with the law of the state.

6. **Nurse is obliged to work harmoniously with the members of the health team.**
   6.1 Appreciates the team efforts in rendering care.
   6.2 Cooperates, coordinates and collaborates with the members of the health team to meet the needs of the people.

7. **Nurse commits to reciprocate the trust invested in nursing profession by society.**
   7.1 Demonstrates personal etiquettes in all dealings.
   7.1 Demonstrates professional attributes in all dealings.

INC CODE OF PROFESSIONAL CONDUCT FOR NURSES

1. **Professional Responsibility and Accountability**
   Nurse:
   1.1 Appreciates sense of self-worth and nurtures it.
   1.2 Maintains standards of professional conduct reflecting credit upon the profession.
   1.3 Carries out responsibilities within the framework of the professional boundaries.
   1.4 Is accountable for maintaining practice standards set by the Indian Nursing Council.
   1.5 Is accountable for own decisions and actions.
   1.6 Is compassionate.
   1.7 Is responsible for continuous improvement of current practices.
   1.8 Provides adequate information to individuals that allows them to make informed choices.
   1.9 Practices healthful behavior.

2. **Nursing Practice**
   Nurse:
   2.1 Provides care in accordance with set standards of practice.
   2.2 Treats all individuals and families with human dignity in providing physical, psychological, emotional, social and spiritual aspects of care.
   2.3 Respects individuals and families in the context of traditional and cultural practices and discourages harmful practices.
   2.4 Presents realistic picture truthfully in all situations for facilitating autonomous decision-making by individuals and families.

2.5 Promotes participation of individuals and significant others in the care.

2.6 Ensures safe practices.

2.7 Consults, coordinates, collaborates and follows up appropriately when individual care needs exceed the nurse's competence.

3. **Communication and Interpersonal Relationships**

Nurse:

3.1 Establishes and maintains effective interpersonal relationship with individuals, families and communities.

3.2 Upholds the dignity of team members and maintains effective interpersonal relationship with them.

3.3 Appreciates and nurtures professional role of team members.

3.4 Cooperates with other health professionals to meet the needs of the individuals, families and communities.

4. **Valuing Human Being**

Nurse:

4.1 Takes appropriates action to protect individuals from harmful ethical practice.

4.2 Considers relevant facts while taking conscience decisions in the best interest of individuals.

4.3 Encourages and supports individuals in their right to speak for themselves and issues affecting their health and welfare.

4.4 Respects and supports choices made by individuals.

5. **Management**

Nurse:

5.1 Ensures appropriate allocation and utilization of available resources.

5.2 Participates in supervision and education of students and other formal care providers.

5.3 Uses judgment in relation to individual competence while accepting and delegating responsibility.

5.4 Facilitates conducive work culture in order to achieve institutional objectives.

5.5 Communicates effectively following appropriate channels of communication.

5.6 Participates in performance appraisal.

5.7 Participates in evaluation of nursing services.

5.8 Participates in policy decisions, following the principles of equity and accessibility of services.

5.9 Works with individuals to identify their needs and sensitizes policy makers and funding agencies for resource allocation.

6. **Professional Advancement**

Nurse:

6.1 Ensures the protection of the human rights while pursuing the advancement of knowledge.

6.2 Contributes to the development.

6.3 Participates in determining and implementing quality care.

6.4 Takes responsibility for updating own knowledge and competencies.

6.5 Contributes to the care of professional knowledge by conducting and participating in research.

INTERNATIONAL COUNCIL FOR NURSES (ICN) CODE OF ETHICS

An international code of ethics for nurses was first adopted by the International Council for Nurses (ICN) in 1953. It has been revised and reaffirmed from time to time. It has been revised and reaffirmed at various times since, most recently with this review and revision were completed in 2021 (Fig. 3.1).

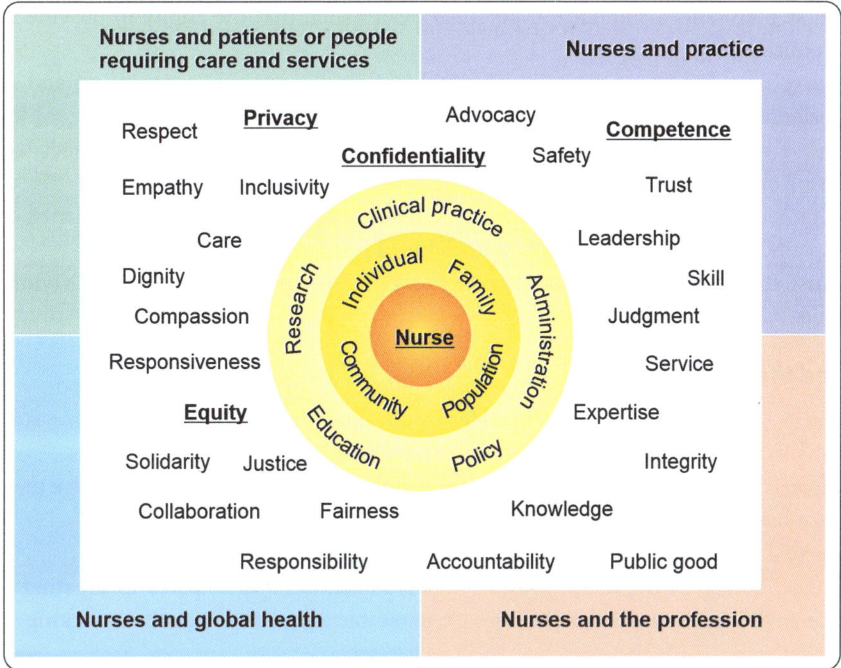

Figure 3.1: ICN code of ethics for nurses—Professional values 2021

The ICN code of ethics for nurses has four principal elements that outline the standards of ethical conduct.

Elements ICN Code of Ethics

Nurses and People

- The nurse's primary professional responsibility is toward people requiring nursing care.
- While providing care, the nurse promotes an environment in which the human rights, values, customs and spiritual beliefs of the individual, family and community are respected.
- The nurse ensures that the individual receives accurate, sufficient and timely information in a culturally appropriate manner on which to base consent for care and related treatment.
- The nurse holds in confidence personal information and uses judgment while sharing patient's information.
- The nurse shares with society the responsibility for initiating and supporting action to meet the health and social needs of the public, in particular those of vulnerable populations.
- The nurse advocates for equity and social justice in resource allocation, access to healthcare and other social and economic services.
- The nurse demonstrates professional values such as respectfulness, responsiveness, compassion, trustworthiness and integrity.

Nurses and Practice

- The nurse carries personal responsibility and accountability for nursing practice and for maintaining competence by continual learning.

- The nurse maintains a standard of personal health such that the ability to provide care is not compromised.
- The nurse uses judgment regarding individual competence while accepting and delegating responsibility.
- The nurse maintains standards of personal conduct at all times, which reflect well on the profession and enhance its image and public confidence.
- While providing care, the nurse must ensure that the use of technology and scientific advances is compatible with the safety, dignity and rights of people.
- The nurse strives to foster and maintain a practice culture promoting ethical behavior and open dialogue.

Nurses and the Profession

- The nurse assumes a major role in determining and implementing acceptable standards of clinical nursing practice, management, research and education.
- The nurse is active in developing a core of research-based professional knowledge that supports evidence-based practice.
- The nurse is active in developing and sustaining a core of professional values.
- The nurse, acting through the professional organization, participates in creating a positive practice environment and maintaining safe, equitable social and economic working conditions in nursing.
- The nurse practices to sustain and protect the natural environment and is aware of its consequences on health.
- The nurse contributes to an ethical organizational environment and challenges unethical practices and setting.

Nurses and Coworkers

- The nurse sustains a collaborative and respectful relationship with coworkers in nursing and other fields.
- The nurse takes appropriate actions to safeguard individuals, families and communities when their health is endangered by a coworker and any other person.
- The nurse takes appropriate actions to support and guide coworkers to advance ethical conduct.

Revised ICN Code of Ethics

Revised ICN code of ethics in 2021 is as follows:

1. **Nurses and Patients or other People Requiring Care or Services**
    1.1 Primary professional responsibility of nurses is toward people requiring nursing care and services now or in the future, whether individuals, families, communities or populations (hereinafter referred to as either 'patients' or 'people requiring care').
    1.2 Nurses promote an environment in which the human rights, values, customs, religious and spiritual beliefs of the individual, families and communities are acknowledged and respected by everyone. Nurses' rights are included under human rights and should be upheld and protected.
    1.3 Nurses ensure that the individual and family receive understandable, accurate, sufficient and timely information in a manner appropriate to the patient's culture, linguistic, cognitive and physical needs, and psychological state on which to base consent for care and related treatment.

1.4   Nurses hold in confidence personal information and respect the privacy, confidentiality and interests of patients in the lawful collection, use, access, transmission, storage and disclosure of personal information.

1.5   Nurses respect the privacy and confidentiality of colleagues and people requiring care and uphold the integrity of the nursing profession in person and in all media, including social media.

1.6   Nurses share with society the responsibility for initiating and supporting action to meet the health and social needs of all people.

1.7   Nurses advocate for equity and social justice in resource allocation, access to healthcare and other social and economic services.

1.8   Nurses demonstrate professional values such as respect, justice, responsiveness, care, compassion, empathy, trustworthiness and integrity. They support and respect the dignity and universal rights of all people, including patients, colleagues and families.

1.9   Nurses facilitate a culture of safety in healthcare environments, recognizing and addressing threats to people and safe care in health practices, services and settings.

1.10   Nurses provide evidence-informed, person-centered care, recognizing and using the values and principles of primary healthcare and health promotion across the lifespan.

1.11   Nurses ensure that the use of technology and scientific advances is compatible with the safety, dignity and rights of people. In the case of artificial intelligence or devices, such as care robots or drones, nurses ensure that care remains person-centered and that such devices support and do not replace human relationships.

Applying the Elements of the Code #1: Nurses and Patients or People Requiring Care or Services		
Nurses, nurse leaders and nurse managers	**Educators and researchers**	**National nurses' associations**
Provide people-focused, culturally appropriate care that respects human rights and is sensitive to the values, customs and beliefs of people without prejudice or unjust discrimination.	In curricula, include content on cultural norms, safety and competence, ethics, human rights, equity, human dignity, justice, disparities and solidarity as the basis for access to healthcare. Design studies to explore human rights issues.	Develop position statements, standards of practice and guidelines that support human rights and ethical standards.
Participate in continuing education on ethical issues, ethical reasoning and ethical conduct. Encourage open dialogue among all stakeholders.	Design curricula to encompass currently peer reviewed and published approaches to nursing ethics. Provide teaching and learning opportunities for ethical issues, ethical principles and reasoning, and ethical decision-making. This includes respect for autonomy, nonmaleficence, beneficence and justice.	Establish standards for ethics education and provide continuing ethics education for nurses.
Ensure informed consent for nursing and/or medical care. This includes the right to choose or refuse treatments.	Educate about respect for autonomy, informed consent, privacy and confidentiality. Respect research participants' right to refuse to participate in or withdraw from studies without prejudice.	Provide guidelines for human participants in research, position statements, relevant documentation and continuing education related to informed consent for nursing and medical care.

Contd...

Applying the Elements of the Code #1: Nurses and Patients or People Requiring Care or Services		
Nurses, nurse leaders and nurse managers	**Educators and researchers**	**National nurses' associations**
Exercise professional ethical judgment in the use of information, health records and reporting systems, whether electronic or paper-based, to ensure protection of human rights, confidentiality and privacy in accordance with patient preferences and community safety and in compliance with any relevant laws.	In curricula, include accuracy, confidentiality and privacy on the use of media, reporting and recording systems, whether images, recordings or comments. Be familiar with the use of required reporting for extreme emergencies.	Prepare guidelines and standards of practice on appropriate use of information and reporting systems that ensure protection of human rights, confidentiality, privacy, and mandated reporting mechanisms for public health outbreaks or extreme emergencies.
Communicate to appropriate supervisors and/or authorities any risks, inappropriate behaviors or misuse of technologies that threaten people's safety, and provide facts supporting this. Nurses need to be involved when technology is developed, and observe and report risks with technology and scientific advancements.	Include in curriculum and conduct research on what constitutes safe care that respects dignity and rights and considers new technology.	Lobby governments, health organizations, medical device and pharmaceutical companies to include nurses during research and development of technology for patient use.
Meet nurses' ethical obligations and responsibilities and actively affirm the values and ideals of the profession.	In curricula, include professional values and ideals, ethical responsibilities and obligations, and ethical frameworks with worldviews. Contribute to and disseminate emphasis on ethical research guidelines. Design studies to explore human rights issues.	Express the values and ideals of nursing in their foundational documents and incorporate into national codes of ethics for nurses.
Develop and monitor safety at the workplace.	Teach and facilitate learning about attributes, risk factors and skills to ensure practice environments that are healthy, safe and sustainable for everyone in the healthcare setting.	Influence employers to promote healthy and safe workplaces for nurses and other healthcare workers. Provide guidelines that assure a safe environment and healthy communities. Advocate for clear, accessible, transparent and effective reporting procedures to protect health and safety.

2. **Nurses and Practice**

    2.1 Nurses carry personal responsibility and accountability for ethical nursing practice, and for maintaining competence by engaging in continuous professional development and lifelong learning.

    2.2 Nurses maintain fitness to practice so as not to compromise their ability to provide quality and safe care.

2.3　Nurses practice within the limits of their individual competence and regulated or authorized scope of practice and use professional judgment while accepting and delegating responsibility.

2.4　Nurses value their own dignity, well-being and health. To achieve this requires positive practice environments, characterized by professional recognition, education, reflection, support structures, adequate resourcing, sound management practices and occupational health and safety.

2.5　Nurses maintain standards of personal conduct at all times, which reflect well on the profession and enhance its image and public confidence. In their professional role, nurses recognize and maintain personal relationship boundaries.

2.6　Nurses share their knowledge and expertise and provide feedback, mentoring and support the professional development of student nurses, novice nurses, colleagues and other healthcare providers.

2.7　Nurses are patient advocates, and they maintain a practice culture that promotes ethical behavior and open dialogue.

2.8　Nurses may conscientiously object to participate in particular procedures or nursing or health-related research but must facilitate respectful and timely action to ensure that people receive care appropriate to their individual needs.

2.9　Nurses maintain a person's right to give and withdraw consent to access their personal, health and genetic information. They protect the use of genetic information, and maintain the privacy and confidentiality of genetic information and human genome technologies.

2.10　Nurses take appropriate actions to safeguard individuals, families, communities and populations when their health is endangered by a coworker, any other person, policy, practice or the misuse of technology.

2.11　Nurses are active participants in the promotion of patient safety. They promote ethical conduct when errors or near misses occur, speak up when patient safety is threatened, advocate for transparency, and work with others to reduce the potential of errors.

2.12　Nurses are accountable for data integrity to support and facilitate ethical standards of care.

Applying the Elements of the Code #2: Nurses and Practice		
Nurses, nurse leaders and nurse managers	Educators and researchers	National nurses' associations
Pursue professional development through reading and study. Request and participate in continuing education to enhance knowledge and skills.	Teach and facilitate learning the value and obligation of lifelong learning and competence to practice. Explore current concepts and innovative teaching methods for theory and practice.	Develop a range of continuing education opportunities, through journals, media, conferences and distance education, that reflect advances in nursing theory and practice.
Initiate continuing education and participate in workplace governance, systems for professional performance, appraisal and systematic renewal of licensure to practice. Monitor, promote and evaluate fitness to practice in nursing staff.	Conduct and disseminate research that explores links between continual learning and competence to practice.	Promote national policies for high-quality nurse education and educational requirements for continued authorization to practice.

Contd...

Applying the Elements of the Code #2: Nurses and Practice		
Nurses, nurse leaders and nurse managers	**Educators and researchers**	**National nurses' associations**
Seek a work-life balance, ongoing personal growth, and maintain a healthy lifestyle.	Teach obligations to self as well as obligations to patients, the importance of fitness to practice, and using evidence-informed care. In curricula, include promoting resilience at the workplace.	Lobby for working environments that promote healthy lifestyle standards for nurses. Provide guidelines on safe and decent work conditions for nurses.
Foster interprofessional collaboration for managing conflict and tensions. Promote an environment of shared ethical values. To improve quality of care and safety, fear of reprisal must be extinguished. This will create a more open, transparent culture that embraces crucial conversations for advancing health for all.	Teach methods and skills of situational assessment and conflict management as well as the roles and values of other healthcare disciplines.	Inform other disciplines and the public about the roles of nurses and the values of the nursing profession. Promote a positive image of nursing. Champion work environments and conditions that are free from abuse, harassment and violence.
Develop appropriate professional relationships with patients and colleagues; exercise professional judgment and decline gifts or bribes and avoid conflicts of interest.	Maintain and teach professional boundaries and skills to safeguard them. Teach identification of and methods to avoid conflicts of interest.	Set standards for professional boundaries and establish processes for the expression of recognition and gratitude.
Assure continuity of care for the patient when exercising conscientious objection, where an action may cause harm or is morally objectionable to the nurse.	Encourage self-reflection and teach frameworks and processes of conscientious objection.	Develop standards and guidelines for refusal of participation in specific medical procedures. Include guidance on conscientious objection in national codes of ethics.

3. **Nurses and the Profession**

   3.1 Nurses assume major leadership role in determining and implementing evidence-informed, acceptable standards of clinical nursing practice, management, research and education.

   3.2 Nurses and nursing scholars are active in expanding research-based, current professional knowledge that supports evidence-informed practice.

   3.3 Nurses are active in developing and sustaining the core of professional values.

   3.4 Nurses, through their professional organizations, participate in creating a positive and constructive practice environment where practice encompasses clinical care, education, research, management and leadership. This includes environments which facilitate a nurse's ability to practice to their optimal scope of practice and to deliver safe, effective and timely healthcare, in working conditions which are safe as well as socially and economically equitable for nurses.

   3.5 Nurses contribute to positive and ethical organizational environments and challenge unethical practices and settings. Nurses collaborate with nursing colleagues, other (health) disciplines and relevant communities to engage in the ethical creation, conduct and dissemination of peer reviewed and ethically responsible research and practice development as they relate to patient care, nursing and health.

3.6   Nurses engage in the creation, dissemination and application of research that improves outcomes for individuals, families and communities.

3.7   Nurses prepare for and respond to emergencies, disasters, conflicts, epidemics, pandemics, social crises and conditions of scarce resources. The safety of those who receive care and services is a responsibility shared by individual nurses and the leaders of health systems and organizations. This involves assessing risks and developing, implementing and resourcing plans to mitigate these.

Applying the Elements of the Code #3: Nurses and the Profession		
Nurses, nurse leaders and nurse managers	**Educators and researchers**	**National nurses associations**
Collaborate with colleagues to support the conduct, dissemination and use of research related to patient care, nursing and health.	Teach research methodology, ethics and evaluation. Conduct, disseminate, utilize and evaluate research to study and advance nursing knowledge.	Develop position statements, guidelines, policy and standards informed by nursing research and scholarly inquiry.
Promote participation in national nurses' associations to create solidarity and cooperation to promote favorable socioeconomic and working conditions for nurses.	Emphasize to learners the nature, function and importance of professional nursing associations and international nursing collaboration.	Communicate the importance of membership in professional nursing organizations and promote participation in national nurses' associations.
Practice ethical behaviors and develop strategies to deal with moral distress during emergent crises, such as pandemics or conflicts.	Prepare students for local response to global issues with a broader vision of solidarity and the common good. Include health disparities, particularly for infants, frail elderly, prisoners, economically disadvantaged, trafficked, displaced persons and refugees.	Collaborate with global organizations to address current and emergent social justice issues.
Develop guidelines for workplace issues, such as bullying, violence, sexual harassment, fatigue, safety, and local incident management. Participate in studies regarding ethics and ethical workplace issues in every setting.	Teach identification of unhealthy work environments and skills to develop resilient and healthy workplace communities. Conduct research on ethical workplace issues across the profession.	Influence, pressure and negotiate for fair and decent working conditions. Develop position statements and guidelines to address workplace issues.
Prepare for and respond to emergencies, disasters, conflicts, epidemics, pandemics and conditions of scarce resources.	Ensure that curricula include essential elements of caring for people and populations in high-risk, challenging environments.	Advocate and lobby governments and health organizations to prioritize; and protect the health, safety and well-being of healthcare workers while responding to health emergencies.

Contd...

Applying the Elements of the Code #3: Nurses and the Profession		
Nurses, nurse leaders and nurse managers	**Educators and researchers**	**National nurses associations**
Practice nondiscrimination against colleagues from other cultures and countries regardless of nationality, race, ethnicity or language.	Teach the principles of the WHO Code of Practice on International Recruitment of Health Personnel to support the ethical recruitment of nurses.	Promote the ethical recruitment of nurses and work with government and licensing boards to reduce barriers to employment for migrant nurses.

4. **Nurses and Global Health**

　4.1　Nurses value healthcare as a human right, affirming the right to universal access to healthcare for all.

　4.2　Nurses uphold the dignity, freedom and worth of all human beings and oppose all forms of exploitation, such as human trafficking and child labor.

　4.3　Nurses lead or contribute to sound health policy development.

　4.4　Nurses contribute to population health and work toward the achievement of the United Nations Sustainable Development Goals (UNSDGs).

　4.5　Nurses recognize the significance of the social determinants of health. They contribute to, and advocate for, policies and programs that address them.

　4.6　Nurses collaborate and practice to preserve, sustain and protect the natural environment and are aware of the health consequences of environmental degradation, e.g., climate change. They advocate for initiatives that reduce environmentally harmful practices to promote health and well-being.

　4.7　Nurses collaborate with other health and social care professions and the public to uphold principles of justice by promoting responsibility in human rights, equity and fairness and by promoting the public good and a healthy planet.

　4.8　Nurses collaborate across countries to develop and maintain global health and to ensure policies and principles for this.

Applying the Elements of the Code #4: Nurses and Global Health		
Nurses, nurse leaders and nurse managers	**Educators and researchers**	**National nurses' associations**
Participate in human rights efforts, such as detecting and preventing trafficking, helping vulnerable populations, providing universal education, and mitigating hunger and poverty.	Ensure that curricula include human rights, SDGs, universal access to care, culturally appropriate care, civic responsibility, equity, and social and environmental justice.	Collaborate with nursing regulatory bodies, voluntary organizations, and global agencies to develop position statements and guidelines that support human rights, environmental justice and international peace.
Educate oneself and colleagues about global health, including current and emergent technologies. Advocate for the ethical use of technology and scientific advances compatible with safety, dignity, privacy, confidentiality and human rights.	Seek opportunities to evaluate the short and long-term ethical consequences of the use of diverse technologies and emerging practices, including innovative equipment, robotics, genetics and genomics, stem cell technologies and organ donation.	Contribute to legislation and policies on the ethical use of technology and scientific advances adapted to the health and social norms and context of the country.

Contd...

Applying the Elements of the Code #4: Nurses and Global Health		
Nurses, nurse leaders and nurse managers	**Educators and researchers**	**National nurses' associations**
Acquire and disseminate knowledge about the negative effects of climate change on people's health and on the planet.	Teach about the facts and consequences of climate change on health and the many opportunities to support climate health at policy and institutional levels.	Participate in the development of legislation to reduce the impact of hospitals and the healthcare industry on the environment and address climate changes that negatively affect the health of populations.
Support the ethical and proficient use of social media and technologies to improve population health consistent with the values of the nursing profession.	Participate in developing, implementing and evaluating new and emerging technologies, including social media, for prevention initiatives, public health education, and the health and well-being of populations. Prepare curricula and engage in research in support of the UN SDGs.	Update knowledge and increase awareness about the UN SDGs for population health and actively strategize nursing participation in achieving these goals.
Act on local and global issues that affect health, such as poverty, food security, shelter, immigration, gender, class, ethnicity, race, environmental health, dignified work, and education.	Educate about sociopolitical and economic issues that affect health, including gender, ethnicity, race, culture, inequality and discrimination. Research sociopolitical factors that contribute to individual and population health and illness.	Collaborate with other national and international nursing organizations to formulate policies and legislations that address the socioeconomic determinants of health.
Embed the concepts of peace, peace diplomacy and peace building into everyday practice.	Educate and research for peace diplomacy and peace building in communities and globally.	Collaborate globally, nationally and regionally with governments and nursing agencies to further the ends of global peace and justice and ameliorate the causes of illness.

FURTHER READINGS

- Code of Ethics for Nurses in India; Code of Professional Conduct for Nurses in India [online] Available from https://hmis.ap.nic.in/APNMC/pdfs/ethics.pdf [Last accessed August, 2023].
- International Council of Nurses (2002). Nursing definitions. [online] Available from https://www.icn.ch/nursing-policy/nursing-definitions [Last accessed August, 2023].
- World Health Organization (2020). Social determinants of health. [online] Available from https://www.who.int/gender-equity-rights/understanding/sdh-definition/ [Last accessed August, 2023].
- World Health Organization (2021). Primary healthcare: key facts. [online] Available from https://www.who.int/news-room/fact-sheets/detail/primary-health-care [Last accessed August, 2023].

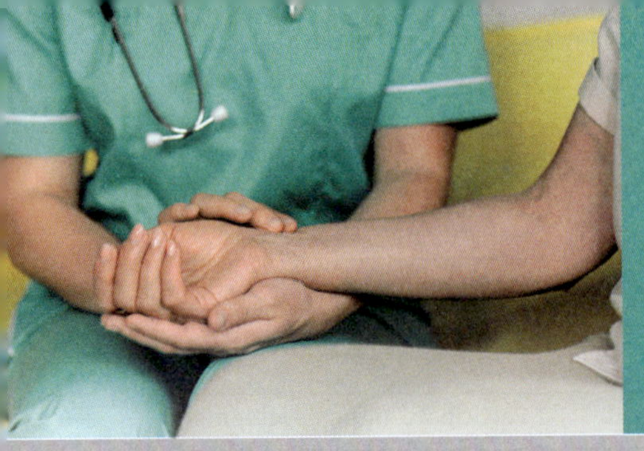

LONG ANSWER QUESTIONS

1. Explain different types of code of ethics.
2. Describe the main purposes of code of ethics.
3. Explain the principal elements of the ICN code of ethics.

SHORT ANSWER QUESTIONS

1. What are the uses of code of ethics?
2. Define the following:
   - i. INC code of ethics
   - ii. Ethics
   - iii. Coworkers
   - iv. Confidentiality
   - v. Values
   - vi. Personal information

MULTIPLE CHOICE QUESTIONS

1. **Which of the following is an ethical principle that guides nursing practice?**
   - a. Autonomy
   - b. Utilitarianism
   - c. Virtue
   - d. Care

2. **What is the ANA code of ethics for nurses?**
   - a. A set of legal rules that nurses must follow.
   - b. A set of moral values that nurses must uphold.
   - c. A set of professional standards that nurses must adhere to.
   - d. A set of ethical frameworks that nurses must apply.

3. **What is informed consent in nursing practice?**
   - a. The process of obtaining permission from a patient to perform a specific procedure or treatment.
   - b. The process of providing information to a patient about the risks and benefits of a specific procedure or treatment.
   - c. The process of ensuring that a patient understands and agrees to a specific procedure or treatment.
   - d. The process of respecting a patient's right to refuse or withdraw from a specific procedure or treatment.

4. **Nursing ethics is defined by:**
   - a. Moral principles and values
   - b. Written rules
   - c. Policy and procedures
   - d. Standards of care

5. **Which of the following options defines the standards of care?**
   - a. How the patient prefers to be taken care of.
   - b. What an ordinary, prudent nurse with similar education and nursing experience would do in similar circumstances.
   - c. The hospital's policy and procedures.
   - d. The expectations of the medical director.

ANSWER KEY

1. a **2.** a **3.** c **4.** a **5.** b

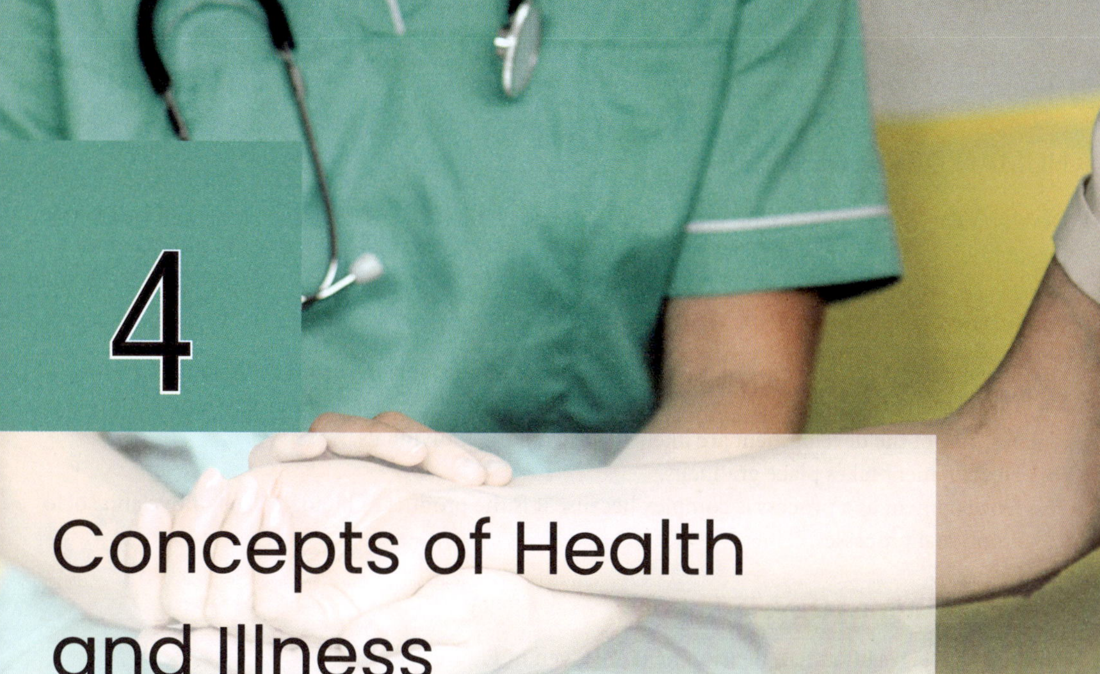

4

Concepts of Health and Illness

LEARNING OBJECTIVES

After the completion of the chapter, the readers will be able to:
- Discuss concepts of health.
- Know GAS and Stuart Stress Adaptation Model.

CHAPTER OUTLINE

- Human Development
- Concepts of Health and Illness
- Factors Affecting Health
- Dimensions of Health
- Determinants of Health

KEY TERMS

Adaptation: It is the change that takes place as a result of the response to a stressor.

Distress or negative stress: Uncontrollable, prolonged or overwhelming stress is destructive.

Eustress or positive stress: Manageable stress which can lead to growth and enhanced competence.

Homeostasis: It refers to a steady state within the body and various physiologic mechanisms within the body respond to internal changes to maintain a relative constancy in the internal environment.

Maladaptive coping: Strategies that cause further problems.

Resilience: Resistant quality that permits a person to recover quickly and thrive in spite of adversity.

Stress: It is a condition in which the human system responds to changes in its normal balanced state.

Stressor: It is anything that is perceived as challenging, threatening or demanding.

HUMAN DEVELOPMENT

Development is the pattern of movement or change that begins at conception and continues throughout the life span which includes growth (may be positive and negative) and decline.

Principles of Human Development

- Development is relatively orderly and can be proximodistal pattern and cephalocaudal pattern.
- While the pattern of development is likely to be similar, the outcomes of development process and rate of the development are likely to vary among individuals.
- Development takes place gradually.
- Development as a process is complex because it is the product of biological, cognitive and socio emotional processes.

Stages of Human Development

The various stages of human development are given in Figure 4.1.

Prenatal development: Conception occurs and development begins there are three stages of prenatal development:

1. Germinal
2. Embryonic
3. Fetal

All of the major structure of the body are forming and the health of the meter is of primary concern.

The influences of nature (genetics) and nature (Nutrition) and teratogens which are environ mental factors during pregnancy that can lead to birth defects) are evident.

- **Birth:** After 36–40 weeks following fertilization, when the baby is fully formed, it is ready to exit the mother's uterus and enter the world. Throughout this stage, the baby begins its journey as a single cell and proceeds to multiply into many cells, forming various organs and body parts necessary for human life.

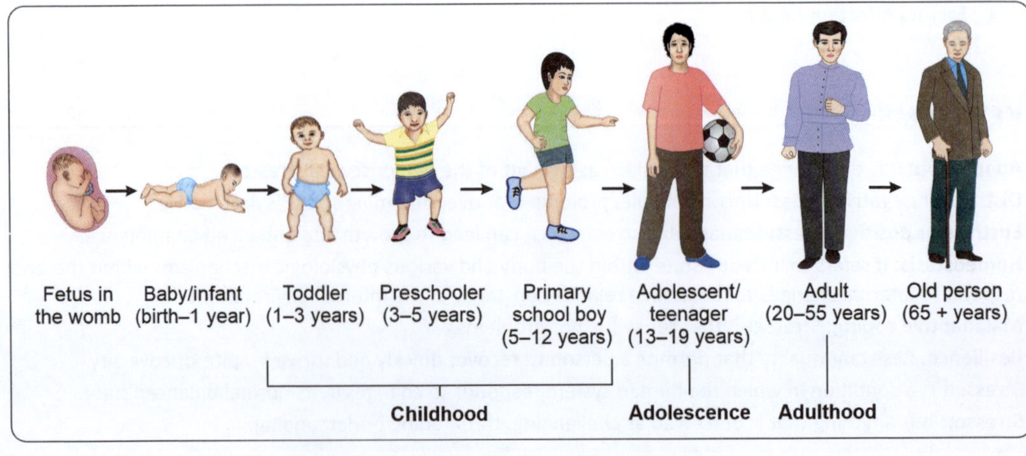

Figure 4.1: Stages of human life development

- **Infancy:** Infancy is categorized as lasting from birth through the first year of life. At this point, the baby exits the mother's uterus. It can breathe, its heart can beat, and other organs can operate efficiently without the assistance of the mother. Although the infant is completely dependent upon its parents and caregivers for survival.
- **Childhood:** Childhood can be divided into:
    - Early childhood (age 1–6 years)
    - Middle childhood (age 6–8 years)
    - Late childhood (age 8–10 years)

  For the first 2 years of childhood, the child is called a toddler. During this time, the child learns how to walk, talk and be more self-sufficient. These skills continue to expand during rest of the childhood and socialization takes place. Childhood is the foundation on which adolescence and later adulthood is built.
- **Adolescence:** Adolescence stage is between age 12 and 18 and is a critical turning point because it is when puberty takes place. The biological event of puberty unleashes a powerful set of changes in the adolescent body that reflect themselves in a teenager's sexual, emotional, cultural and spiritual passion. In adolescence, the boy's voice changes and the menstrual cycle begins in the girls. Children start separating from their parents and become more independent.
- **Adulthood:** It is the longest stage. Adulthood is when human beings are fully grown. At the end of adulthood, the body begins to deteriorate. Adulthood can be divided into:
    - Early adulthood (age 20–35 years)
    - Midlife (age 35–55 years)
    - Mature adulthood (age 60 + years)
    - Late adulthood (age 80 + years)

Erikson Stages of Psychosocial Development

Erikson articulated stages of psychosocial development through which a healthy developing human should pass, from infancy to late adulthood. These stages have been given in Figure 4.2.

- **Stage 1: Infancy (psychological crisis "trust versus mistrust"):** Trust versus mistrust is the earliest psychosocial stage that occurs during the first year. During this stage the infant is

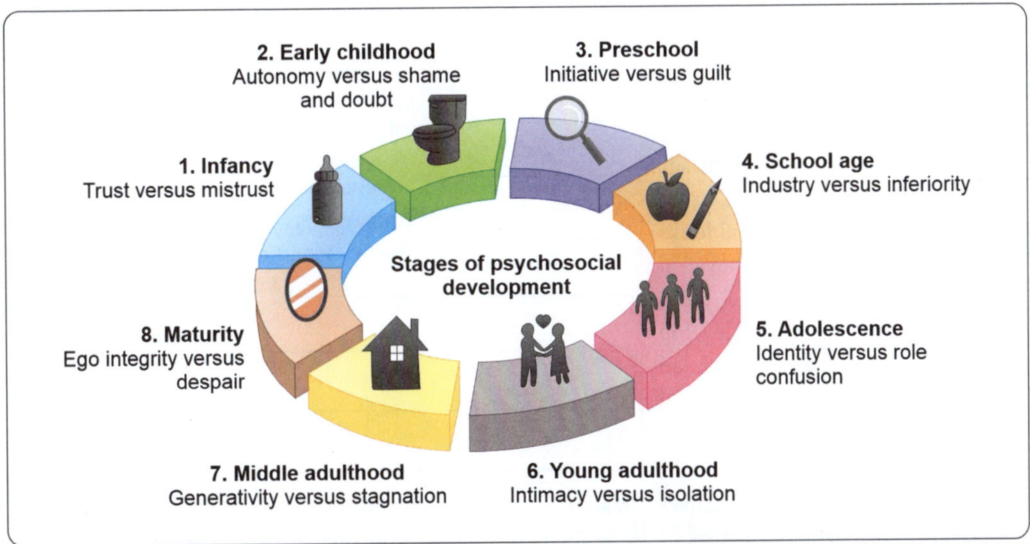

Figure 4.2: Erikson stages of psychosocial development

uncertain about the world in which they live. To resolve these feelings of uncertainty the infant looks toward their primary caregivers for stability and consistency of care.

- **Stage 2: Early childhood autonomy versus (shame and doubt):** At this stage, the child develops physically and becomes more moveable. It is critical that parents allow their children to explore the limits of their abilities within an encouraging environment which is to be learnt from failure.
- **Stage 3: Preschool initiative versus (guilt age 3–5 years):** This age is centered on developing a sense of self-initiative. Children who are allowed and encouraged to engage in self-directed play, emerge with a sense of strong initiative, while those who are discouraged from these activities may begin to feel a sense of guilt over their self-initiated activities.
- **Stage 4: School age industry (competence) versus inferiority (age 5–12 years):** During middle childhood (ages 6–11 years), children enter the psychosocial stage. As children engage in social interaction with friends and academic activities at school, they begin to develop a sense of pride and accomplishment in their work and abilities. Children who are praised and encouraged develop a sense of competence, while those who are discouraged are left with a sense of inferiority.
- **Stage 5: Adolescence identity versus role confusion (age 12–18 years):** This stage is particularly critical in which a strong identity serves as a basis for finding future direction in life. Those who find a sense of self and personal identity feel secure, independent and ready to face the future, while those who remain confused may feel lost, insecure and unsure of their place in the world.
- **Stage 6: Young adulthood intimacy versus isolation (age 18–40 years):** This stage centered on forming intimate relationship with other people. By successfully forming loving relationships with other people, individuals are able to experience love and enjoy intimacy. Those who fail may feel isolated.
- **Stage 7: Middle adulthood generativity versus stagnation (age 40–65 years):** Psychological conflict becomes centered on the need to create things that will outlast the individual. Raising a family, working and contributing to the community are all ways that people develop a sense of purpose. Those who fail to find ways to contribute may feel useless and become stagnant and feel unproductive.
- **Stage 8: Maturity ego integrity versus despair (age 65 + years):** This stage begins around the age of 65 and lasts until death. During this period, the individual looks back on life. Those who have led an unproductive life, feel guilt, dissatisfaction and develop despair and those who have led a productive life, feel a sense of peace, wisdom and fulfillment.

Figure 4.3 represent Erikson's eight psychological stages and the tenses most relevant at particular stages of the life span.

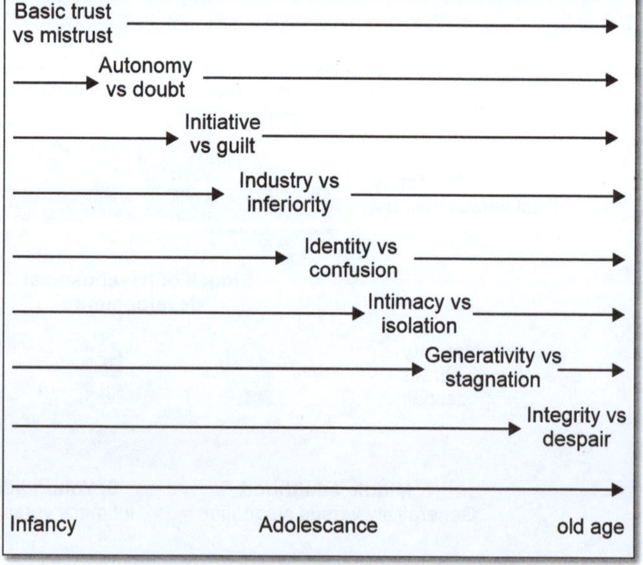

Figure 4.3: Erikson's eight psychological stages

CONCEPTS OF HEALTH AND ILLNESS

- As per World Health Organization (WHO), 1948, health is a state of complete physical, mental and social well-being and not merely an absence of disease or infirmity. A condition of quality of the human organism expressing the adequate functioning of the organism in given conditions, genetic or environmental.
- In 1984, WHO revised the definition of health as "the extent to which an individual or group is able to realize aspirations and satisfy needs and to change or to cope with the environment". Health is a resource for everyday life, not the objective of living. It is a positive concept, emphasizing social and personal resources, as well as physical capacities.

Health is referred to as the ability to maintain homeostasis and recover from insults. Mental, intellectual, emotional and social health are referred to a person's ability to handle stress, to acquire skills, to maintain relationships, all of which form resources for resiliency and independent living. Three dimensions of good health are shown in Figure 4.4.

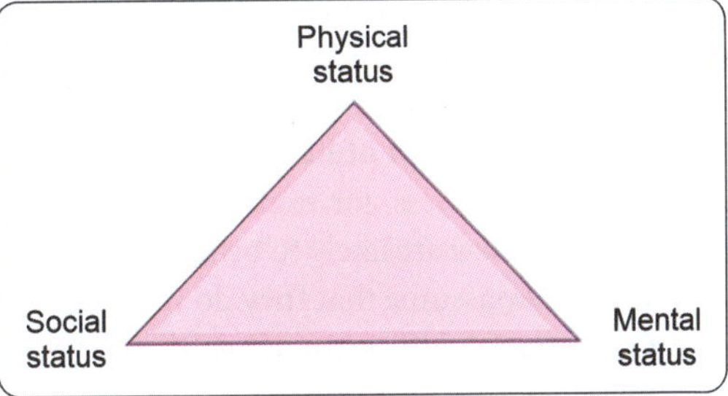

Figure 4.4: Three dimensions of good health

Various Concepts of Health

Biomedical Concept

Traditionally, health has been viewed as an "absence of disease" and if one is free from the disease, then the person is considered healthy. This concept has the basis in the "germ theory of disease". The medicine viewed the human body as a machine, disease as a consequence of the breakdown of the machine and one of the doctor's tasks is to repair the machine.

Drawback: The criticism leveled against the concept is that it has minimized the role of environment, social, psychological and cultural determinants of health.

Ecological Concept

Health is viewed as a dynamic equilibrium between human being and environment and disease as a maladjustment of the human organism to environment.

Health implies the relative absence of pain and discomfort and a continuous adaptation and adjustment to the environment, to ensure optimal function. Human's ecological and cultural adaptations determine the occurrence of disease.

Drawback: The ecological concept raises two issues:

1. Imperfect human
2. Imperfect environment

Psychological Concept

Health is not only biomedical phenomenon but it is also influenced by social, psychological, cultural, economic and political factors of the people concerned. Psychological concept views health as both a biological and social phenomenon.

Holistic Concept

The holistic model is a synthesis of biomedical, ecological and psychosocial concept. It recognizes the role of social, economic, political and environmental influences on health. Holistic concept views that health implies a sound mind in a sound body, in a sound family, in a sound environment. This emphasizes promotion and protection of health. A holistic concept of health is the belief that being healthy means being without any physical disorders or diseases or being emotionally comfortable. People with this view are likely to label themselves as ill when they experience a wide range of unpleasant feelings, and not just physical discomfort or pain.

- **Positive concept of health:** A positive concept of health is the belief that being healthy is a state achieved only by continuous effort. People with this belief take active steps to maintain their health. According to this view, people who do not take action to maintain their own health cannot be healthy.
- **Negative concept of health:** A negative concept of health is the view that being healthy is the absence of illness, for example, not having any symptoms of diseases, pain or distress. People with this view are likely to believe that good health is normal and take it for granted that they are well. They assume that they do not need to take any special actions to keep healthy.
- **Operational definition of health:** No obvious evidence of disease and that person is functioning normally.
  - Several organs of the body are functioning adequately in themselves, and in relation to one another's philosophy.

Various Concepts of Illness

Illness is a personal state in which the person feels unhealthy or ill. Illness may or may not be related to disease. It is a state in which a person's physical, emotional, intellectual, social, developmental or spiritual functioning is diminished or impaired as compared with previous experience. It is the human experience of disease. Illness is defined as an absence of health or deteriorated rhythm of life, diminished coping, an unsuccessful adjustment to life and a loss of the sense of well-being and vitality.

Psychological Consequences of Illness

- Uncooperativeness
- Hostility
- Paranoid
- Demanding
- Dependent
- Aggression
- Sense of shame
- Guilt, fear, anxiety, regression

Classification of Illness

Illness may be classified as:

- **Acute illness:** Acute illness has a short duration and severity. The signs and symptoms appear abruptly, are intense and often subside after a relevant short period. After acute illness, a person may return to normal level of wellness.
- **Chronic illness:** Chronic illness has a slow onset, persists usually for >6 months and can also affect functioning in any dimension.

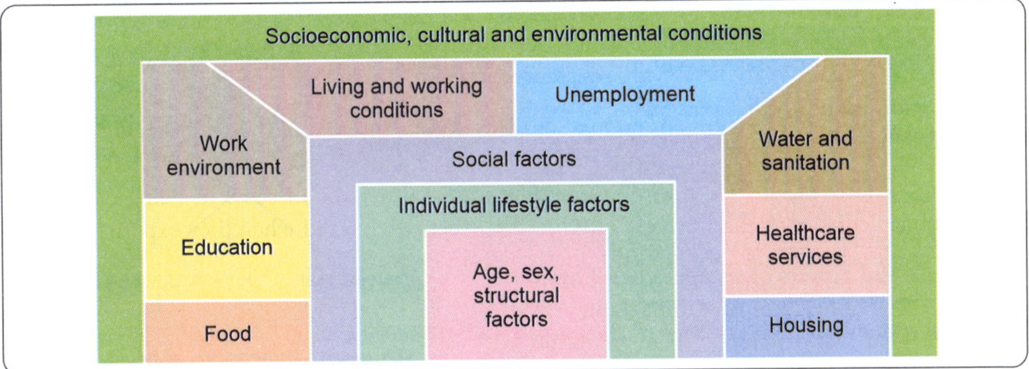

Figure 4.5: Factors affecting health

Precursor of Illness

Precursors of illness are the factors which impose on the individuals to lead toward illness spectrum.

- Hereditary factors
- Behavioral factors
- Environmental factors

FACTORS AFFECTING HEALTH

Many factors combine together to affect the health of individuals and communities as shown in Figure 4.5. Factors such as residence, relationship, environment, genetics, income and education level, have considerable impact on health. Some of these factors are:

- **Social and economic factors:** It includes superstition, religious and social beliefs.
- **Environmental factors:** The environment in which a person lives can also affect his/her health. The environment may be internal or external.
- **Personal factors:** Personal factors also affect our health like eating, sleeping, tension and stress. These can make a healthy person ill.
- **Heredity factors:** Some hereditary diseases like diabetes mellitus (DM) and hemophilia also affect health.

DIMENSIONS OF HEALTH

"Health means absence of disease. A state of complete physical, mental and social well-being, not merely the absence of disease or infirmity."   **—WHO, 1948**

"The extent to which an individual or group, on the one hand is able to realize aspirations and safety needs; and on other hand is able to change or cope with the environment. Health is therefore, seen as a resource for everyday life, not the object of living, it is a positive concept emphasizing social and personal resources, as well as physical capabilities."   **—WHO, 1984**

"Health is a means to an end rather than a fixed state that a person can or should aspire to."   **—Seed house, 1986**

There are many dimensions of health as given in Figure 4.6, which interact in a synergistic manner allowing human beings to engage in the wide array of life experiences.

- **Physical dimensions:** This dimension makes the body systems and organs function efficiently, have high level of resistance and immunity, have muscular strength, flexibility and neuromuscular coordination and balance. Physical characteristics are body weight, visual ability, strength, coordination, level of endurance, level of susceptibility to disease and powers of recuperation. Physical dimension of health is very important.

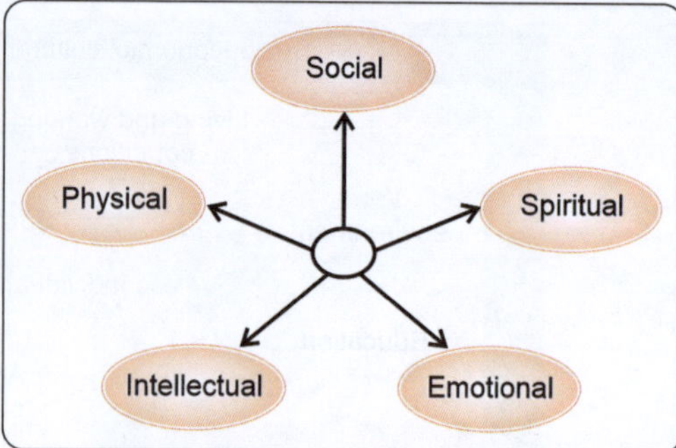

Figure 4.6: Dimensions of health

- **Emotional dimension:** The emotional dimension of health means a person's ability to cope with stress, remain flexible and compromise to resolve conflicts. Emotional dimension focuses on ensuring attention of feelings, thoughts and behavior.
- **Social dimension:** Social dimension includes social skills and insights. This dimension of health focuses on the process of creating and maintaining healthy relationships. This is the ability to make and maintain healthy relationships with other people. Social dimension also includes accepting social standards and norms of behavior.
- **Spiritual dimension:** Spiritual dimension focuses on establishing a purpose in life. It may involve having goals in life. Spirituality includes relationships with other living beings, the nature of human behavior, and need and willingness to serve others. These all are important components of health. By the spiritual dimension, one can develop an expanded perception of the universe.
- **Intellectual dimension:** This dimension of health involves thinking process and learning and making healthy choices. It is an individual's capacity to make decisions that lead to good health. Intellectual dimension focuses on ability and acts on information values and beliefs, and decision-making capacity. In other words, it is a cognitive ability to develop skills and knowledge to enhance one's life.

Wider Dimensions of Health

Wider dimensions of health include:

- **Occupational dimension:** Occupational dimension is the ability to get personal fulfillment from job while maintaining balance in lives. It involves enjoyment and working with manageable workload.
- **Environmental dimension:** Environmental dimension is the ability to recognize own responsibility for the quality of the air, the water and the land that surround us. It is an ability to make a positive impact on the quality of environment. It involves living in harmony with environment, protecting environment, daily habits, awareness of earth's limits and resources.

There are many dimensions to a person's health. These dimensions depend on and influence each other. When one is out of sync, the other is actually affected.

DETERMINANTS OF HEALTH

Determinants are defined as those predisposing factors which influence the health of a particular community.

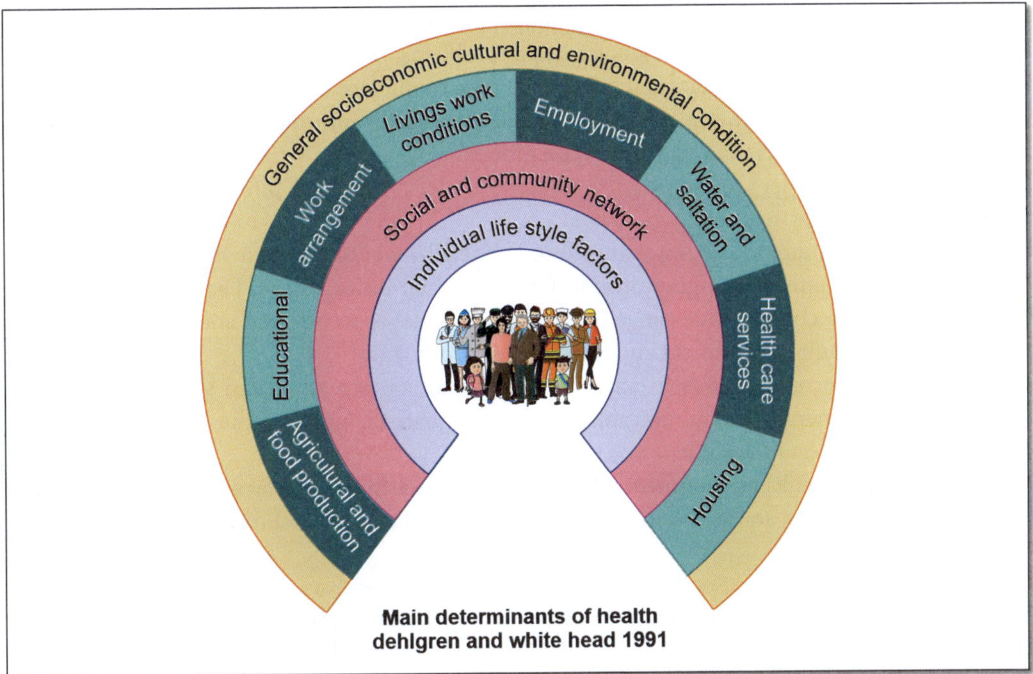

Figure 4.7: Main determinants of health dahlgren and whitehead 1991

Many factors combine together to affect the health of individuals and communities. Whether people are healthy or not, is determined by their circumstances and environment. Almost every characteristic of a society affects the health of its citizens.

The determinants of health (Fig. 4.7) include:

The determinants of health refer to the range of personal, social, economic and environmental factors which determine the health status of individuals or populations.

- The social and economic environment
- The physical environment
- The person's individual characteristics and behavior

Some other determinants are:

- **Early childhood development:** Early childhood development has a formative impact on an adult. Early nutrition, physical development and fitness are important, as is emotional development. If emotional development is positive, it builds resiliency and if negative, it enhances vulnerability. The impact of broken homes, chronic childhood stresses and so forth have nonspecific effects acting mainly to increase emotional vulnerability in adult life.
- **Income and social status:** Higher income and social status are linked to better health. A person's social status is defined by a combination of his/her wealth, education, occupation and lifestyle and by other factors such as ethnicity, personality. Each of these alone or in combination can exert positive or negative influence on a person's health. The association between social status and health is now termed social inequality in health.

Poverty refers to having inadequate resources to meet basic needs for shelter, nutritious food, clothing and education. People living in poverty, lack the resources and opportunities to make choices that promote good health. Being poor may also expose them to inferior physical environment that places them at risk for health problems.

- **Education and literacy:** Education has a more direct influence on health as it affects a person's ability to navigate the healthcare system, to interpret health information and to communicate effectively with physicians and other health professionals.

  Health literacy refers to the patient's ability to understand health information and to follow guidelines for their treatment.

- **Physical environment:** Safe water and clean air, healthy workplaces, safe houses, communities and roads all contribute to good health. Environmental influences on health can be positive or negative and cover a wide range of factors, from global to national and regional to local, including the built environment and the social environment.

  Exposures to contaminants in air, water, food and soil are associated with many chronic diseases and emerging communicable diseases. Climate change and the associated weather extremes also affect the health.

  Design of the built environment also influences health. Overcrowding in housing and community designs are increasingly identified as risk factors for chronic diseases especially respiratory conditions.

- **Social support network:** Social support benefits health in several ways. Support from families, friends and communities is linked to better health. Social support is a source of emotional reassurance and provides a safe place for a person to discuss his problems, which helps him to cope with adversity. Social support provides information and practical support. It can also support people in making healthier behavior choices.

- **Employment, working conditions:** The WHO recognizes fair employment and decent work as a cornerstone of health. Working conditions must be fair. The work stress affects worker's health. It coincides with other determinants, such as income. Work stress arises from a combination of high psychological demands. The occupational diseases are disorders that result from conditions in the workplace, typically from exposures to physical, chemical and perhaps psychological hazards.

- **Genetics:** Inheritance plays a part in determining lifespan healthiness and the likelihood of developing certain illnesses.

- **Gender:** Men and women suffer from different types of diseases at different ages.

- **Culture:** A person's cultural background has an important influence on his/her beliefs, behaviors, perceptions, emotions, language, diet, body image and attitudes to illness and pain. Culture also underpins values, which are deeply held beliefs that define what is desirable and moral.

FURTHER READINGS

- https://www.who.int/news-room/questions-and-answers/item/determinants-of-health
- https://jflowershealth.com/8-dimensions-of-wellness

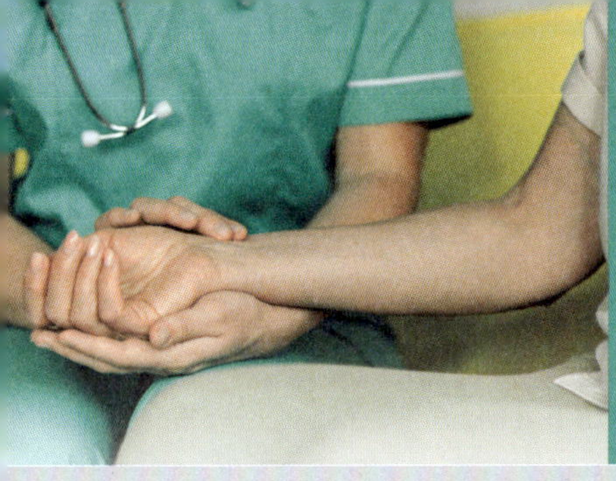

LONG ANSWER QUESTIONS

1. Describe developmental stages of human.
2. Discuss the concepts of health and illness in detail.

SHORT ANSWER QUESTION

1. Define the following:
   a. Factors affecting health
   b. Dimensions of health

MULTIPLE CHOICE QUESTIONS

1. **Which of the following is the World Health Organization's (WHO) definition of health?**
   a. The absence of disease and illness
   b. Complete physical, mental, and social well-being
   c. A state of physical fitness only
   d. The ability to function in society

2. **Which model of health focuses on biological factors as the main determinants of health?**
   a. Biopsychosocial model
   b. Environmental model
   c. Biomedical model
   d. Holistic model

3. **Which of the following best describes "illness"?**
   a. A condition that always requires medical treatment
   b. A subjective experience of feeling unwell
   c. A measurable physiological abnormality
   d. A chronic disease that cannot be cured

4. **Health promotion focuses primarily on:**
   a. Treating diseases in hospitals
   b. Preventing diseases and promoting healthy behaviors
   c. Conducting surgical interventions
   d. Diagnosing diseases through medical tests

5. **Which of the following is NOT a social determinant of health?**
   a. Education level
   b. Genetic predisposition
   c. Income level
   d. Employment status

6. **The ability to recover from illness or adapt to life challenges is known as:**
   a. Resilience
   b. Resistance
   c. Retention
   d. Remission

7. **Which of the following describes a holistic approach to health?**
   a. Focusing solely on curing physical diseases
   b. Considering the complete physical, mental, social, and spiritual aspects of a person
   c. Emphasizing only physical fitness and nutrition
   d. Treating illnesses with pharmaceuticals exclusively

8. **What is "primary prevention" in healthcare?**
   a. Early diagnosis and treatment of disease
   b. Rehabilitation after an illness
   c. Prevention of disease by addressing risk factors
   d. Limiting the progression of an established disease

9. **Chronic diseases are best described as:**
   a. Illnesses that come and go quickly
   b. Long-lasting conditions that can often be controlled but not cured
   c. Diseases caused exclusively by infections
   d. Diseases with a single, identifiable cause

10. **Which of the following terms refers to the difference in health outcomes between different population groups?**
    a. Health equity
    b. Health disparity
    c. Health improvement
    d. Health status

ANSWER KEY

1. b   2. c   3. b   4. b   5. b   6. a   7. b   8. b   9. b
10. b

5

Stress and Adaptation

LEARNING OBJECTIVES

After the completion of the chapter, the readers will be able to:

- Know about the stress and its models.
- Discuss about adaptation of stress.
- Describe Stuart Model of Stress management in nursing.

CHAPTER OUTLINE

- Stress
- Theory of Stress
- Adaptation

KEY TERMS

Coping mechanisms: Strategies used to manage stress, such as problem-solving, emotional support, and relaxation techniques, which can be adaptive or maladaptive.

Cortisol: A hormone released during stress that helps regulate various body functions but can lead to health issues if elevated for long periods.

Distress: Negative stress that can be overwhelming and harmful.

Eustress: Positive stress that can be motivating or improve performance.

Fight-or-flight response: The body's automatic reaction to perceived threats, preparing an individual to either confront or escape the stressor.

Stressors: External or internal factors that cause stress, such as work pressure, financial concerns, or health issues.

STRESS

Stress is a normal physical response to events that make a person feel threatened; or upset their balance in some way. The stress response is the body's way of protection. Stress is the body's reaction to harmful situations whether they are real or perceived. Stress is defined as a response to a stimulus or stressor. As per Selye stress is "a nonspecific response of the body to any kind of demand made on it."

Stress is simply a reaction to a stimulus that disturbs physical or mental equilibrium. In other words, it is an omnipresent part of life. A stressful event can trigger the "fight-or-flight" response, causing hormones such as adrenaline and cortisol to surge through the body.

Definitions

Stress is the way human beings react both physically and mentally to changes, events, and situations in their lives. People experience stress in different ways and for different reasons. The reaction is based on perception of an event or situation. If a situation is negative, one will likely feel distressed—overwhelmed, oppressed, or out of control. Distress is the more familiar form of stress. The other form, eustress, results from a "positive" view of an event or situation, which is why it is also called "good stress."

Symptoms

The symptoms of stress are as follows:

General symptoms
• Headaches
• Fatigue
• Gastrointestinal problems
• Hypertension (high blood pressure)
• Heart problems, such as palpitations
• Inability to focus/lack of concentration
• Sleep disturbances, whether it's sleeping too much or an inability to sleep
• Sweating palms/shaking hands
• Anxiety
• Sexual problems
• Behavioral changes are also expressions of stress
They can include:
• Irritability
• Disruptive eating patterns (overeating or under eating)
• Harsh treatment of others
• Increased smoking or alcohol consumption
• Isolation

> ### Must Know
>
> **Stressors**
> This term is created by Selye to differentiate cause of stress from response to stress. It is any factor that produces stress and disturbs the body's equilibrium.
>
> **Common Stressors**
> The common stressors are:
>
> | | |
> |---|---|
> | Increased academic demands | Being in a new environment like new job |
> | Changes in family relations | Financial responsibilities |
> | Changes in social life | Exposure to new people, ideas, and temptations |
> | Poverty | Unemployment |
> | Physical threats | Threats to our self-image |
> | An important life event | A fight or conflict with a friend/relative/co-worker |
> | Tight deadlines | Loss of something or someone we care for |

Causes of Stress

The most frequent reasons for "stressing out" fall into three main categories:

1. The unsettling effects of change
2. The feeling that an outside force which is challenging or threatening
3. The feeling of lost personal control. Stress is a normal physical response to events that make a person

General causes of stress are tabulated (Table 5.1) as follows.

Clinical Features of Stress

The clinical features of stress are tabulated in Table 5.2.

Stress Cycle

The stress cycle refers to the process by which stress is experienced, managed, and relieved. It typically involves several stages. The stress cycle has been shown in Figure 5.1.

TABLE 5.1:   Causes of stress

External causes of stress	Internal causes of stress
Major life changes	Chronic worry
Relationship difficulties	Rigid thinking, lack of flexibility
Work or school	Negative self-talk
Financial problems	Pessimism
Being too busy	Unrealistic expectations/perfectionism
Children and family	All-or-nothing attitude

TABLE 5.2:   Clinical features of stress

Emotional symptoms	Physical symptoms	Cognitive symptoms	Behavioral symptoms
Agitation, frustration, and moody	Low energy	Constant worrying	Changes in appetite—either not eating or eating too much
Feeling overwhelmed	Headaches	Racing thoughts	Procrastinating and avoiding responsibilities
Having difficulty in relaxing and having quiet mind	Upset stomach, including diarrhea, constipation, and nausea	Forgetfulness and disorganization	Increased use of alcohol, drugs or cigarettes
Feeling bad (low self-esteem), lonely, worthless, and depressed	Aches, pains, and tense muscles	Inability to focus	Exhibiting more nervous behaviors, such as nail biting and pacing
Avoiding others	Chest pain and rapid heartbeat	Being pessimistic or seeing only the negative side	
	Insomnia		
	Frequent colds and infections		
	Loss of sexual desire and/or ability		
	Nervousness and shaking, ringing in the ear, cold or sweaty hands and feet		
	Dry mouth and difficulty swallowing		
	Clenched jaw and grinding teeth		

Consequences of Long-Term Stress

The consequences of long-term stress are mentioned as follows:

- Mental health problems, such as depression, anxiety, and personality disorders.

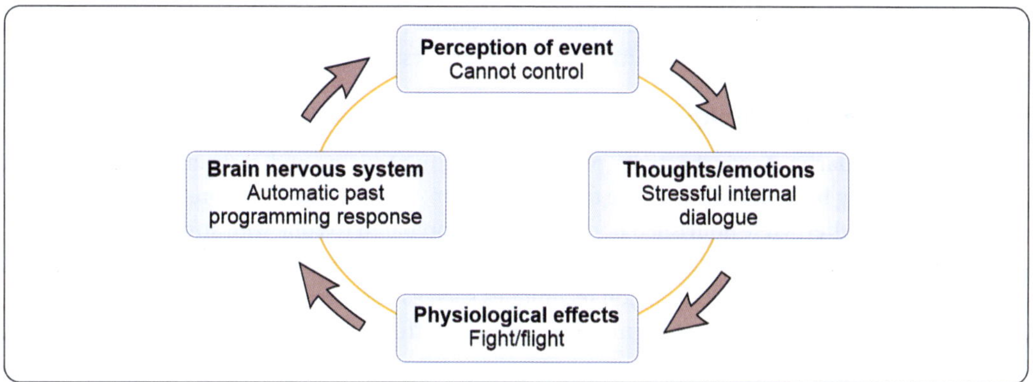

Figure 5.1: Stress cycle

- Cardiovascular diseases, including heart disease, high blood pressure, abnormal heart rhythms, heart attacks and stroke.
- Obesity and other eating disorders.
- Menstrual problems.
- Sexual dysfunction, such as impotence and premature ejaculation in men and loss of sexual desire in both men and women.
- Skin and hair problems, such as acne, psoriasis, and eczema, and permanent hair loss.
- Gastrointestinal problems, such as gastroesophageal reflux disease (GERD), gastritis, ulcerative colitis, and irritable colon.
- Weight problems
- Autoimmune diseases
- Pain of any kind
- Sleep problems

Stress Management

Stress management involves changing the stressful situation, changing reaction when cannot change the stressful situation, taking care, and making time for rest and relaxation.

Four A's for stress relief are: Avoid, Alter, Adapt and Accept.

1. **Avoid:** It is an unnecessary stress. Not all stresses can be avoided, but by learning how to say no, distinguishing between "should" and "must" on to-do list, and steering clear of people or situations that stress out, one can eliminate many daily stressors.
2. **Alter:** To alter the situation. If one cannot avoid a stressful situation, try to alter it. Be more assertive and deal with problems head on. Instead of bottling up feelings and increasing stress, respectfully let others know about one's concerns. Or be more willing to compromise and try meeting others halfway on an issue.
3. **Adapt:** To adapt the stressor. When one cannot change the stressor, try changing self. Reframe problems or focus on the positive things in life. If a task at work has stressed, focus on the aspects of job and enjoy it.
4. **Accept:** To accept the things one cannot change. There will always be stressors in life that people cannot do anything about. Learn to accept the inevitable rather than rail against a situation

and making it even more stressful. Look for the upside of a situation, even the most stressful circumstances can be an opportunity for learning or personal growth.

Stress Management Techniques

- **Exercise regularly:** Physical activity plays a key role in reducing and preventing the effects of stress. Nothing beats aerobic exercise for releasing pent-up stress and tension.
- **Eat a healthy diet:** Well-nourished bodies are better prepared to cope with stress. Start day with a healthy breakfast, reduce caffeine and sugar intake, and cut back on alcohol and nicotine.
- **Set aside relaxation time:** Relaxation techniques such as yoga, meditation, and deep breathing activate the body's relaxation response, a state of restfulness, i.e., the opposite of the stress response.
- **Get plenty of sleep:** Feeling tired can increase stress by causing to think irrationally. Keep cool by getting a good night's sleep.
- **Quick stress relief:** The best way to reduce stress quickly and reliably is by using senses—what people see, hear, smell, taste, and touch—or through movement. By viewing a favorite photo, smelling a specific scent, listening to a favorite music, tasting a piece of gum will relax a person, although it may do nothing but irritate someone else.
- **Emotional connection:** Nothing contributes more to chronic stress than emotional disconnection with ourselves and others. Understanding the influence of emotions on people's thoughts and actions is vital in managing stress. Life doesn't have to be like a rollercoaster ride with extreme ups and downs.
- **Healthy ways to relax and recharge are as follows:**

Go for a walk	Spend time in nature
Call a good friend	Sweat out tension with a good workout
Write in journal	Light scented candles
Take a long bath	Savor a warm cup of coffee or tea
Play with a pet	Get a massage
Work in garden	Listen to music
Curl up with a good book	Watch a comedy

THEORY OF STRESS

Systemic Stress: Selye's Theory of General Adaptation Syndrome (GAS)

Hans Selye (1907–1982) a Hungarian endocrinologist, was first to give a scientific explanation for biological stress. Hans Selye has been regarded as the founder of modern stress theory (Capel & Gurnsey, 1987). One of the first attempts to explain the process of stress related illness was given in Selye (1976) whereby the individual experiences three stages during the stress response. Hans Selye explained his stress model based on physiology and psychobiology as General adaptation syndrome (GAS). His model states that any event that threatens an organism's well-being (a stressor) leads to a three-stage bodily response. One of the first attempts to explain the process of stress related illness was given in Selye (1976) whereby the individual experiences three stages during the stress response (Fig. 5.2).

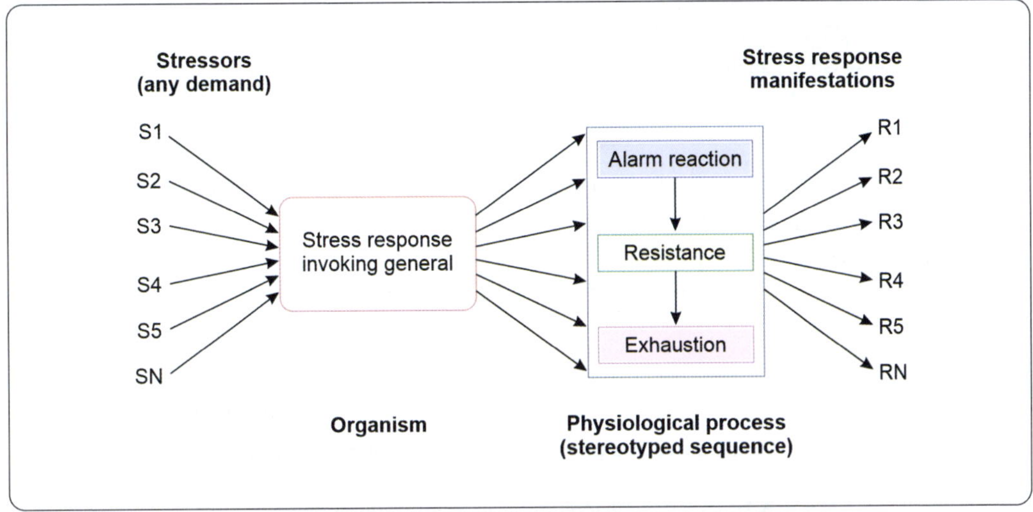

Figure 5.2: Manifestations of stress response to stressors

The popularity of the stress concept in science and mass media stems largely from the work of the endocrinologist Hans Selye. In a series of animal studies, he observed that a variety of stimulus events (e.g., heat, cold, toxic agents) applied intensely and long enough are capable of producing common effects, meaning not specific to either stimulus event. Besides these nonspecific changes in the body, each stimulus produces, of course, its specific effect, heat, for example, produces vasodilatation, and cold vasoconstriction. According to Selye, these non-specifically caused changes constitute the stereotypical, i.e., specific, response pattern of systemic stress. Selye (1976) defines this stress as `a state manifested by a syndrome which consists of all the non-specifically induced changes in a biologic system.'

General Adaptation Syndrome

General adaptation syndrome (GAS) is defined as physiological response of the whole body to stress. It involves several body systems, primarily the autonomic nervous system and the endocrine system. This stereotypical response pattern, called the `General Adaptation Syndrome' (GAS), proceeds in three stages (Figure 5.3) discussed as follows.

Stage 1. Alarm Stage

The alarm reaction comprises an initial shock phase and a subsequent countershock phase. The shock phase exhibits autonomic excitability, an increased adrenaline discharge, and gastro-intestinal ulcerations. The countershock phase marks the initial operation of defensive processes and is characterized by increased adrenocortical activity.

It includes the mobilization of the defense mechanisms of the body or the mind to cope with the stress: "Fight or flight" response (hormonal) sympathetic nervous system is activated. The body's resources get mobilized. There is increased mental energy and alertness. Hormones such as cortisol and adrenalin are released into the bloodstream to meet the threat or danger. If the situation is not resolved, it leads to stage 2.

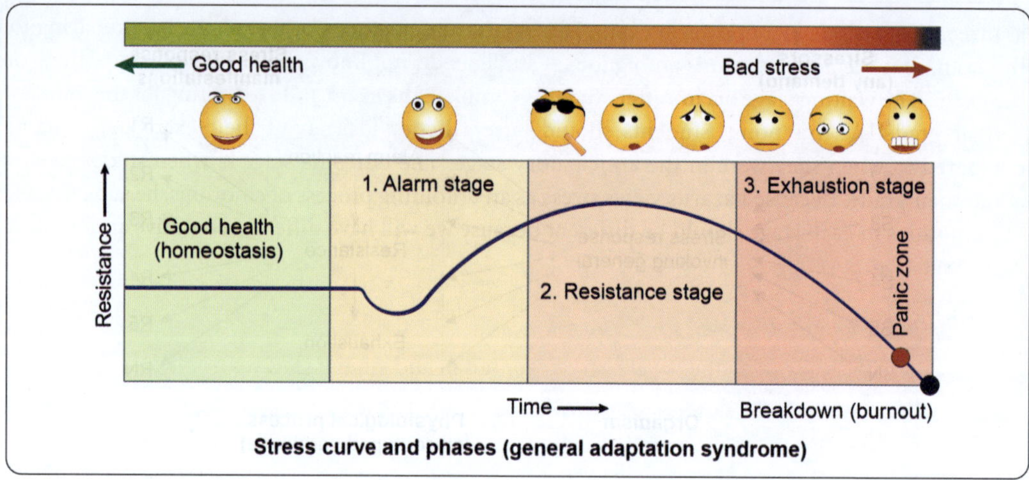

Figure 5.3: Stress curve and phases in general adaptation syndrome

Stage 2. Resistance Stage

If noxious stimulation continues, the organism enters the stage of resistance. In this stage, the symptoms of the alarm reaction disappear, which seemingly indicates the organism's adaptation to the stressor. However, while resistance to the noxious stimulation increases, resistance to other kinds of stressors decreases at the same time. It includes stabilization where a person attempts to adapt to the stressor. Physiological functions of parasympathetic nervous system return to normal levels. while body focuses on resources against the stressor.

Hormone levels, heart rate, BP, breathing and cardiac output return to normal.

Blood glucose levels remain high, cortisol and adrenalin continue to circulate at elevated levels, but outward appearance of organism seems normal.

If successful, body repairs the damage. Body remains on red alert.

However, if stressor remains and person is unable to adapt, the next stage begins.

Stage 3. Exhaustion

If stressor continues beyond body's capacity, body cannot resist the stress, and energy necessary to maintain adaptation is depleted. When the aversive stimulation persists, resistance gives way to the stage of exhaustion. The organism's capability of adapting to the stressor is exhausted, the symptoms of stage 1 reappear, but resistance is no longer possible.

Physiological response is intensified but the person's energy level is compromised and adaptation to the stressor diminishes. Physiological regulation diminishes, organism exhausts resources and becomes susceptible to disease. Irreversible tissue damages appear, and, if the stimulation persists, the organism dies.

Psychological Stress–The Lazarus Theory

Lazarus views stress as a process during which our interpretation of the event causes changes in our emotions. In a classic study, Folkman and Lazarus (1985) assessed undergraduate students' emotions at three time periods of a mid-term exam. During the anticipatory stage, students are preparing for the exam, but the actual exam is ambiguous – students do not know the difficulty or questions on the exam. The waiting stage occurs after students complete the exam and are waiting for the outcome – their grade! At this point, students should have a better idea about their exam performance compared to when they were in the anticipatory stage. The outcome stage is when students learn about their grade. Because Lazarus views stress as an unfolding process of emotions, he suggests that our emotions in each stage should be different because we will have different cognitive appraisals in each stage (Fig. 5.4).

Major Concepts of Lazarus Theory

Three major concepts of this theory are-stress, appraisal, and coping (Fig. 5.5).

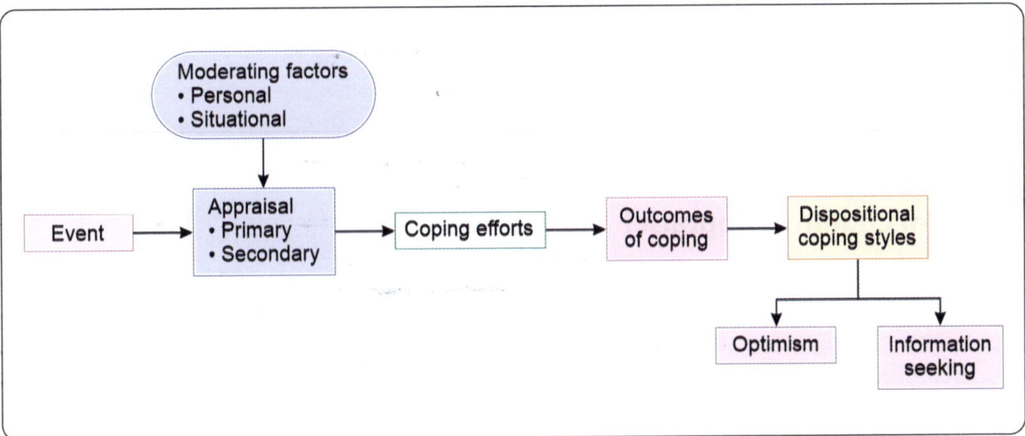

Figure 5.4: Lazarus stress theory model

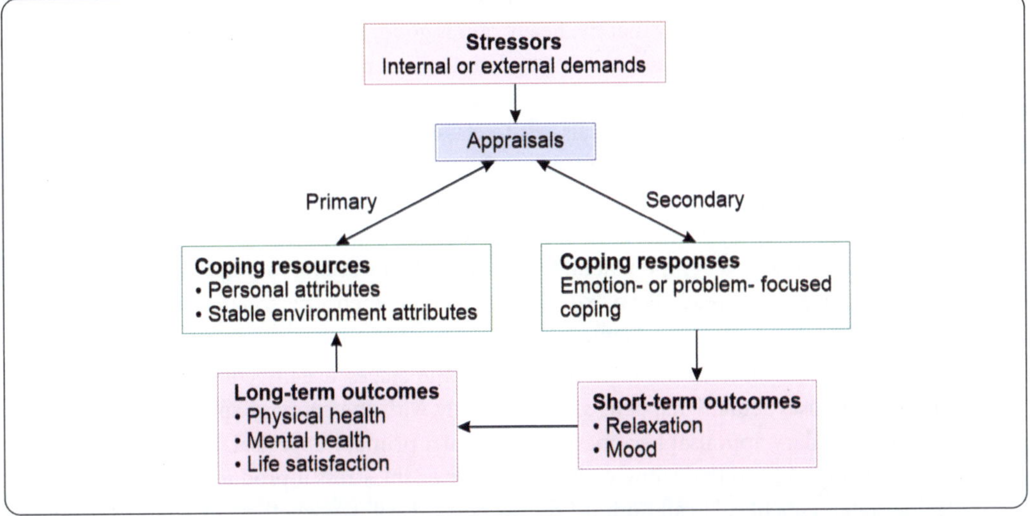

Figure 5.5: Concepts of Lazarus Theory

Stress

Lazarus states that stress is a condition or feeling experienced when a person perceives that the "demands exceed the personal and social resources the individual is able to mobilize." this is called the 'transactional model of stress and coping. Neither the environmental event nor the people's response defines stress, rather the individual's perception of the psychological situation is the critical factor. According to Lazarus, the effect that stress has on a person is based more on that person's feeling of threat, vulnerability and ability to cope than on the stressful event itself. He defines psychological stress as a "particular relationship between the person and environment that is appraised by the person as taxing or exceeding his or her resources and endangering his or her wellbeing."

Cognitive Appraisal

Lazarus stated that cognitive appraisal occurs when a person considers two major factors that majorly contribute in his response to stress. These two factors include:

1. The threatening tendency of the stress to the individual,
2. The assessment of resources required to minimize, tolerate or eradicate the stressor and the stress it produces.

Stages of Cognitive Appraisal

In general, cognitive appraisal is divided into two types or stages: primary and secondary appraisal.
Primary appraisal: In the stage of primary appraisal, an individual tends to ask questions like, "What does this stressor and/or situation mean?", and, "How can it influence me?"

According to psychologists, the three typical answers to these questions are:

1. "this not important",
2. "this is good",
3. "this is stressful".

To better understand primary appraisal, suppose a non-stop heavy rain suddenly pours at your place. You might think that the heavy rain is not important, since you don't have any plans of going somewhere today. Or, you might say that the heavy rain is good, because now you don't have to wake up early and go to school since classes are suspended. Or, you might see the heavy rain as stressful because you have scheduled a group outing with your friends. After answering these two questions, the second part of primary cognitive appraisal is to classify whether the stressor or the situation is a threat, a challenge or a harm-loss. When you see the stressor as a threat, you view it as something that will cause future harm, such as failure in exams or getting fired from job. When you look at it as a challenge, you develop a positive stress response because you expect the stressor to lead you to a higher class ranking, or a better employment. On the other hand, seeing the stressor as a "harm-loss" means that the damage has already been experiences, such as when a person underwent a recent leg amputation, or encountered a car accident.

Secondary appraisal: Unlike in other theories where the stages usually come one after another, the secondary appraisal actually happens simultaneously with the primary appraisal. In fact, there are times that secondary appraisal becomes the cause of a primary appraisal. Secondary appraisals involve those feelings related to dealing with the stressor or the stress it produces.

Uttering statements like, "I can do it if I do my best", "I will try whether my chances of success are high or not", and "If this way fails, I can always try another method" indicates positive secondary appraisal. In contrast to these, statements like, "I can't do it; I know I will fail", "I will not do it because no one believes I can" and, "I won't try because my chances are low" indicate negative secondary appraisal. Although primary and secondary appraisals are often a result of an encounter with a stressor, stress doesn't always happen with cognitive appraisal. One example is when a person gets involved in a sudden disaster, such as an earthquake, and he doesn't have more time to think about it, yet he still feels stressful about the situation.

Coping

Coping is defined as a process of "constantly changing cognitive and behavioral efforts to manage specific external and/or internal demands that are appraised as taxing or exceeding the resources of the person.

There are two forms of coping: Problem-focused coping used when we feel we have control over the situation, thus can manage the source of the problem.

There are four steps to manage this stress:

1. Define the problem,
2. Generate alternative solutions,
3. Learn new skills to dealing with stressors,
4. Reappraise and find new standards of behavior.

Emotion focused coping used when an individual feels as if they cannot manage the source of the problem.

Strategies for regulating stress: It involves gaining strategies for regulating stress.

- Avoiding (I am not going to school),
- Distancing (yourself from the stress, 'it doesn't matter'),
- Acceptance (I failed that exam, but I have 4 other subjects),
- Seeking Medical Support,
- Turning to alcohol.

Lazarus (1991) distinguishes 15 basic emotions:

Nine of these are negative (anger, fright, anxiety, guilt, shame, sadness, envy, jealousy, and disgust), whereas four are positive (happiness, pride, relief, and love). (Two more emotions, hope and compassion, have a mixed valence.)

At a molecular level of analysis, the anxiety reaction, for example, is based on the following pattern of primary and secondary appraisals: there must be some goal relevance to the encounter. Furthermore, goal incongruence is high, i.e., personal goals are thwarted. Finally, ego- involvement concentrates on the protection of personal meaning or ego- identity against existential threats. At a more molar level, specific appraisal patterns related to stress or distinct emotional reactions are described as core relational themes. The theme of anxiety, for example, is the confrontation with uncertainty and existential threat. The core relational theme of relief, however, is 'a distressing goal-incongruent condition that has changed for the better or gone away' (Lazarus 1991). Coping is intimately related to the concept of cognitive appraisal and, hence, to the stress relevant person-environment transactions. Most approaches in coping research follow Folkman and Lazarus, who define coping as 'the cognitive and behavioral efforts made to master, tolerate, or reduce external and internal demands and conflicts among them.'

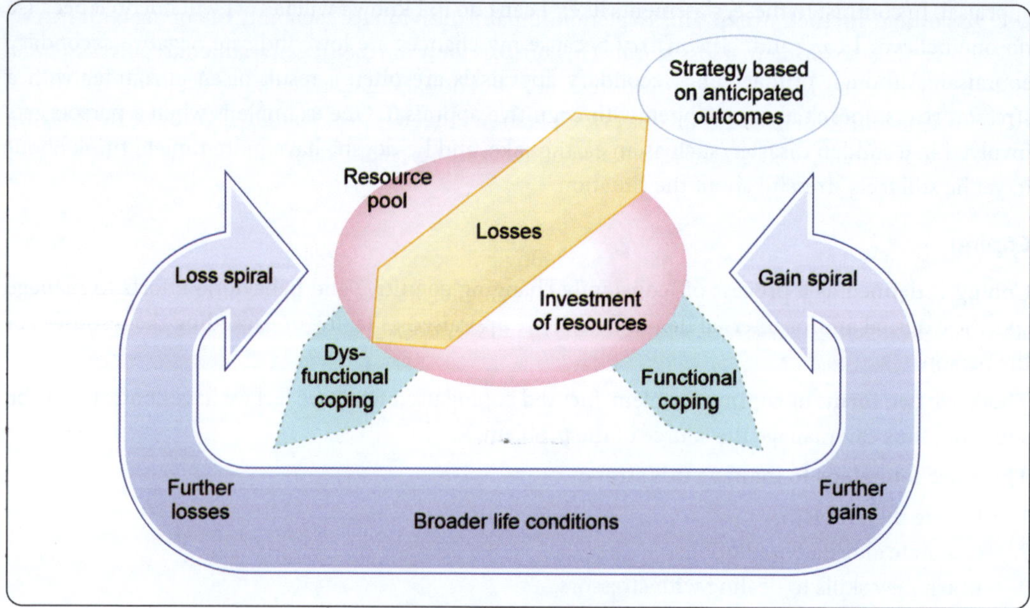

Figure 5.6: Resource theory of stress

Resource Theory of Stress - Stevan E. Hobfoll

Resource theory of stress is an important concept in psychology and organizational behavior. It proposes that stress occurs when individuals perceive that they lack the resources to cope with the demands placed upon them.

This theory was developed by Stevan E. Hobfoll in 1989 and is also known as the Conservation of **Resources (COR) theory:** It emphasizes the importance of resource management in stress prevention and coping (Fig. 5.6).

Principles

Hobfoll and co-workers outlined a number of testable hypotheses (called principles) derived from basic assumptions of COR (Hobfoll et al. 1996).

- **Loss of resources is the primary source of stress:** This principle contradicts the fundamental assumption of approaches on critical life events (cf. Holmes and Rahe 1967) that stress occurs whenever individuals are forced to readjust themselves to situational circumstances, may these circumstances be positive (e.g., marriage) or negative (e.g., loss of a beloved person). In an empirical test of this basic principle, Hobfoll and Lilly (1993) found that only loss of resources was related to distress.
- **Resources act to preserve and protect other resources:** Self-esteem is an important resource that may be beneficial for other resources. Hobfoll and Leiberman (1987), for example, observed that women who were high in self-esteem made good use of social support when confronted with stress, whereas those who lacked self-esteem interpreted social support as an indication of personal inadequacy and, consequently, misused support.

- **Following stressful circumstances, individuals have an increasingly depleted resource pool to combat further stress:** This depletion impairs individuals' capability of coping with further stress, thus resulting in a loss spiral. This process view of resource investment requires to focus on how the interplay between resources and situational demands changes over time as stressor sequences unfold. In addition, this principle shows that it is important to investigate not only the effect of resources on outcome, but also of outcome on resources.

Key Points

- **Resources:** These can be physical, psychological, social, or material.
- **Stress:** Results from an imbalance between demands and available resources.
- **Conservation:** People strive to obtain, retain, and protect their resources.
- **Loss:** The threat of resource loss or actual loss is the primary source of stress.

Types of Resources

- **Object resources:** Physical items like a house or car
- **Condition resources:** Status, relationships, tenure
- **Personal resources:** Skills, self-esteem, optimism
- **Energy resources:** Time, money, knowledge

Resource Loss vs. Gain: The theory posits that resource loss has a more significant impact than resource gain. People are more sensitive to losses, which can trigger a defensive state to protect remaining resources.

Resource caravans: Resources tend to aggregate. Those with more resources are better positioned to gain more, while those lacking resources may struggle to acquire them.

Applications

- Workplace stress management
- Trauma recovery
- Burnout prevention
- Organizational change management

Cox's Theory of Stress

According to Cox (1978, 1985) the individual becomes stressed when a discrepancy occurs between the perceived level of the stressful demands and his/her perceived ability to respond to and to cope with the demands. There is thus an imbalance between a perceived demand and a perceived capacity to cope (Fig. 5.7).

- Cox (1985) notes that the classic stressful situation is one in which the person's resources are not well matched to the level of demand and where there are constraints on coping and little social support. Stress, itself, is an individual psychological state. It is to do with the person's perception of the work environment and the emotional experience of it.
- Cox (1978, 1985) maintains that perception plays an important role in recognizing stressors. The individual's ability to cope with environmental—threats or adverse events is also emphasized. This view would suggest that if the individual can perceive environmental and psychological demands made on him, he can learn (for example, through counselling as a form of intervention)

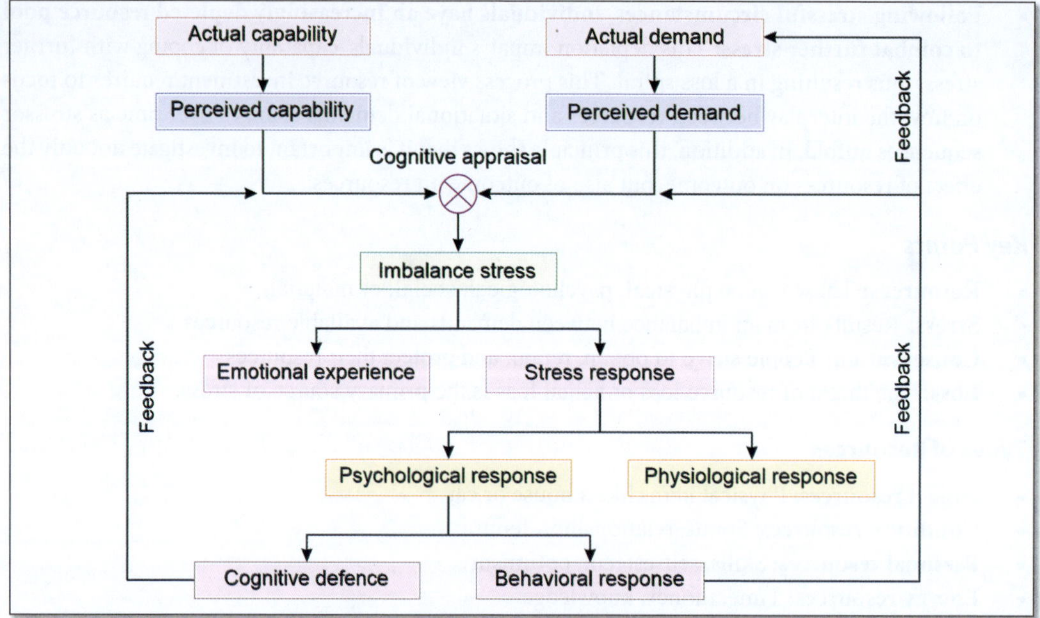

Figure 5.7: Cox model of stress and adaptation

to recognize which are the best resources to call upon when confronted with perceived stressful demands.

- Cox (1985) emphasizes that the stress phases experienced by the individual involve a complex interactive process with various levels of appraisal, emotion and response, with the immediate response to a stressful situation being in the form of negative emotion, propelling the individual into flight or fight action.
- Cox (1978, 1985) maintains that stress is an imbalance between a perceived demand and a perceived capability, with the demands changing at various levels of appraisal during the phases of the stress process. An appraisal of capability takes into account external resources as well as internal capabilities.

In using the capabilities, the individuals make an assessment of the social support available (external factors) and appraises his or her internal strengths or limitations in order to deal with the stressor.

ADAPTATION

Adaptation is the evolutionary process whereby an organism becomes better able to live in its habitat or habitats. The Hedonic Adaptation to Positive and Negative Experiences (HAPNE) model, developed in collaboration with Ken Sheldon, posits that adaptation proceeds via two separate paths, such that initial well-being gains or drops corresponding to a positive or negative life change, e.g., relationship startup vs. breakup.

Indicators of Positive Adaptation

(Adapted from Callista Roy)

Physiological Functions

- **Oxygenation:** This includes stable processes of ventilation, stable pattern of gas exchange, adequate transport of gases and adequate processes of compensation.
- **Nutrition:** This includes stable digestive processes, adequate nutritional pattern for body requirements, metabolic and other nutritive needs and altered means of Ingestion.
- **Elimination:** It includes effective homeostatic bowel processes, stable pattern of bowel elimination, effective processes of urine formation, stable pattern of urine elimination and effective coping strategies for altered elimination.
- **Activity and rest:** Integrated processes of mobility, adequate recruitment of compensatory movement processes during inactivity, effective pattern of activity and rest, effective sleep pattern and effective environmental changes for altered sleep conditions constitutes activity and rest.
- **Protection:** Intact skin, effective processes of immunity, effective healing response, adequate secondary protection for changes in skin integrity and immune status are all included in protection.
- **Senses:** This includes effective processes of sensation, effective integration of sensory input into information, stable patterns of perception, i.e., interpretation and appreciation of input and effective coping strategies for altered sensation.
- **Fluid and electrolytes:** This includes water balance stability of salts in body fluids, balance of acid/base status and effective chemical buffer regulation.

Neurological Functions

Neurological functions include effective processes of arousal/attention, sensation/perception; coding, concept formation, memory, language; planning, motor response, integrated thinking and feeling processes, plasticity, and functional effectiveness of developing, aging, and altered nervous system.

Endocrine Functions

Effective hormonal regulation of metabolic and body processes, effective hormonal regulation of reproductive development, stable patterns of closed loop, negative feedback, hormone systems, stable patterns of cyclical hormone rhythms for effective coping strategies for stress are included in endocrine functions.

Self-Concepts

- **Physical self:** Positive body image, effective sexual function, psychic integrity with physical growth, adequate compensation for bodily changes, effective coping strategies for loss, effective process of life closure are all important aspects of physical self.
- **Personal self:** Stable pattern of self-consistency, effective integration of self-ideal, effective processes of moral-ethical-spiritual growth, functional self-esteem and effective coping strategies for threats to self are all included in personal self of a person.

Role Functions

The role function includes effective processes of role transition, integration of instrumental and expressive role behaviors, integration of primary, secondary, and tertiary roles, stable pattern of role mastery and effective processes for coping with changed role.

Interdependence

Interdependence includes stable pattern of giving and receiving, nurturing, affectional adequacy, effective pattern of aloneness and relating and effective coping strategies for separation and loneliness.

Stuart Stress Adaptation Model

Stuart Stress Adaptation Model is a model of psychiatric nursing care, which integrates biological, psychological, sociocultural, environmental, and legal-ethical aspects of patient care into a unified framework for practice (Fig. 5.8). Dr. Stuart's theory model includes psychiatric nursing care, which integrates various aspects of patient care into a unified framework for practice. Her Stress Adaptation Model of health and wellness provides a consistent nursing-oriented framework (Stuart, 2009).

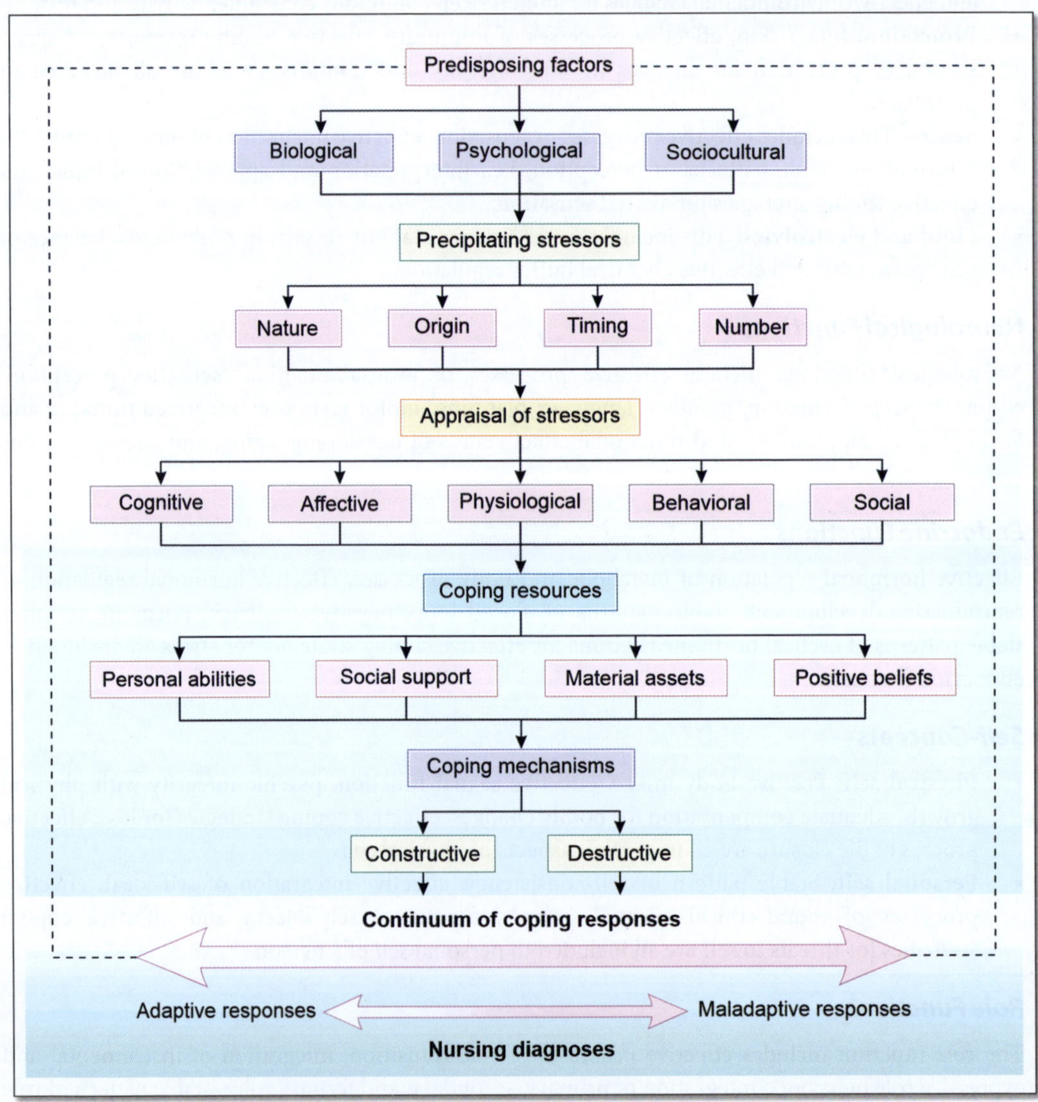

Figure 5.8: Stuart's stress adaptation model of health and wellness

Dr Gail Stuart's Stress Adaptation Model of health and wellness provides a:

- Consistent nursing-oriented framework, with clear explanations of biological, psychological, sociocultural, environmental, and legal-ethical components.
- Structure for thinking, observing, and interpreting what is seen. Conceptual nursing models are frames of reference within which patients, their environment and health states, and nursing activities are described.

Approaches

- **Biopsychosocial approach:** A holistic perspective that integrates biological, psychological and sociocultural aspects of care.
- **Predisposing factors:** Risk factors such as genetic all background.

Assumptions

- Nature is in order as a social hierarchy from the simplest unit to the most complex and the individual is a part of family, group, community, society and the larger biosphere.
- Nursing care is provided within a biological, psychological, sociocultural, environmental and legal-ethical context.
- Health/illness and adaptation/maladaptation (nursing world view) are two distinct continuums.
- The model includes the primary, secondary and tertiary levels of prevention by describing four discrete stages of psychiatric treatment: Crisis, acute, maintenance and health promotion.
- Nursing care is based on the use of the nursing process and the standards of care and professional performance for psychiatric nurses (Fig. 5.9).

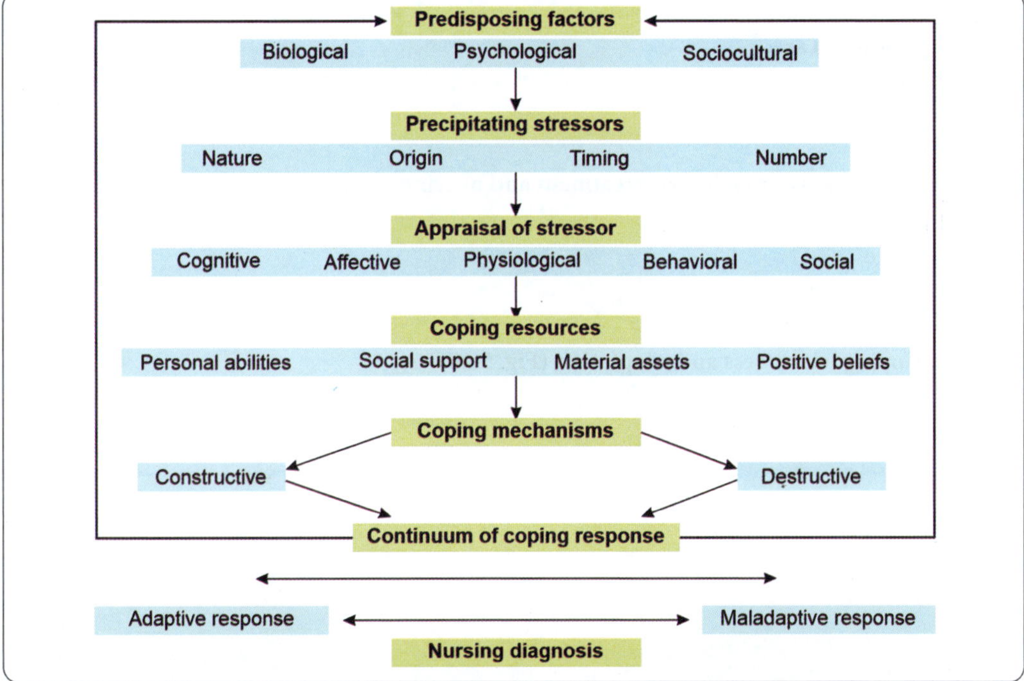

Figure 5.9: Stuart stress adaptation model in psychiatric nursing

Major Concepts of the Stress Model

- **Biopsychosocial approach:** A holistic perspective that integrates biological, psychological, and sociocultural aspects of care.
- **Predisposing factors:** Risk factors such as the genetic background.
- **Precipitating stressors:** Stimuli that the person perceives as challenging such as life events.
- **Appraisal of stressor:** An evaluation of the significance of a stressor.

Coping resources: The coping resources are options or strategies that:

- Help determine what can be done as well as what is at stake
- Adaptation or maladaptation
- Levels of prevention (Primary, Secondary, Tertiary).

Four Stages of Psychiatric Treatment and Nursing Care

1. Crisis stage
2. Acute stage
3. Maintenance stage
4. Health promotion stage and conclusion

Predisposing Factors

- **Precipitating stressors:** Stimuli that the person perceive as challenging such as life events.
- **Appraisal of stressor:** An evaluation of the significance of a stressor.
- **Coping resources:** Options or strategies that help determine what can be done as well as what is at stake.

Levels of prevention are:

- Primary
- Secondary
- Tertiary

Example: Four stages of psychiatric treatment and nursing care:

1. Crisis stage
2. Acute stage
3. Maintenance stage
4. Health promotion stage

Example: Coping with stress and adaptation (Fig. 5.10).

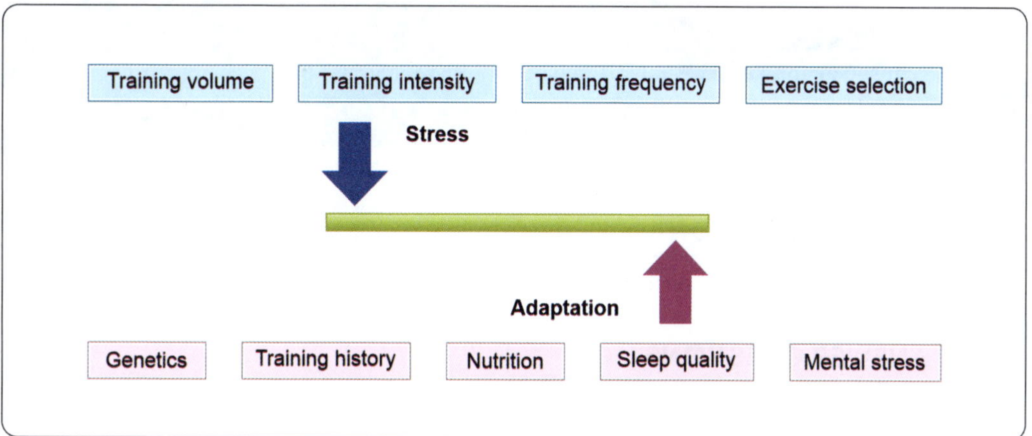

Figure 5.10: Example of coping with stress in nursing

FURTHER READINGS

- https://psycnet.apa.org/record/1996
- https://www.ncbi.nlm.nih.gov/books/

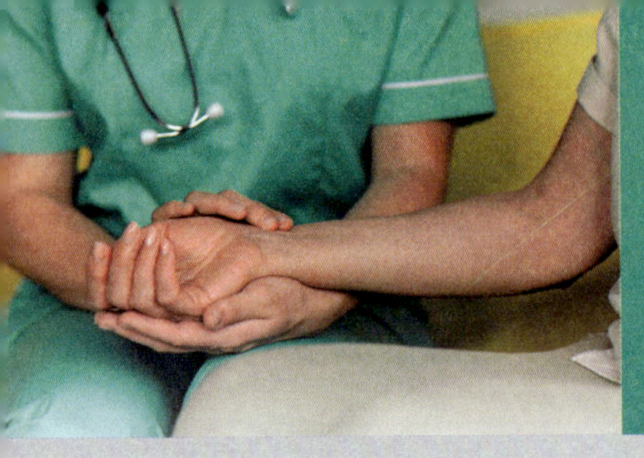

LONG ANSWER QUESTION

1. What is stress and adaptation? Discuss in detail.

SHORT ANSWER QUESTIONS

1. Stress management
2. Stuart Stress Adaptation Model
3. General Adaptation syndrome

MULTIPLE CHOICE QUESTIONS

1. **A nursing student finds that she comes down with a sinus infection toward the end of every semester. When this occurs, which stage of stress is the student most likely experiencing?**
   a. Alarm reaction stage
   b. Stage of resistance
   c. Stage of exhaustion
   d. Fight-or-flight stage

2. **Meditation has been shown to be an effective stress management technique. When meditation is effective, what should a nurse expect to assess?**
   a. An achieved state of relaxation
   b. An achieved insight into ones feelings
   c. A demonstration of appropriate role behaviors
   d. An enhanced ability to problem-solve

3. **When an individual's stress response is sustained over a long period of time, which physiological effect of the endocrine system should a nurse anticipate?**
   a. Decreased resistance to disease
   b. Increased libido
   c. Decreased blood pressure
   d. Increased inflammatory response

4. **Which symptom should a nurse identify as typical of the fight-or-flight response?**
   a. Pupil constriction
   b. Increased heart rate
   c. Increased salivation
   d. Increased peristalsis

5. **The 'Stress' word was originally used by Selye in.........**
   a. 1936
   b. 1946
   c. 1956
   d. 1996

6. **According to Selye, ... is the pressure experienced by an individual in response to life demands.**
   a. Stress
   b. Constipation
   c. Blood pressure
   d. Heart attack

7. **Which of the following is an internal stressor that stimulate proceeding or precipitating a change?**
   a. Trauma
   b. Peer pressure
   c. Fear
   d. All of these

ANSWER KEY

1. c **2.** a **3.** a **4.** b **5.** a **6.** a **7.** d

6

Legal and Ethical Aspects of Nursing

LEARNING OBJECTIVES

After the completion of the chapter, the readers will be able to:
- Discuss the legal issues in nursing.
- Know about the ethical issues in nursing.
- Explain patient's rights.

CHAPTER OUTLINE

- Legal Aspects of Nursing
- Some Legal Aspects of Nursing Practice
- Safe Practices for Nurses
- Ethics in Nursing
- Ethical Principles
- Sources of Ethical Distress
- Ethical Dilemmas
- Some other Issues Faced by Nurses
- Charter of Patients' Rights for Adoption by NHRC

KEY TERMS

Constitutional laws: Constitutional laws are a set of basic laws that define and limit the powers of government.

Informed consent: Informed consent is an agreement by a patient to accept a course of treatment or a procedure after being fully informed of it.

Law: Law can be defined as the rules made by humans which regulate social conduct in a formally prescribed and legally binding manner.

Malpractice: Malpractice refers to the behavior of a professional person's wrongful conduct, improper discharge of professional duties or failure to meet the standards of acceptable care which results in harm to another person.

Negligence (breach of duty): Negligence is the failure of an individual to provide care that a reasonable person would ordinarily use in similar circumstances.

Tort law: Tort law is the enforcement of duties and rights, independent of contractual agreements.

LEGAL ASPECTS OF NURSING

Definition

Law can be defined as the rules made by humans which regulate social conduct in a formally prescribed and legally binding manner. Laws are rules of conduct enforced by the Government. Laws consist of broad, interpretative principles based on reasons, traditional justice and common sense.

Nurses should have complete knowledge regarding the law of the state(s) in which they are licensed to practice.

Functions of Law in Nursing

- It provides a framework for establishing a legal nursing action for clients.
- It differentiates the nurse's responsibilities from other healthcare professionals.
- It helps to establish the boundaries of independent nursing actions.
- It assists in maintaining a standard of nursing practice by making nurses accountable under the law.

Sources of Law

The sources of law are shown in Figure 6.1.

Types of Law

Public Law

Public law deals with an individual's relationship with the state. Sources of public law are as follows:

- **Constitution:** Constitutional laws are a set of basic laws that define and limit the powers of government. Nurse maintains rights as an individual.
- **Administration:** Administrative laws are developed by groups who are appointed in governmental administrative agencies.

Civil Law

Civil law deals with crimes against a person or persons in such legal matters as: Contracts and Torts.

Contract Law

Contract law is the enforcement of agreements among private individuals. Employment contract is an example of contract law.

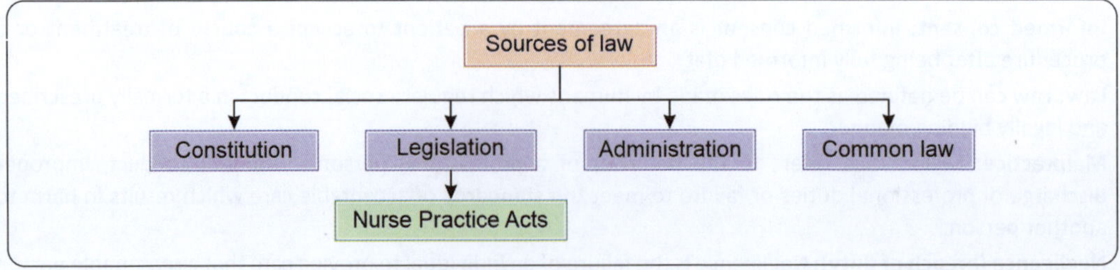

Figure 6.1: Sources of law

Tort Law

Tort law is the enforcement of duties and rights, independent of contractual agreements. It is a civil wrong committed on a person or property stemming from either a direct invasion of some legal rights of a person.

> **Nursing Consideration**
>
> Nursing practice falls under both public and civil law. In all states, nurses are bound by rules and regulations stipulated by the law as determined by the legislature. Public laws are designed to protect the public, when these laws are broken. A nurse can be punished by paying a fine or losing her/his license. Civil laws deal with problems occurring between a nurse and a client.

Different types of torts are shown in Figure 6.2. Torts can be intentional or unintentional which are as follows:

Intentional Torts

- **Assault and battery:**
  - Assault is defined as intentionally putting another person in reasonable apprehension of an imminent harmful or offensive contact. Assault is the intentional and unlawful offer to touch a person in an offensive, insulting or physically intimidating manner.

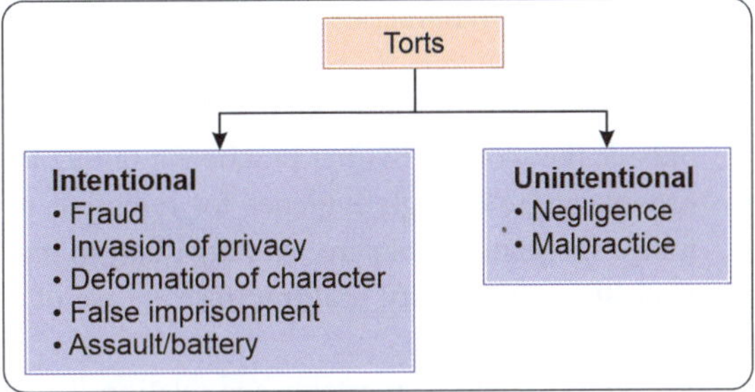

Figure 6.2: Types of torts

  - **Battery** is the offensive or harmful touching of someone without their expressed or implied consent. Many nursing duties, such as administering medication or assisting a patient to the restroom, require close proximity or physical contact with a patient. It is imperative to be well-versed on what constitutes battery and nurse must ensure to obtain the necessary consent to follow their duties, since patients have the right to refuse help and treatment.
- **False imprisonment:** False imprisonment is an intentional tort. False imprisonment is defined as an act of restraining and confining the person to a bounded area. An example of possible false imprisonment in healthcare is the use of restraints. Restraints can be physical, chemical or verbal. Nurses must vigilantly follow healthcare agency policies related to the use of physical restraints and monitor clients who are restrained. Chemical restraints include the administration of PRN medications and require clear documentation supporting their use. Verbal threats to keep an individual in an inpatient environment can also qualify as false imprisonment and should be avoided.
- **Breaching privacy and confidentiality:** Breaching privacy and confidentiality are intentional torts. Confidentiality is the right of an individual to have personal, identifiable medical information, referred to as protected health information, kept private. All types of patient information should only be shared with healthcare team members who are actively providing care to them. Some examples of breaching the privacy and confidentiality of patients are as follows:
  - Gossiping or talking about patients where other people can overhear.
  - Mishandling medical records or leaving medical records unsecured.
  - Illegally or unauthorized accessing of patient files.
  - Sharing information with unauthorized people.

- Texting or e-mailing patient's information on an unencrypted device.
- Sharing information on social media.

Unintentional Torts

- **Negligence (breach of duty):** Negligence is the failure of an individual to provide care that a reasonable person would ordinarily use in similar circumstances. Negligence is a general term that denotes conduct lacking in due care, carelessness, and a deviation from the standard of care that a reasonable person would use, in a particular set of circumstances. Negligence tends to arise from a mistake or carelessness that causes the patient unintended harm. For example, accidentally administering the incorrect medication or forgetting to document the nursing observations of patients, may be considered negligence.

- **Malpractice:** Malpractice refers to the behavior of a professional person's wrongful conduct, improper discharge of professional duties or failure to meet the standards of acceptable care which results in harm to another person. For example, a nurse performing the procedure is outside the scope of his/her practice or failing to closely follow a physician's patient-monitoring orders can be enough evidence for a patient to enforce charges. When nurses choose not to follow the standard of care, they are likely to make mistakes resulting in patient harm or injury.

  Conditions to satisfy malpractice: A case of malpractice must satisfy these four conditions which are as follows:

  1. **Duty:** There is an established relationship, such as the nurse–patient relationship.
  2. **Breach of duty:** The professional fails to provide a reasonable standard of care, according to professional practice guidelines or what another nursing professional would provide in a similar circumstance.
  3. **Damages:** The patient sustained injuries or harm.
  4. **Causation:** There is a proven link between the injuries or harm experienced by the patient and the nurse's actions or inactions.

Safe practices for nurses and nursing students to avoid negligence and malpractice:

To avoid being sued for negligence or malpractice, and to avoid the risk of losing their nursing license, it is essential for nurses and nursing students to follow the scope and standards of nursing practice care set forth by their state's Nurse Practice Act, and employer's policies, procedures, and protocols.

Examples of nurse's breach of duty that can be viewed as negligence include:

- **Failure to assess:** Nurses should assess for all potential nursing problems/diagnoses, not just those directly affected by the medical disease. For example, all patients should be assessed for fall risk and appropriate fall precautions must be implemented.
- **Insufficient monitoring:** Some conditions require frequent monitoring by the nurse, such as risk for falls, infection, confusion, and self-injury.
- **Failure to communicate:**
  - **Lack of documentation:** A basic rule of thumb in a court of law is that if an assessment or action was not documented, it will considered not done. Nurses must document all assessments and interventions, in addition to the specific type of patient documentation called a nursing care plan.
  - **Lack of provider notification:** In case of changes in patient's condition a nurse should immediately communicated with the healthcare provider based on the patient's status.

Documentation of provider notification should include—the date, time, and person notified and follow-up actions taken by the nurse.

- **Failure to follow protocols:** Government health agencies have rules for reporting certain behaviors or concerns. For example, a nurse is required to report suspicion of patient, child or elder abuse based on data gathered during an assessment, and notification of diseases.

SOME LEGAL ASPECTS OF NURSING PRACTICE

Nurses need to understand and apply legal aspects in their various roles. Nurse as an advocate of client should ensure the client's right to informed consent.

Confidentiality

The patient's privacy is consistent with the Hippocratic oath and with the law as part of the constitutional right to privacy. The professional verse should assure the patient of confidentiality.

Informed Consent

- Informed consent is an agreement by a patient to accept a course of treatment or a procedure after being fully informed of it.
- Consents are either expressed or implied. Expressed consent could be oral or written.
- If the procedure is more invasive, written permission is needed.
- Implied consent exists when the client's nonverbal behavior indicates agreement such as in positioning their body for an injection or while taking vital signs.
- Informed consent must be voluntary.
- The consent must be given by a patient who is capable and competent to understand. Children, unconscious patients, and mentally ill patients cannot provide consent.
- The patient must be given enough information for decision-making.

Nursing Considerations

Information to be given to a patient for informed consent:
- Diagnosis that requires treatment
- Purpose of treatment
- What patient can feel or experience
- Benefits of the treatment
- Possible risks
- Advantages and disadvantages of alternatives to treatment

Delegation

Delegation is the transfer of responsibility for the performance of an activity from one person to another retaining accountability for the outcome. When delegation is to occur, the nurse must be very careful.

Violence, Abuse and Neglect

- Violent behavior may include domestic violence, human abuse and sexual abuse.
- Neglect is the absence of care to maintain the health and safety of a patient.

Advocacy

The professional nurse has the duty to:
- Pronate what is left for the patient.
- Ensure that the patient's needs are met.
- Protect the patient's rights.

Must Know

Malpractice allegations:

- Failure to communicate
- Failure to maintain safety
- Improper technique
- Failure to monitor and report
- Medication errors
- Failure to follow policy
- Wrong and poor documentation
- Improper use of equipment

SAFE PRACTICES FOR NURSES

- Practice according to current standards of practice and institution policies.
- Stick to organizational policies and procedures.
- Document in a manner that permits accurate reconstruction of patient assessments and the sequence of events, especially when notifying providers regarding clinical concerns.
- Maintain competence through continuing education, participation in professional conferences, seminars, CNEs, membership in professional organizations, and subscribing to professional journals.
- Maintain professional boundaries. Personal relationships with patients or with their families must be prohibited for juries and can be viewed as evidence of departure from professional standards.
- Engage the chain of command with patient concerns and pursue concerns to resolution.

ETHICS IN NURSING

Ethics in nursing involve the application of moral principles to everyday practice. These moral principles guide nurses in making decisions that promote the well being of their patients and the integrity of the profession.

Ethics involve doing good and causing no harm. Ethics in nursing is something which depends on individual interpretation. It is based on individual's morals and values. Nursing ethics is a unique field which is concerned with how broadly societal issues affect health and wellness—means nurse's endeavor to maintain awareness of aspects of social justice that affects well-being; and to advocate for a change. Nurses are responsible for the ethics of their practice (Fig. 6.3). Following are the primary values of nursing ethics:

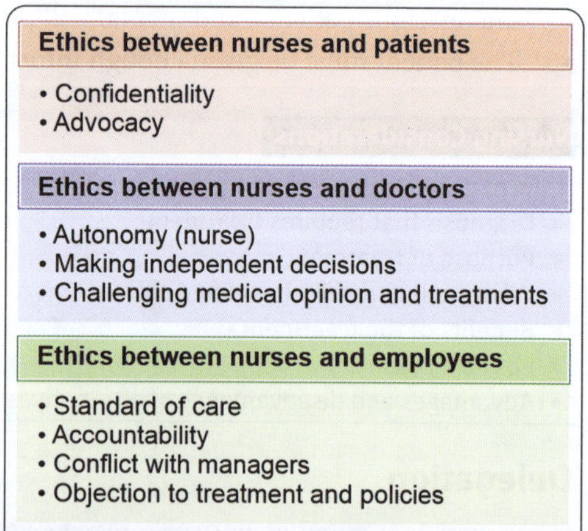

Ethics between nurses and patients

- Confidentiality
- Advocacy

Ethics between nurses and doctors

- Autonomy (nurse)
- Making independent decisions
- Challenging medical opinion and treatments

Ethics between nurses and employees

- Standard of care
- Accountability
- Conflict with managers
- Objection to treatment and policies

Ethics between nurses and the profession

- Political action
- Strikes
- Professionalism

Figure 6.3: Nursing ethics

- Providing safe, compassionate, competent and ethical care.
- Promoting health and well-being.
- Promoting and respecting informed decision-making.
- Preserving dignity.
- Ensuring privacy and confidentiality.
- Promoting justice.
- Being accountable.

Role of Ethics in Nursing Practice

> **Mnemonics**
>
> To abide by a good nursing practice with ethics, you can remember the mnemonic **"CODE"**.
> **C:** Courage to be moral requires
> **O:** Obligations to honor (what is right)
> **D:** Danger to manage
> **E:** Expression and action

Ethics involve recognizing the values and beliefs of patients, respecting their autonomy, well being and avoiding harm:

- **Maintaining patient trust safety and dignity:** Nurses can establish trust with patient by ethical principles. Nurse provide them competent care. Nurses can promote patient dignity by respecting their beliefs, values and cultural background.
- **Upholding nursing standards:** Ethical principles guide nurses to provide compassionate and competent care and adhere to professional boundaries.
- **Building a good relationship:** Nurses who follow ethical standards build and good reputation and they can earn patients trust.

ETHICAL PRINCIPLES

Ethical principles provide decision-based criteria in relation to ethical dilemmas. Ethical principles are tabulated in Table 6.1. Ethics inform our judgments and values and help individuals decide on how to act. Secondary ethical principles can be incorporated with the primary principles.

TABLE 6.1: Ethical principles
Primary ethical principles
Beneficence
Nonmaleficence
Respect for autonomy
Fairness
Truthfulness and honesty
Justice
Secondary ethical principles
Veracity
Confidentiality
Fidelity

Primary Ethical Principles

- **Beneficence:** Beneficence is doing or actively promoting good. It is done by:
    - Providing health benefits to the patients.
    - Balancing benefits and risks of harm.
    - Ensuring how a patient can be helped.
- **Nonmaleficence:** Nonmaleficence is doing no harm to clients. This is done by doing the following interventions:
    - Avoid deliberate harm while performing nursing duties.
    - Inform patients about risks and benefits.
- **Respects for autonomy:** It is an individual's right of autonomy and freedom of decision-making.
    - Patient should be able to make decisions about their care. Respect for autonomy involves concepts of informed consent including advance directives.
    - Informed consent is a method that promotes and respects a person's autonomy.
    - Informed consent is the idea that a person must be fully informed about and understand the potential benefits and risks of their choice of treatment.

- **Justice and fairness:** Justice is being fair to all and giving equal treatment, including distributing benefits, risks and costs equally. It is the promotion of equity or fairness in every situation a nurse encounters. Examples of justice are as follows:
  - Ensuring fair allocation of resources (appropriate staffing).
  - Determining the order in which patient should be treated (priority treatments for the clients in pain).
- **Autonomy:** Autonomy is the principle that recognizes the patient's right to make their own healthcare decisions. Nurses can provide autonomy to patients by providing all necessary information for informed decision making, understanding that each patient has unique values, preferences and circumstances. This involves clear communication about treatment options, outcomes and risks ensuring that patients are fully aware of their choices and can consent or refuse care.

Secondary Ethical Principles

- **Veracity:** Veracity is telling the truth and not intentionally deceiving or misleading clients.
- **Privacy and confidentiality:** Confidentiality is the prohibition of some disclosure of information gained in certain relationships without the consent of the original source of the information. All personal information released must be authorized by the patient. Privacy is a right of limited physical or informational accessibility.
- **Fidelity:** Fidelity is being loyal and faithful commitments and accountable for responsibilities. It is the duty to keep promises.

SOURCES OF ETHICAL DISTRESS

- Harm to patient (pain and suffering)
- Treatment of patient as object
- Policy constraints
- Medical prolongation of dying without information
- Brain death
- Inadequate staffing
- Cost

ETHICAL DILEMMAS

Ethical dilemmas arise when two or more ethical principles are in conflict.

Such dilemmas can be addressed by applying principles on a case by case bases once all available data are gathered and analyzed. Ethical dilemmas can be presented before ethical committees to provide guidance.

Ethical committees identify, examine and promote resolution of ethical issues and dilemmas by:
- Protecting the patient's rights.
- Protecting the staff and the organization.
- Reviewing decisions regarding clinical practice and standards of practice.
- Improving the quality of care and services.
- Serving as educational resources to staff.
- Building a consensus on ethical issues with professional organizations.

Examples of ethical dilemmas
- Unsafe nurse to patient ratio.
- Nonresponse by physician.
- Inappropriate orders.

SOME OTHER ISSUES FACED BY NURSES

- Job safety
- Shortage of staff
- Workplace mental violence
- Workplace health hazards
- Long working hours
- Less recognition of work
- Non-nursing roles
- Poor work environment
- Nurse burnout

CHARTER OF PATIENTS' RIGHTS FOR ADOPTION BY NHRC

Patients' Rights are Human Rights!

In India, there are various legal provisions related to Patient's Rights which are scattered across different legal documents, e.g., The Constitution of India, Article 21, Indian Medical Council (Professional Conduct, Etiquette and Ethics) Regulations 2002, The Consumer Protection Act 1986, Drugs and Cosmetic Act 1940, Clinical Establishment Act 2010 and rules and standards framed therein; various judgments given by Hon'ble Supreme Court of India and decisions of the National Consumer Disputes Redressal Commission. This Charter of Patient's Rights adopted by the National Human Rights Commission draws upon all relevant provisions, inspired by international charters and guided by national level provisions, with the objective of consolidating these into a single document, thereby making them publicly known in a coherent manner. There is an expectation that this document will act as a guidance document for the Union Government and State Governments to formulate concrete mechanisms so that Patient's Rights are given adequate protection and operational mechanisms are set up to make these rights functional and enforceable by law. This is especially important and is an urgent need at the present juncture because India does not have a dedicated regulatory like other countries and the existing regulations in the interest of patients, governing the healthcare delivery system is on the anvil, some States have adopted the National Clinical Establishments Act 2010, certain other States have enacted their own State level legislations like the Nursing Homes Act to regulate hospitals, while a few other States are in the process of adopting/developing such regulations.

The Charter of Patient's Rights has been drafted with the hope that it shall be incorporated by policy makers in all existing and emerging regulatory legislations concerning the healthcare sector. This charter would also enable various kinds of healthcare providers to actively engage with this framework of patient's rights to ensure their observance, while also benefiting from the formal codification of patient's responsibilities. Another objective of this Charter is to generate widespread public awareness and educate citizens regarding what they should expect from their governments and healthcare providers—about the kind of treatment they deserve as patients and human beings, in healthcare settings. NHRC firmly believes that informed and aware citizens can play a vital role in elevating the standard of healthcare, when they have guidance provided by codified rights, as well as awareness of their responsibilities (Table 6.2).

TABEL 6.2:		Rights of patients and associated duty bearers
Sl. no.	**Rights of patients**	**Description of rights and associated duty bearers**
1.	**Right to information**	Every patient has a right to adequate relevant information about the nature, cause of illness, provisional/confirmed diagnosis, proposed investigations and management, and possible complications To be explained at their level of understanding in language known to them. The treating physician has a duty to ensure that this information is provided in simple and intelligible language to the patient to be communicated either personally by the physician, or by means of his/her qualified assistants. Every patient and his/her designated caretaker have the right to factual information regarding the expected cost of treatment based on evidence. The hospital management has a duty to communicate this information in writing to the patient and his/her designated caretaker. They should also be informed about any additional cost to be incurred due to change in the physical condition of the patient or line of treatment in writing. On completion of treatment, the patient has the right to receive an itemized bill, to receive an explanation for the bill(s) regardless of the source of payment or the mode of payment, and receive payment receipt(s) for any payment made. Patients and their caretakers also have a right to know the identity and professional status of various care providers who are providing service to him/her and to know which Doctor/Consultant is primarily responsible for his/her care. The hospital management has a duty to provide this information routinely to all patients and their caregivers in writing with an acknowledgement.
2.	**Right of records and reports**	Every patient or his caregiver has the right to access originals/copies of case papers, indoor patient records, investigation reports (during period of admission, preferably within 24 hours and after discharge, within 72 hours). This may be made available wherever applicable after paying appropriate fees for photocopying or allowed to be photocopied by patients at their cost. The relatives/caregivers of the patient have a right to get discharge summary or in case of death, death summary along with original copies of investigations. The hospital management has a duty to provide these records and reports and to instruct the responsible hospital staff to ensure provision of the same are strictly followed without fail.
3.	**Right to emergency medical care**	As per Supreme Court, all hospitals both in the government and in the private sector are duty bound to provide basic Emergency Medical Care, and injured persons have a right to get Emergency Medical Care. Such care must be initiated without demanding payment/advance and basic care should be provided to the patient irrespective of paying capacity. It is the duty of the hospital management to ensure provision of such emergency care through its doctors and staff, rendered promptly without compromising on the quality and safety of the patients.
4.	**Right to informed consent**	Every patient has a right that informed consent must be sought prior to any potentially hazardous test/treatment (e.g., invasive investigation/surgery/chemotherapy) which carries certain risks. It is the duty of the hospital management to ensure that all concerned doctors are properly instructed to seek informed consent, that an appropriate policy is adopted and that consent forms with protocol for seeking informed consent are provided for patients in an obligatory manner. It is the duty of the primary treating doctor administering the potentially hazardous test/treatment to explain to the patient and caregivers the main risks that are involved in the procedure, and after giving this information, the doctor may proceed only if consent has been given in writing by the patient/caregiver or in the manner explained under Drugs and Cosmetic Act Rules 2016 on informed consent.

Contd...

Sl. no.	Rights of patients	Description of rights and associated duty bearers
5.	**Right to confidentiality, human dignity and privacy**	All patients have a right to privacy, and doctors have a duty to hold information about their health condition and treatment plan in strict confidentiality, unless it is essential in specific circumstances to communicate such information in the interest of protecting other or due to public health considerations. Female patients have the right to presence of another female person during physical examination by a male practitioner. It is the duty of the hospital management to ensure presence of such female attendants in case of female patients. The hospital management has a duty to ensure that its staff upholds the human dignity of every patient in all situations. All data concerning the patient should be kept under secured safe custody and insulated from data theft and leakage.
6.	**Right to second opinion**	Every patient has the right to seek second opinion from an appropriate clinician of patients'/caregivers' choice. The hospital management has a duty to respect the patient's right to second opinion, and should provide to the patients caregivers all necessary records and information required for seeking such opinion without any extra cost or delay. The hospital management has a duty to ensure that any decision to seek such • Annexure 8 of standards for Hospital level 1 by National Clinical Establishments Council set up as per Clinical Establishment Act 2010 • The Consumer Protection Act, 1986–8 second opinion by the patient/caregivers must not adversely influence the quality of care being provided by the treating hospital as long as the patient is under care of that hospital. Any kind of discriminatory practice adopted by the hospital or the service providers will be deemed as Human Rights' violation.
7.	**Right to transparency in rates, and care according to prescribed rates wherever relevant**	Every patient and their caregivers have a right to information on the rates to be charged by the hospital for each type of service provided and facilities available on a prominent display board and a brochure. They have a right to receive an itemized detailed bill at the time of payment. It would be the duty of the Hospital/Clinical Establishment to display key rates at a conspicuous place in local as well as English language, and to make available the detailed schedule of rates in a booklet form to all patients/caregivers. Every patient has a right to obtain essential medicines as per India Pharmacopeia, devices and implants at rates fixed by the National Pharmaceutical Pricing Authority (NPPA) and other relevant authorities. Every patient has a right to receive healthcare services within the range of rates for procedures and services prescribed by Central and State Governments from time to time, wherever relevant. However, no patient can be denied choice in terms of medicines, devices and standard treatment guidelines based on the affordability of the patients' right to choice. Every hospital and clinical establishment has a duty to ensure that essential medicines under NLEM as per Government of India and World Health Organisation, devices, implants and services are provided to patients at rates that are not higher than the prescribed rates or the maximum retail price marked on the packaging
8.	**Right to nondiscrimination**	Every patient has the right to receive treatment without any discrimination based on his or her illnesses or conditions, including HIV status or other health condition, religion, caste, ethnicity, gender, age, sexual orientation, linguistic or geographical/social origins. The hospital management has a duty to ensure that no form of discriminatory behavior or treatment takes place with any person under the hospital's care. The hospital management must regularly orient and instruct all its doctors and staff regarding the same.

Contd...

Sl. no.	Rights of patients	Description of rights and associated duty bearers
9.	**Right to safety and quality care according to standards**	Patients have a right to safety and security in the hospital premises. They have a right to be provided with care in an environment having requisite cleanliness, infection control measures, safe drinking water as per BIS/FSSAI Standards and sanitation facilities. The hospital management has a duty to ensure safety of all patients in its premises including clean premises and provision for infection control. Patients have a right to receive quality healthcare according to currently accepted standards, norms and standard guidelines as per National Accreditation Board for Hospitals (NABH) or similar. They have a right to be attended to, treated and cared for with due skill, and in a professional manner in complete consonance with the principles of medical ethics. Patients and caretakers have a right to seek redressal in case of perceived medical negligence or damaged caused due to deliberate deficiency in service delivery. The hospital management and treating doctors have a duty to provide quality healthcare in accordance with current standards of care and standard treatment guidelines and to avoid medical negligence or deficiency in service delivery system in any form.
10.	**Right to choose alternative treatment options if available**	Patients and their caregivers have a right to choose between alternative treatment/management options, if these are available, after considering all aspects of the situation. This includes the option of the patient refusing care after considering all available options, with responsibility for consequences being borne by the patient and his/her caregivers. In case a patient leaves a healthcare facility against medical advice on his/her own responsibility, then notwithstanding the impact that this may have on the patient's further treatment and condition, this decision itself should not affect the observance of various rights mentioned in this charter. The hospital management has a duty to provide information about such options to the patient as well as to respect the informed choice of the patient and caregivers in a proper recorded manner with due acknowledgement from the patient or the caregivers on the communication and the mode.
11.	**Right to choose source for obtaining medicines and tests**	When any medicine is prescribed by a doctor or a hospital, the patients and their caregivers have the right to choose any registered pharmacy of their choice to purchase them. Similarly when a particular investigation is advised by a doctor or a hospital, the patient and his caregiver have a right to obtain this investigation from any registered diagnostic centre/laboratory having qualified personnel and accredited by National Accreditation Board for Laboratories (NABL). It is the duty of every treating physician/hospital management to inform the patient and his caregivers that they are free to access prescribed medicines/investigations from the pharmacy/diagnostic centre of their choice. The decision by the patient/caregiver to access pharmacy/diagnostic centre of their choice must not in any ways adversely influence the care being provided by the treating physician or hospital.
12.	**Right to proper referral and transfer, which is free from perverse commercial influences**	A patient has the right to continuity of care, and the right to be duly registered at the first healthcare facility where treatment has been sought, as well as at any subsequent facilities where care is sought. When being transferred from one healthcare facility to another, the patient/caregiver must receive a complete explanation of the justification for the transfer, the alternative options for a transfer and it must be confirmed that the transfer is acceptable to the receiving facility. The patient and caregivers have the right to be informed by the hospital about any continuing healthcare requirements following discharge from the hospital. The hospital management has a duty to ensure proper referral and transfer of patients regarding such a shift in care. In regard to all referrals of patients, including referrals

Contd...

Sl. no.	Rights of patients	Description of rights and associated duty bearers
		to other hospitals, specialists, laboratories or imaging services, the decision regarding facility to which referral is made must be guided entirely by the best interest of the patient. The referral process must not be influenced by any commercial consideration such as kickbacks, commissions, incentives, or other perverse business practices.
13.	**Right to protection for patients involved in clinical trials**	Every person/patient who is approached to participate in a clinical trial has a right to due protection in this context. All clinical trials must be conducted in compliance with the protocols and Good Clinical Practice Guidelines issued by Central Drugs Standard Control Organisation, Directorate General of Health Services, Govt. of India as well as all applicable statutory provisions of Amended Drugs and Cosmetics Act, 1940 and Rules, 1945, including observance of the following provisions related to patients rights: • Participation of patients in clinical trials must always be based on informed consent, given after provision of all relevant information. The patient must be given a copy of the signed informed consent form, which provides him/her with a record containing basic information about the trial and also becomes documentary evidence to prove their participation in the trial. • A participant's right to agree or decline consent to take part in a clinical trial must be respected and her/his refusal should not affect routine care. • The patient should also be informed in writing about the name of the drug/intervention that is undergoing trial along with dates, dose and duration of administration. • At all times, the privacy of a trial participant must be maintained and any information gathered from the participant must be kept strictly confidential. • Trial participants who suffer any adverse impact during their participation in a trial are entitled to free medical management of adverse events, irrespective of relatedness to the clinical trial, which should be given for as long as required or till such time as it is established that the injury is not related to the clinical trial. In addition, financial or other assistance must be given to compensate them for any impairment or disability. In case of death, their dependents have the right to compensation. • Ancillary care may be provided to clinical trial participants for nonstudy/trial related illnesses arising during the period of the trial. This could be in the form of medical care or reference to facilities, as may be appropriate. • Institutional mechanisms must be established to allow for insurance coverage of trial related or unrelated illnesses (ancillary care) and award of compensation wherever deemed necessary by the concerned Ethics Committee. • After the trial, participants should be assured of access to the best treatment methods that may have been proven by the study. Any doctor or hospital who is involved in a clinical trial has a duty to ensure that all these guidelines are followed in case of any persons/patients involved in such a trial.
14.	**Right to protection of participants involved in biomedical and medical research**	Every patient who is taking part in biomedical research shall be referred to as research participant and every research participant has a right to due protection in this context. Any research involving such participants should follow the National Ethical Guidelines for Biomedical and Health Research Involving Human Participants, 2017 laid down by Indian council for Medical Research and should be carried out with prior approval of the Ethics Committee. Documented informed consent of the research participants should be taken. Additional safeguards should

Contd…

Sl. no.	Rights of patients	Description of rights and associated duty bearers
		be taken in research involving vulnerable population. Right to dignity, right to privacy and confidentiality of individuals and communities should be protected. Research participants who suffer any direct physical, psychological, social, legal or economic harm as a result of their participation are entitled, after due assessment, to financial or other assistance to compensate them equitably for any temporary or permanent impairment or disability. The benefits accruing from research should be made accessible to individuals, communities and populations whenever relevant. Any doctor or hospital who is involved in biomedical and health research involving patients has a duty to ensure that all these guidelines are followed in case of any persons/patients involved in such research.
15.	**Right to take discharge of patient, or receive body of deceased from hospital**	A patient has the right to take discharge and cannot be detained in a hospital, on procedural grounds such as dispute in payment of hospital charges. Similarly, caretakers have the right to the dead body of a patient who had been treated in a hospital and the dead body cannot be detailed on procedural grounds, including nonpayment/dispute regarding payment of hospital charges against wishes of the caretakers. The hospital management has a duty to observe these rights and not to indulge in wrongful confinement of any patient, or dead body of patient, treated in the hospital under any circumstances.
16.	**Right to patient education**	Patients have the right to receive education about major facts relevant to his/her condition and healthy living practices, their rights and responsibilities, officially supported health insurance schemes relevant to the patient, relevant entitlements in case of charitable hospitals, and how to seek redressal of grievances in the language the patients understand or seek the education. The hospital management and treating physician have a duty to provide such education to each patient according to standard procedure in the language the patients understand and communicate in a simple and easy to understand manner.
17.	**Right to be heard and seek redressal**	Every patient and their caregivers have the right to give feedback, make comments, or lodge complaints about the healthcare they are receiving or had received from a doctor or hospital. This includes the right to be given information and advice on how to give feedback, make comments, or make a complaint in a simple and user-friendly manner. Patients and caregivers have the right to seek redressal in case they are aggrieved, on account of infringement of any of the above mentioned rights in this charter. This may be done by lodging a complaint with an official designated for this purpose by the hospital/healthcare provider and further with an official mechanism constituted by the government such as Patients rights Tribunal Forum or Clinical establishments regulatory authority as the case may be. All complaints must be registered by providing a registration number and there should be a robust tracking and tracing mechanism to ascertain the status of the complaint resolution. The patient and caregivers have the right to a fair and prompt redressal of their grievances. Further, they have the right to receive in writing the outcome of the complaint within 15 days from the date of the receipt of the complaint. Every hospital and clinical establishment has the duty to set up an internal redressal mechanism as well as to fully comply and cooperate with official redressal mechanisms including making available all relevant information and taking action in full accordance with orders of the redressal body as per the Patient's Right Charter or as per the applicable existing laws.

Contd...

Sl. no.	Rights of patients	Description of rights and associated duty bearers
	References	**References** • Annexure 8 of standards for Hospital level 1 by National Clinical Establishments Council set up as per Clinical Establishment Act 2010 • Patients Charter by National Accreditation Board for Hospitals (NABH) • The Consumer Protection Act, 1986 • MCI Code of Ethics section 1.3.2 • Central Information Commission judgment, Nisha Priya Bhatia Vs. Institute of HB&AS, GNCTD, 2014 • Supreme court judgment Parmanand Katara v. Union of India (1989) 2) Judgment of National Consumer Disputes Redressal Commission Pravat Kumar Mukherjee v. Ruby General Hospital & Others (2005) • MCI Code of Ethics sections 2.1 and 2.4 • Article 21 of the Constitution 'Right to Life • Drugs and Cosmetic Act 1940, Rules 2016 on Informed Consent • Section 9(i) and 9(ii) of Clinical establishments (Central Government) Rules 2012 • Various Drug price control orders • Drugs Price Control Order (DPCO) section 3 of the Essential Commodities Act, 1955 • World Health Organisation – Referral Notes • Various IPHS documents • Protocols and Good Clinical Practice Guidelines issued by Central Drugs Standard Control Organisation, Directorate GeneralHealth Services, Govt. of India • Amended Drugs and Cosmetics Act, 1940 and Rules, 1945 especially schedule • National Ethical Guidelines for Biomedical and Health Research Involving Human Participants, Indian Council of Medical Research, New Delhi, 2017 • World Medical Assembly Declaration of Helsinki: Ethical Principles for Medical Research Involving Human Subjects • World Medical Assembly Declaration of Helsinki: Ethical Principles for Medical Research Involving Human Subjects available at • www.wma.net/en/30publications/ 10policies/b3/17c.pdf 3) • Drugs & Cosmetic Act, Rules 2016 on Clinical Trails

Responsibilities of Patients and Caretakers

Along with promoting their rights, patients and caretakers should follow their responsibilities so that hospitals and doctors can perform their work satisfactorily.

- Patients should provide all required health related information to their doctor, in response to the doctor's queries without concealing any relevant information, so that diagnosis and treatment can be facilitated.
- Patients should cooperate with the doctor during examination, diagnostic tests and treatment, and should follow doctor's advice, while keeping in view their right to participate in decision making related to treatment.
- Patients should follow all instructions regarding appointment time, cooperate with hospital staff and fellow patients, avoid creating disturbance to other patients, and maintain cleanliness in the hospital.

- Patients should respect the dignity of the doctor and other hospital staff as human beings and as professionals. Whatever the grievance may be, patient / caregivers should not resort to violence in any form and damage or destroy any property of the hospital or the service provider.
- The Patients should take responsibility for their actions based on choices made regarding treatment options, and in case they refuse treatment.

FURTHER READINGS

- Berman A, Snyder S, Frandsen G. Kozier and Erb's Fundamentals of Nursing: Concepts, Process, and Practice, 10th edition. Upper Saddle River, NJ: Pearson Prentice Hall; 2015.
- Chhugani M, James MM. Challenges faced by nurses in India—the major workforce of the healthcare system. Nurse Care Open Access J. 2017;2(4):112-4.
- Nursing Fundamentals. [online] Available from https://wtcs.pressbooks.pub/nursingfundamentals/chapter [Last accessed August, 2023].
- Potter PA, Perry AG, Stockert PA, Hall A. Fundamentals of Nursing, 11th edition. Philadelphia: Elsevier; 2022.
- University of Texas at Arlington. Experience a transformative education online. [online] Available from https://academicpartnerships.uta.edu/ [Last accessed August, 2023].
- Wisconsin Technical College System. Nursing: Mental health and community concepts. [online] Available from https://wtcs.pressbooks.pub/nursingmhcc/chapter/5-5-patient-rights [Last accessed August, 2023].
- https://main.mohfw.gov.in/sites/default/files/PatientCharterforcomments.pdf

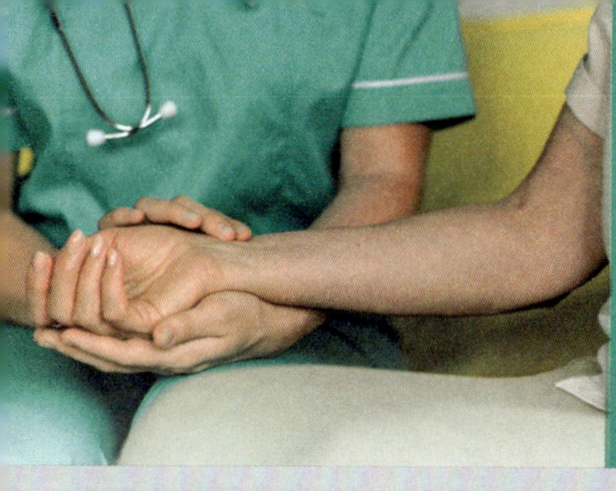

LONG ANSWER QUESTIONS

1. What are the legal aspects of nursing? Describe the types of laws.
2. What are the ethical principles? Discuss ethical issues in nursing.

SHORT ANSWER QUESTIONS

1. Write the different types of tort.
2. Write about the informed consent.
3. Write the functions of laws in nursing.

MULTIPLE CHOICE QUESTIONS

1. **Which of the following is an ethical principle that guides nursing practice?**
   a. Autonomy
   b. Utilitarianism
   c. Virtue
   d. Care

2. **A nurse is caring for a patient who is refusing treatment for their condition. The patient's family is pressuring the nurse to persuade the patient to accept treatment. What should the nurse do?**
   a. Persuade the patient to accept treatment to satisfy the family's wishes.
   b. Respect the patient's autonomy and allow them to refuse treatment.
   c. Seek a court order to force the patient to accept treatment.
   d. Consult with another nurse to determine the best course of action.

3. **Which of the following is an example of an ethical dilemma in nursing?**
   a. A nurse has to decide whether to report a colleague who made a medication error.
   b. A nurse has to decide whether to follow a patient's advance directive or a family's request.
   c. A nurse has to decide whether to accept a gift from a grateful patient.
   d. A nurse has to decide whether to join a union or not.

4. **What is moral distress in nursing?**
   a. The feeling of being unable to act according to one's moral values.
   b. The feeling of being uncertain about what is morally right.
   c. The feeling of being conflicted between two or more moral values.
   d. The feeling of being harmed by someone else's immoral actions.

5. **Which of the following is an example of applying the principle of justice in nursing practice?**
   a. Providing equal access to healthcare for all patients regardless of their social status.
   b. Providing individualized care for each patient according to their needs and preferences.
   c. Providing compassionate care for all patients regardless of their diagnosis or prognosis.
   d. Providing truthful information to all patients regardless of their ability to understand.

6. **What is informed consent in nursing practice?**
    a. The process of obtaining permission from a patient to perform a specific procedure or treatment.
    b. The process of providing information to a patient about the risks and benefits of a specific procedure or treatment.
    c. The process of ensuring that a patient understands and agrees to a specific procedure or treatment.
    d. The process of respecting a patient's right to refuse or withdraw from a specific procedure or treatment.

7. **Which of the following is an example of an ethical issue related to confidentiality in nursing practice?**
    a. A nurse shares a patient's medical record with another nurse who is not involved in the patient's care.
    b. A nurse discusses a patient's condition with the patient's family without the patient's consent.
    c. A nurse reports a suspected case of child abuse to the appropriate authorities without the parent's consent.
    d. A nurse refuses to disclose a patient's HIV status to another healthcare provider who is at risk of exposure.

7

Metaparadigm of Nursing

LEARNING OBJECTIVES

After the completion of the chapter, the readers will be able to:
- Discuss theories of nursing.
- Importance of nursing theories for a nurse.

CHAPTER OUTLINE

- Nursing Theories
- Self-Care Deficit Theory: Dorothea E. Orem
- Betty Neuman's Systems Model
- Hildegard Peplau's Interpersonal Relations
- Sister Callista Roy's Adaptation Model
- Florence Nightingale's Environment Theory
- Imogene King's Theory of Goal Attainment

KEY TERMS

Concept: Concepts are often called the building blocks of theories. They are primarily the vehicles of thought that involve images.

Conceptual framework: A conceptual framework is a group of related ideas, statements or concepts. It is often used interchangeably with the conceptual model and with grand theories.

Domain: The domain is the perspective or territory of a profession or discipline.

Metaparadigm: A metaparadigm is the most general statement of discipline and functions as a framework in which the more restricted structures of conceptual models develop. Most of the theoretical work in nursing is focused on articulating relationships among four major concepts: Person, environment, health and nursing.

Models: Models are representations of the interaction among and between the concepts showing patterns. They present an overview of the theory's thinking and may demonstrate how theory can be introduced into practice.

Paradigm: A paradigm refers to a pattern of shared understanding and assumptions about reality and the world, worldview or widely accepted value system.

Philosophy: These are beliefs and values that define a way of thinking and are generally known and understood by a group or discipline.

Process: Processes are organized steps, changes or functions intended to bring about the desired result.

Proposition: Propositions are statements that describe the relationship between the concepts.

Theory: A belief, policy or procedure proposed or followed as the basis of action. It refers to a logical group of general propositions used as principles of explanation. Theories are also used to describe, predict or control phenomena.

NURSING THEORIES

A theory is a system of ideas that is proposed to explain a given phenomenon. The nursing practice must be based on nursing theories. This is what makes the nursing discipline a profession. The nursing theories provide direction and guidance for structuring professional nursing practice, education and research. They also differentiate the focus of nursing from other professions. Nursing theories serve to guide assessment, intervention, and evaluation of nursing care. They provide a rationale for collecting reliable and valid data about the health status of clients, which is essential for effective decision-making and implementation. Nursing theories enhance the autonomy of nursing by defining its own independent functions.

Metaparadigm

A metaparadigm is a concept that is extremely general, one that serves to define an entire world of thought. Originates from two Greek words: Meta, meaning "with" and paradigm, meaning "pattern". It is the most global conceptual or philosophical framework of a discipline or profession. "Meta" means "that which is behind", in Greek, and refers to that which undergirds something else, serving as a conceptual basis.

Types of Metaparadigms

There are four types of metaparadigms in nursing which are as follows:

1. Person

This paradigm refers to the sick individual not as a "patient", but as a "subject", a person in the full sense of the word. This includes families and social groups that have come to define the person as such. This person is unique and autonomous and should be treated as such. A real person is not a mere object of professional care and surveillance.

Human beings are viewed as open energy fields with unique life experiences. As energy fields, they are greater than and different from the sum of their parts and cannot be predicted from knowledge of their parts. Humans as holistic beings, are unique, dynamic, sentient, and multidimensional, capable of abstract reasoning, creative, can appreciate esthetic values and have a sense of self-responsibility. Language, empathy, caring and other abstract patterns of communication are aspects of an individually high level of complexity and diversity and enable one to increase knowledge of self and environment. Humans are viewed as valued persons to be respected, nurtured and understood with the right to make informed choices regarding their health.

The nursing client is an open system, continually changing in a mutual process with the changing environment. Recipients of nursing actions may be well or ill; and include individuals, families and communities.

2. Health

Like all meta-concepts, health is immensely general. Meta-concept does not deal with health in a strictly clinical manner. Further, it concerns nurses as medical professionals. It defines "health" in abstract terms in which health is "negotiated" and "contextual", in the words of Slevin, health is not an absolute concept, but exists in the context of the health problems of the individual.

Health is a dynamic process. It is the synthesis of wellness and illness and is defined by the perception of the client across the life span. This view focuses on the entire nature of the client in physical, social, esthetic, and moral realms. Health is contextual and relational.

- Wellness, in this view, is the lived experience of congruence between one's possibilities and one's realities and is based on caring and feeling cared for.
- Illness is defined as the lived experience of loss or dysfunction that can be mediated by caring relationships. Inherent in this conceptualization is each client's approach to stress and coping. The degree or level of health is an expression of the mutual interactive process between human beings and their environment.

3. Environment

Environment is the landscape and geography of human social experience, the setting or context of experience as everyday life and includes variations in space, time and quality. This geography includes personal, social, national, global, and beyond. Environment also includes societal beliefs, values, mores, customs, and expectations. Environment serves to explain healthcare and nursing specifically. It is little less than the totality of things that impact the recovery of the patient. Home life, mental state, addictions, physical pain, chances of relapse, rewarding work and a host of other variables come to define the context of recovery. All of these clearly impact recovery or even the patient's desire for recovery. This also includes social and cultural dimensions such as religious beliefs and general attitudes toward death and suffering. The environment is an energy field in mutual process with the human energy field and is conceptualized as the arena in which the nursing client encounters aesthetic beauty, caring relationships, threats to wellness and the lived experiences of health. Dimensions that may affect health include physical, psychosocial, cultural, historical and developmental processes as well as the political and economic aspects of the social world.

4. Nursing

Nursing is an academic discipline and a practice profession. It is the art and science of holistic healthcare guided by the values of human freedom, choice, and responsibility. Nurses use critical thinking and clinical judgment to provide evidence-based care to individuals, families, aggregates, and communities to achieve an optimal level of client wellness in diverse nursing settings/contexts. Clinical judgment skills are therefore essential for professional nursing practice. Human caring as the moral ideal of nursing is the central focus of professional practice. It involves concern and empathy, and a commitment to the client's lived experience of human health and the relationships among wellness, illness, and disease.

Nursing itself is a meta-theory that seeks to help contextualize nursing. It is the paradigm of compassion, the reason why nurses become nurses: To help and ease suffering. It is an intensely ethical and emotional paradigm that goes to the root of nursing as a profession with its own set of rewards.

Importance of Nursing Theories

Nursing theories provide the foundations of nursing practice, generate further knowledge, and indicate which direction nursing should develop in the future.   **—Brown, 1964**

By providing nurses a sense of identity, nursing theory can help patients, managers, and other healthcare professionals to acknowledge and understand the unique contribution that nurses make to the healthcare service.   **—Draper, 1990**

In many cases, nursing theories guide knowledge development and direct education, research, and practice, although each influences the others.   **—Fitzpatrick and Whall, 2005**

Nursing theories:

- Aim to define, describe, predict and explain the phenomenon of nursing.
- Help us to decide what we know and what we need to know.
- Help us to distinguish what should form the basis of practice by explicitly describing nursing.
- Facilitate better patient care, enhanced professional status for nurses and improved communication between nurses.
- Analyze and explain what nurses do.
- Establish a unique body of knowledge.
- Maintain professional boundaries of the nursing profession.
- Help recognize what should set the foundation of practice by explicitly describing nursing.
- Help nurses to understand their purpose and role in the healthcare setting.
- Serve as a rationale or scientific reasons for nursing interventions and give nurses the knowledge base necessary for acting and responding appropriately in nursing care situations.
- Prepare the nurses to reflect on the assumptions and question the nursing values, thus further defining nursing and increasing the knowledge base.
- Maintain and preserve professional limits and boundaries of nursing profession.
- Help in guiding research and informing evidence-based practice.
- Provide a common language and terminology for nurses to use in communication and practice.
- Serve as a basis for the development of nursing education and training programs.

Characteristics of Theories

Theories are:

- Interrelated concepts in such a way as to create a different way of looking at a particular phenomenon.
- Logical in nature.
- Generalizable.
- Basis of hypotheses that can be tested.
- Increasing the general body of knowledge within the discipline through the research implemented to validate them.
- Used by practitioners to guide and improve their practice.
- Consistent with other validated theories, laws and principles but will leave open unanswered questions that need to be investigated.

SELF-CARE DEFICIT THEORY: DOROTHEA E. OREM

Self-care deficit theory (Fig. 7.1) developed as a result of Dorothea E. Orem working toward her goal of improving the quality of nursing. The model interrelates concepts in such a way as to create a

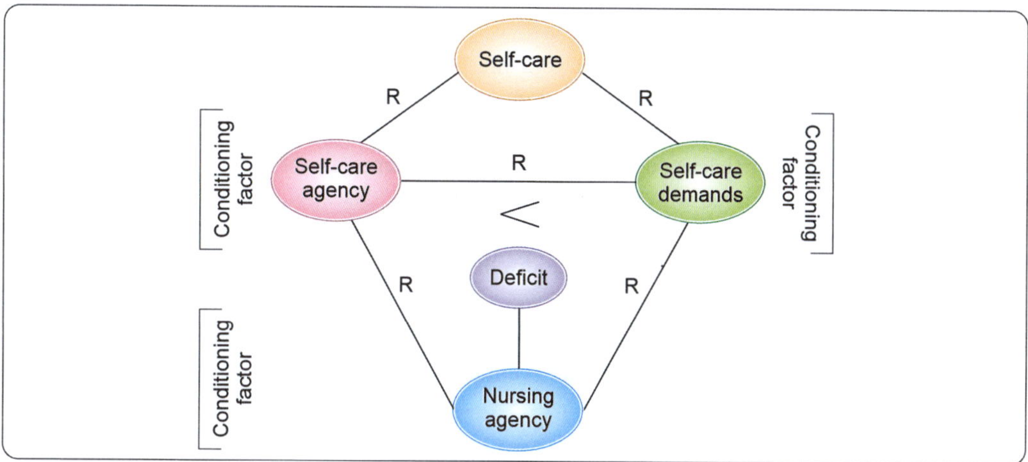

Figure 7.1: Orem's self-care model

different way of looking at a particular phenomenon. The theory is relatively simple, but generalizable to apply to a wide variety of patients. It can be used by nurses to guide and improve practice, but it must be consistent with other validated theories, laws and principles.

Assumptions of Orem's Theory

The major assumptions of Orem's Self-Care Deficit Theory are as follows:

- People should be self-reliant, and responsible for their care as well as others in their family who need care.
- People are distinct individuals.
- Nursing is a form of action. It is an interaction between two or more people.
- Successfully meeting universal and development self-care requisites is an important component of primary care prevention and ill health.
- A person's knowledge of potential health problems is needed for promoting self-care behaviors.
- Self-care and dependent care are behaviors learned within a sociocultural context.

Components of Orem's Theory

Orem's theory is comprised of three related parts:

1. Theory of Self-Care

The theory of self-care includes:

- **Self-care:** It is the practice of activities that an individual initiates and performs on his/her own behalf to maintain life, health and well-being.
- **Self-care agency:** It is a human ability that is "the ability for engaging in self-care", conditioned by age, developmental state, life experience, sociocultural orientation, health and available resources.
- **Therapeutic self-care demand:** It is the total self-care actions to be performed over a specific duration to meet self-care requisites by using valid methods and related sets of operations and actions.
- **Self-care requisites:** They include the categories of universal, developmental, and health deviation self-care requisites.

Requirements of Self-Care

Universal self-care requisites are associated with life processes as well as the maintenance of the integrity of human structure and functioning. Orem's theory identifies these requisites, also called activities of daily living or ADLs, as:

- The maintenance of sufficient intake of air, food, and water.
- Provision of care associated with the elimination process.
- A balance between activities and rest as well as between solitude and social interaction.
- The prevention of hazards to human life and well-being.
- The promotion of human functioning.

Developmental self-care requisites are associated with developmental processes. They are generally derived from a condition or associated with an event.

Applications of Orem's Self-Care Theory

Health deviation self-care is required in conditions of illness, injury or disease. These include:

- Seeking and securing appropriate medical assistance.
- Being aware of and attending to the effects and results of pathologic conditions.
- Effectively carrying out medically prescribed measures.
- Modifying self-concepts to accept oneself as being in a particular state of health and in specific forms of healthcare.
- Learning to live with the effects of pathologic conditions.

2. Theory of Self-Care Deficit

The second part of the theory, self-care deficit specifies when nursing is needed. According to Orem, nursing is required when an adult is incapable or limited in the provision of continuous, effective self-care. The theory identifies five methods of helping—acting for and doing for others; guiding others; supporting others; providing an environment promoting personal development in relation to meet future demands; and teaching other.

3. Theory of Nursing Systems

The theory of nursing systems describes how the patient's self-care needs will be met by the nurse, the patient or by both. Orem identifies three classifications of nursing system to meet the self-care requisites of the patient:

1. Wholly compensatory system
2. Partly compensatory system
3. Supportive-educative system

Orem's approach to the nursing process provides a method to determine the self-care deficits and then to define the roles of patient or nurse to meet the self-care demands.

The nursing process in this model has three parts.

1. First is the assessment, which collects data to determine the problem or concern that needs to be addressed.
2. Second step is the diagnosis and creation of a nursing care plan.
3. The third and final step of the nursing process is implementation and evaluation.

The nurse sets the healthcare plan into motion to meet the goals set by the patient and his/her healthcare team and, when finished, evaluate the nursing care by interpreting the results of the implementation of the plan.

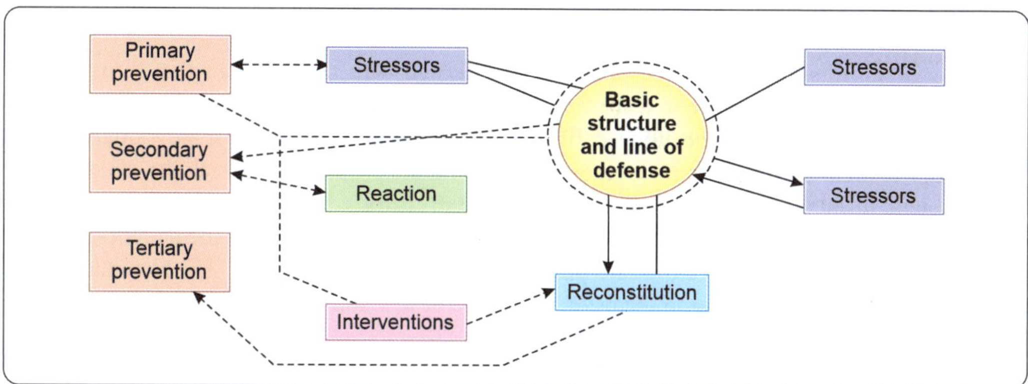

Figure 7.2: Betty Neuman's systems model

BETTY NEUMAN'S SYSTEMS MODEL

Betty Neuman's System Model (Fig. 7.2) provides a comprehensive holistic and system-based approach to nursing that contains an element of flexibility. The theory focuses on the response of the patient system to actual or potential environmental stressors and the use of primary, secondary and tertiary nursing prevention intervention for retention, attainment, and maintenance of patient wellness.

- **Primary prevention** is applied in patient assessment and intervention, in identification and reduction of possible or actual risk factors.
- **Secondary prevention** relates to symptomatology following a reaction to stressors, appropriate ranking of intervention priorities, and treatment to reduce their noxious effects.
- **Tertiary prevention** relates to adjustive processes taking place as reconstitution begins, and maintenance factors move them back in a cycle toward primary prevention.

Assumptions of Betty Neuman's Systems Model

The basic assumptions of the model are:

- Each patient system is a unique composite of factors and characteristics within a range of responses contained in a basic structure.
- May known, unknown, and universal stressors exist. Each differs in their potential for upsetting a client's usual stability level.
- Each patient has evolved a normal range of responses to the environment referred as the normal line of defense. It can be used as a standard by which to measure health deviation.
- The particular interrelationships of patient variables, at any point of time can affect the degree to which a client is protected by the flexible line of defense against possible reaction to stressors.
- When the flexible line of defense is incapable of protecting the patient against an environmental stressor, that stressor breaks through the line of defense.
- The client is a dynamic composite of the interrelationships of the variables, whether in a state of illness or wellness. Wellness is on a continuum of available energy to support the system in a state of stability.
- Each patient has implicit internal resistance factor known as IOR, which functions to stabilize and realign the patient to the usual state of wellness.
- The patient is in dynamic, constant energy exchange with the environment.

Nursing is a Unique Profession–Neuman

Neuman views nursing as a unique profession concerned with the variables that influences the response the patient might have to a stressor. Nursing also addresses the whole person, giving the theory a holistic perspective. The model defines nursing as "actions which assist individuals, families and groups to maintain a maximum level of wellness, and the primary aim is stability of the patient-client system, through nursing interventions to reduce stressors."

Neuman also says the nurse's perception must be assessed in addition to the patient's, since the nurse's perception will influence the care plan he/she sets up for the patient. The Neuman systems model views the role of nursing in terms of the degree of reaction to stressors as well as the use of primary, secondary and tertiary interventions.

Nursing Process in Neuman's Systems Model

According to Neuman's Systems Model, nursing process has six steps, each with specific categories of data about the patient (Fig. 7.3). It begins with the assessment of the patient, which looks at actual and potential stressors; conditions and strengths of basic factors and energy sources; characteristics

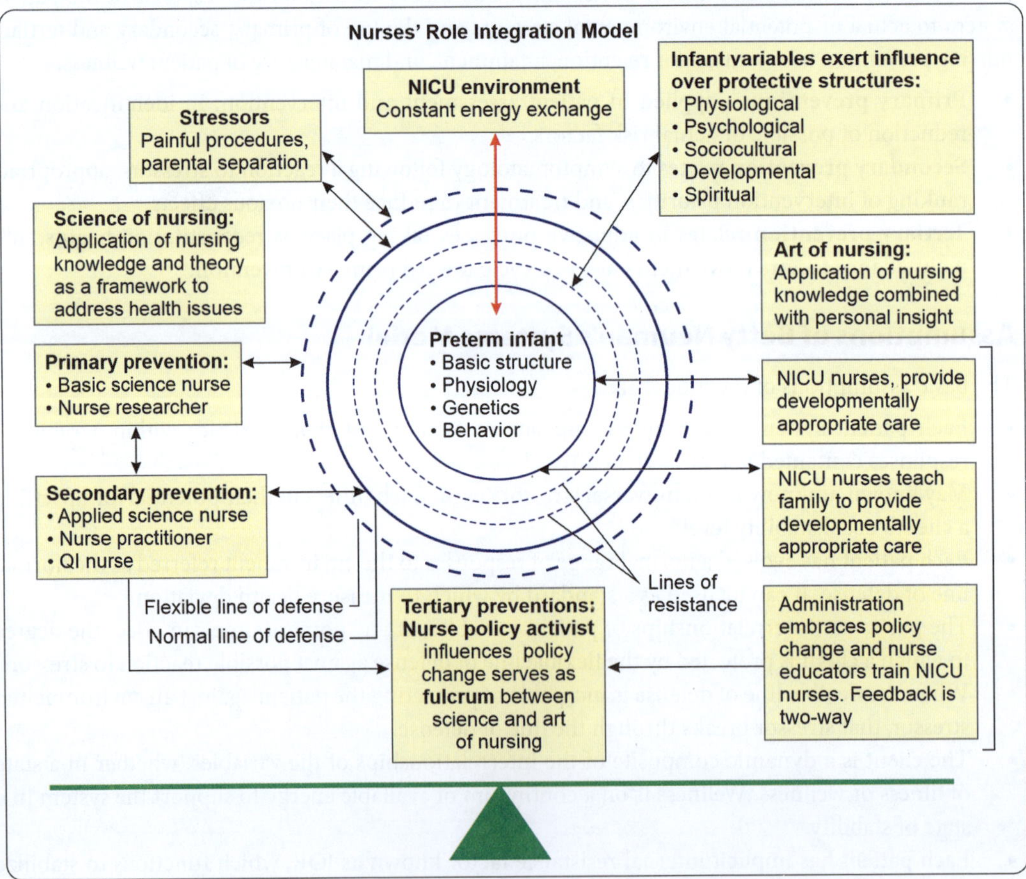

Figure 7.3: Betty Neuman's systems model—Nurse's role in NICU

of flexible and normal lines of defense, lines of resistance, degree of reaction and potential for reconstitution; interaction between the patient and his/her environment; life process and coping factors for optimal wellness; and the perceptual difference between the care giver and the patient.

Next is that the nurse makes a diagnosis by interpreting the data collected. The data includes health-seeking behaviors, activity intolerance, ineffective coping and ineffective thermoregulation. The third step in the nursing process is to set goals. The ultimate goal is to keep the client system stable. From the goals, a plan is created, which focuses on strengthening lines of defense and resistance. That plan is implemented using primary, secondary and tertiary preventions. Finally, the nursing process is evaluated to determine whether or not balance was restored and a stable state maintained.

Components of Betty Neuman's Systems Model

In this model, each concentric circle or layer is made up of the five variable areas which are considered and these occur simultaneously in each client's concentric circles. These are as follows:

1. **Physiological**—refers to bodily structure and function.
2. **Psychological**—refers to mental processes, functioning and emotions.
3. **Sociocultural**—refers to relationships; and social/cultural functions and activities.
4. **Spiritual**—refers to the influence of spiritual beliefs.
5. **Developmental**—refers to life's developmental processes.

Basic Structure of Energy Resources

Central core: This is otherwise known as the central core, and is made up of the basic survival factors common to all organisms. These include the following:

- **Normal temperature range:** Body temperature regulation ability.
- **Genetic structure:** Hair color and body features.
- **Response pattern:** Functioning of body systems homeostatically.
- Organ strength or weakness.
- Ego structure.
- Knowns or commonalities—value system.

The person's system is an open system—dynamic and constantly changing and evolving. Stability, or homeostasis, occurs when the amount of energy that is available exceeds that being used by the system. A homeostatic body system is constantly in a dynamic process of input, output, feedback and compensation, which leads to a state of balance.

Flexible lines of defense: It is the outer boundary to the normal line of defense, the line of resistance and the core structure.

- Keeps the system free from stressors and is dependent on the amount of sleep, nutritional status as well as the quality and quantity of stress an individual experiences.
- If the flexible line of defense fails to provide adequate protection to the normal line of defense, the lines of resistance get activated.

Normal line of defense: Represents client's usual wellness level. It can change over the time in response to coping or responding to the environment, which includes intelligence, attitudes, problem solving and coping abilities. Example is skin which is generally smooth and fair may eventually form callous over the times.

Lines of resistance: The last boundary that protects the basic structure.

- It protects the basic structure and becomes activated when environmental stressors invade the normal line of defense. An example is that when a certain bacterium enters our system, there is an increase in leukocyte count to combat infection.
- If the lines of resistance are effective, the system can reconstitute and if the lines resistance are not effective, the resulting energy loss can result in death.

Stressors

Stressors are capable of producing either a positive or negative effect on the client system. It is an environmental force which can potentially affect the stability of the system:

- **Intrapersonal:** Occurs within person, for example, infection, thoughts and feelings.
- **Interpersonal:** Occurs between individuals, for example, role expectations.
- **Extrapersonal:** Occurs outside the individual, for example, job or finance concerns.

Reaction to Stressors

A person's reaction to stressors depends on the strength of the lines of defense. When the lines of defense fail, the resulting reaction depends on the strength of the lines of resistance.

Reconstitution: As part of the reaction, a person's system can adapt to a stressor, an effect known as reconstitution. Reconstitution is the increase in energy that occurs in relation to the degree of reaction to the stressor which starts after initiation of treatment for invasion of stressors. It may expand the normal line of defense beyond its previous level, stabilize the system at a lower level or return it to the level that existed before the illness.

Nursing interventions: Nursing interventions focus on retaining or maintaining system stability. By means of primary, secondary and tertiary interventions, the person (or the nurse) attempts to restore or maintain the stability of the system. Prevention is the primary nursing intervention. It focuses on keeping stressors and the stress response from having a detrimental effect on the body.

- **Primary prevention:** Primary prevention focuses on protecting the normal line of defense and strengthening the flexible line of defense. This occurs before the system reacts to a stressor and strengthens the person (primarily the flexible line of defense) to enable him to better deal with stressors and also manipulates the environment to reduce or weaken stressors. It includes health promotion and maintenance of wellness.
- **Secondary prevention:** Secondary prevention focuses on strengthening internal lines of resistance, reducing the reaction of the stressor and increasing resistance factors in order to prevent damage to the central core. This occurs after the system reacts to a stressor. This includes appropriate treatment of symptoms to attain optimal client system stability and energy conservation.
- **Tertiary prevention:** Tertiary prevention focuses on readaptation and stability and protects reconstitution or return to wellness after treatment. This occurs after the system has been treated through secondary prevention strategies. Tertiary prevention offers support to the client and attempts to add energy to the system or reduce energy needed in order to facilitate reconstitution.

HILDEGARD PEPLAU'S INTERPERSONAL RELATIONS

Hildegard Peplau published her Theory of Interpersonal Relations in 1952 and in 1968, interpersonal techniques became the crux of psychiatric nursing. The Theory of Interpersonal Relations is a middle-range descriptive classification theory as shown in Figure 7.4.

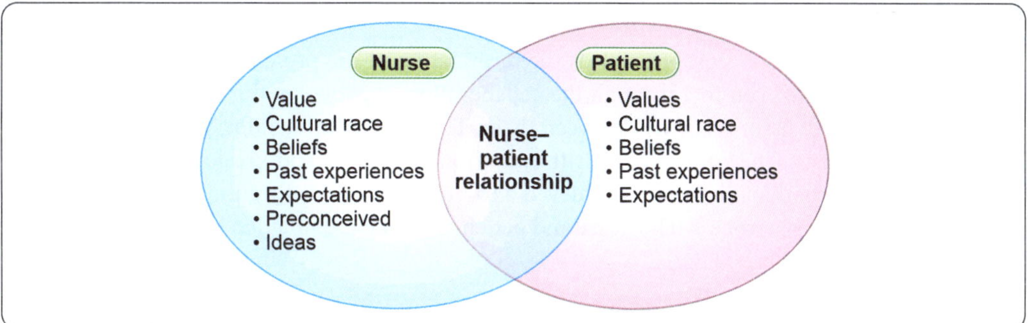

Figure 7.4: Hildegard Peplau's theory of interpersonal relations

Components of Theory of Interpersonal Relations

- **Person** is a developing organism that tries to reduce anxiety caused by needs.
- **Environment** consists of existing forces outside of the person, and put in the context of culture.
- **Health** is a word symbol that implies forward movement of personality and other human processes toward creative, constructive, productive, personal, and community living.

Phases of Theory of Interpersonal Relations

The nursing model identifies four sequential phases in the interpersonal relationship: Orientation, identification, exploitation and resolution.

1. Orientation Phase

The orientation phase defines the problem. It starts when the nurse meets the patient and the two are strangers. After defining the problem, the orientation phase identifies the type of service needed by the patient. The patient seeks assistance, tells the nurse what he/she needs, asks questions and shares preconceptions and expectations based on past experiences. Essentially, the orientation phase is the nurse's assessment of the patient's health and situation.

2. Identification Phase

The identification phase includes the selection of the appropriate assistance by a professional. In this phase, the patient begins to feel if he/she belongs, and feels capable of dealing with the problem which decreases the feeling of helplessness and hopelessness. The identification phase is the development of a nursing care plan based on the patient's situation aid goals.

3. Exploitation Phase

The exploitation phase uses professional assistance for problem-solving alternatives. The advantages of the professional services used are based on the needs and interests of the patients. In the exploitation phase, the patient feels like an integral part of the helping enlivenment and may make minor requests or use attention-getting techniques. When communicating with the patient, the nurse should use interview techniques to explore, understand and adequately deal with the underlying problem. The nurse must also be aware of the various phases of communication since the patient's independence is likely to fluctuate.

4. Resolution Phase

The final phase is the resolution phase. It is the termination of the professional relationship since the patient's needs have been met through the collaboration of patient and nurse. They must sever their relationship and dissolve any ties between them. This can be difficult for both if psychological dependence still exists. The patient may drift away from the nurse and breaks the bond between them. A healthier emotional balance is achieved and both become mature individuals. This is the evaluation of the nursing process. The nurse and patient evaluate the situation based on the goals set and whether or not they met.

Goal of Psychodynamic Nursing

The goal of psychodynamic nursing is to help understand one's own behavior, help others identify the difficulties faced and apply principles of human relations to the problems that come up at all experience levels. Peplau explains that nursing is therapeutic because it is a healing art, assisting a patient who is sick or in need of healthcare. It is also an interpersonal process because of the interaction between two or more individuals who have a common goal. The nurse and patient work together so both become mature and knowledgeable in the care process.

Role of a Nurse in Hildegard Peplau's Nursing Theory

The nurse has a variety of roles in Hildegard Peplau's nursing theory. The six main roles are: Stranger, teacher, resource person, counselor, surrogate and leader.

1. **As a stranger**, the nurse receives the patient in the same way the patient meets a stranger in other life situations. The nurse should create an environment that builds trust.
2. **As a teacher**, the nurse imparts knowledge in reference to the needs or interests of the patient.
3. **As a resource person**, the nurse is providing specific information needed by the patient that helps the patient understand a problem or situation.
4. **As a counselor**, the nurse helps the patient understand and integrate the meaning of current life situations as well as provide guidance and encouragement in order to make changes.
5. **As a surrogate**, the nurse helps the patient clarify the domains of dependence, interdependence and independence and acts as an advocate for the patient.
6. **As a leader**, the nurse helps the patient take on maximum responsibility for meeting his/her treatment goals.

Additional roles of a nurse include technical expert, consultant, tutor, socializing and safety agent, environment manager, mediator, administrator, record observer and researcher.

SISTER CALLISTA ROY'S ADAPTATION MODEL

The Adaptation Model of Nursing (Fig. 7.5) was developed by Sister Callista Roy in 1976. Roy became convinced of the importance of describing the nature of nursing as a service to society. This prompted her to begin developing her model with the goal of nursing being to promote adaptation. She first began organizing her theory of nursing as she developed course curriculum for nursing students. She introduced her ideas as a basis for an integrated nursing curriculum.

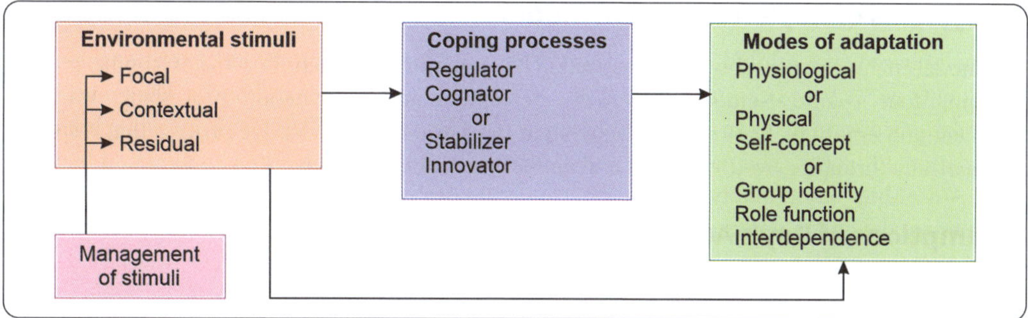

Figure 7.5: Sister Callista Roy's adaptation model of nursing

Factors Influencing Development of Roy's Adaptation Model of Nursing

The factors that influences the development of the model include—family, education, religious background, mentors and clinical experience. Roy's model asks the questions:

- Who is the focus of nursing care?
- What is the target of nursing care?
- When is nursing care indicated?

Key Concepts of Roy's Adaptation Model

Roy explained that adaptation occurs when people respond positively to environmental changes, and it is the process and outcome of individuals and groups who use conscious awareness, self-reflection, and choice to create human and environmental integration. The key concepts of Roy's Adaptation Model are made up of four components:

1. **Person:** According to Roy's model, a person is a biopsychosocial being in constant interaction with a changing environment. He/she uses innate and acquired mechanisms to adapt. The model includes people as individuals as well as in groups such as families, organizations and art communities. This also includes society as a whole.
2. **Health:** The adaptation model states that health is an inevitable dimension of a person's life, and is represented by a health illness continuum. Health is also described as a state and process of being and becoming integrated and whole.
3. **Environment:** All conditions, circumstances and surroundings influence affect the development and behavior of people and groups with particular consideration to mutuality of person and earth resources, including focal, contextual, and residual stimuli.
   The environment has three components:
   i. Focal, which is internal or external and immediately confronts the person.
   ii. Contextual, which is all stimuli present in the situation that all contribute to the effect of the focal stimulus
   iii. Residual, whose effects in the current situation are not clear.
4. **Nursing:** To promote adaptations for individuals/groups thus contributing the quality of life.

Subsystems of Roy's Adaptation Model

The model includes two subsystems, as well. The cognator subsystem is a major coping process involving four cognitive-emotive channels—perceptual and information processing, learning, judgment and emotion. The regulator subsystem is a basic type of adaptive process that responds automatically through neural, chemical and endocrine coping channels.

Assumptions of Roy's Adaptation Model

Explicit assumptions: The Adaptive Model makes ten explicit assumptions:

1. The person is a biopsychosocial being.
2. The person is in constant interaction with a changing environment.
3. To cope with a changing world, a person uses coping mechanisms, both innate and acquired, which are biological, psychological and social in origin.
4. Health and illness are inevitable dimensions of a person's life.
5. In order to respond positively to environmental changes, a person must adapt.
6. A person's adaptation is a function of the stimulus he is exposed to and his adaptation level.
7. The person's adaptation level is such that it comprises a zone indicating the range of stimulation that will lead to a positive response.
8. The person has four modes of adaptation—physiologic needs, self-concept, role function and interdependence.
9. Nursing accepts the humanistic approach of valuing others' opinions and perspectives. Interpersonal relations are an integral part of nursing.
10. There is a dynamic objective for existence with the ultimate goal of achieving dignity and integrity.

Implicit assumptions: There are also four implicit assumptions which state:

1. A person can be reduced to parts for study and care.
2. Nursing is based on causality.
3. A patient's values and opinions should be considered and respected.
4. A state of adaptation frees a person's energy to respond to other stimuli.

Adaptive Modes in Roy's Adaptation Model

The goal of nursing is to promote adaptation in the four adaptive modes. Nurses also promote adaptation for individuals and groups in the four adaptive modes, thus contributing to health, quality of life and dying with dignity by assessing behaviors and factors that influence adaptive abilities and by intervening to enhance environmental interactions. The four adaptive modes of Roy's Adaptation Model are—physiologic needs, self-concept, role function and interdependence.

Nursing Process in Roy's Adaptation Model

The Adaptation Model includes a six-step nursing process:

1. The first level of assessment, which addresses the patient's behavior.
2. The second level of assessment, which addresses the patient's stimuli.
3. Diagnosis of the patient.
4. Setting goals for the patient's health.
5. Intervention to take actions in order to meet those goals.
6. Evaluation of the result to determine if goals were met.

FLORENCE NIGHTINGALE'S ENVIRONMENT THEORY

As the founder of modern nursing, Florence Nightingale's Environment Theory (Fig. 7.6) changed the nursing practice. She served as a nurse during the Crimean War and at that time she observed a correlation between the patients who died and their environmental conditions. As a result of her observations, the Environment Theory of nursing was born. Nightingale explained in her book, Notes on Nursing "What it is, What it is Not?" The model of nursing that were developed by Nightingale, who is considered the first nursing theorist, contains elements that have not changed since the establishment of the modern nursing profession.

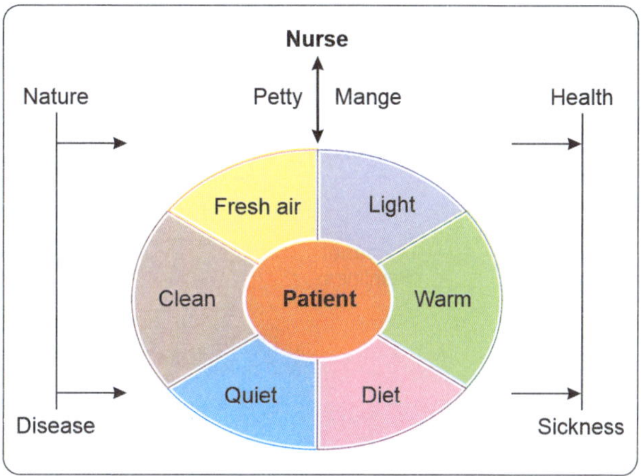

Figure 7.6: Florence Nightingale's environment theory

Although this theory was pioneering at the time it was created, the principles it applies are timeless.

Assumptions of Environment Theory

The seven assumptions made in the Environment Theory, focus on taking care of the patient's environment in order to reach health goals and cure illness. These assumptions are as follows:

1. Natural laws.
2. Mankind can achieve perfection.
3. Nursing is a calling.
4. Nursing is an art and a science.
5. Nursing is achieved through environmental alteration.
6. Nursing requires a specific educational base.
7. Nursing is distinct and separate from medicine.

Focus of Nursing in Environment Theory

Alter the patient's environment: The focus of nursing in this model is to alter the patient's environment in order to affect change in his/her health. The environmental factors that affect health, as identified in the theory, are—fresh air, pure water, sufficient food supplies, efficient drainage, cleanliness of the patient and environment and light (particularly direct sunlight). If any of these areas is lacking, the patient may experience diminished health. A nurse's role in a patient's recovery is to alter the environment in order to gradually create the optimal conditions for the patient's body to heal itself. In some cases, this would mean minimal noise and in other cases it could mean a specific diet. All of these areas can be manipulated to help the patient meet his/her health goals and get healthy.

Focus on the care of the patient rather than nursing process: The Environment Theory of nursing is a patient care theory. It focuses on the care of the patient rather than the nursing process, the relationship between patient and nurse or the individual nurse. In this way, the model must be adapted to fit the needs of individual patients. The environmental factors affect different patients in a unique way toward their situations and illnesses. The nurse must address these factors on a case-to-case basis in order to make sure that the factors are altered in a way that best care for an individual patient and his/her needs are provided.

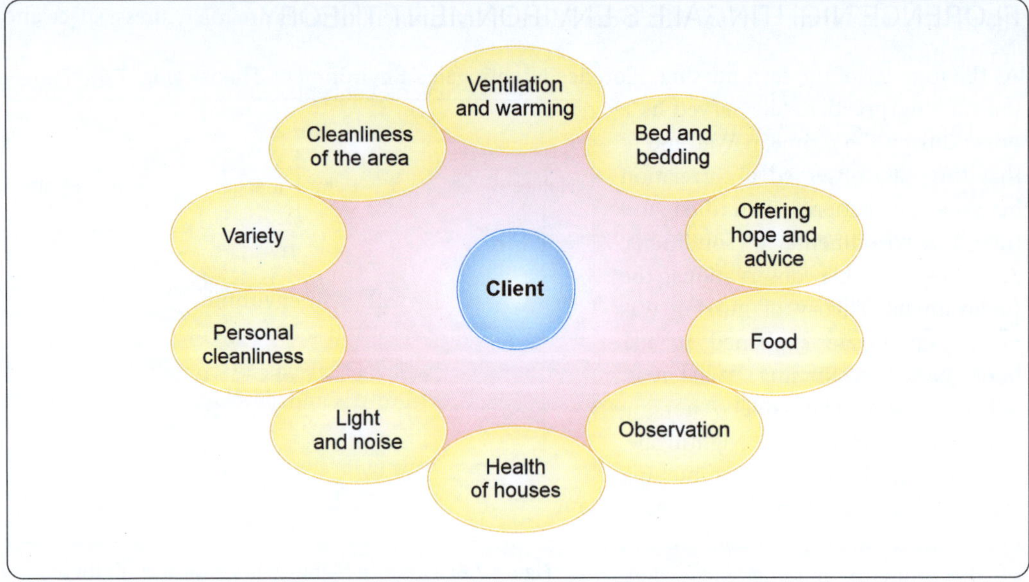

Figure 7.7: Nightingale's canons—major concepts

Concepts of Environment Theory

The ten major concepts of the Environment Theory (Fig. 7.7) are also identified as Nightingale's Canons.

Nursing According to Nightingale's Theory of Environment

According to Nightingale, nursing is separate from medicine. The goal of nursing is to put the patient in the best possible condition in order for nature to act.

- Nursing is "the activities that promote health which occur in any caregiving situation."
- Health is "not only to be well, but to be able to use well every power we have."

Nightingale's theory addresses disease on a literal level, explaining it as the absence of comfort. The environment paradigm in Nightingale's model is understandably the most important aspect. Her observations taught her that unsanitary environments contribute greatly to ill health and that the environment can be altered in order to improve conditions for a patient and allow healing to occur.

IMOGENE KING'S THEORY OF GOAL ATTAINMENT

The Theory of Goal Attainment (Fig. 7.8) in which a patient grows and develops to attain certain life goals.

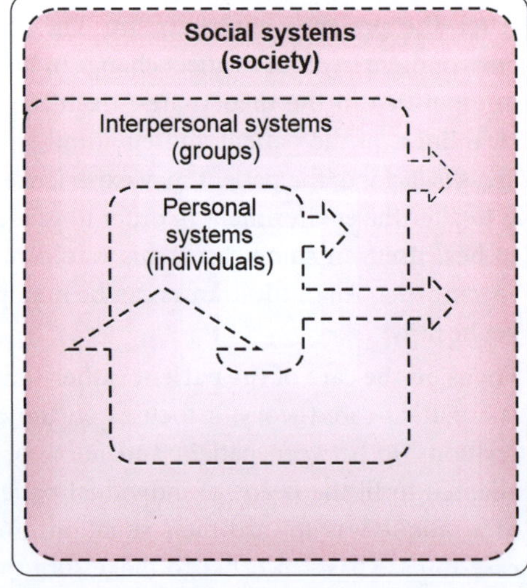

Figure 7.8: Imogene theory of goal attainment

The theory explains that factors which can affect the attainment of goals are roles, stress, space and time. It includes:

- Several basic assumptions
- Three interacting systems
- Several concepts relevant for each system

Basic Assumptions

- Nursing focuses on the care of human being.
- Nursing goal is the healthcare of individuals and groups.
- Human beings are open systems interacting constantly with their environment.
- Interacting systems: Personal system, interpersonal system and social system.
- Concepts are given for each system:
  - **Concepts for personal system:** Perception, self-growth and development, body image, space and time.
  - **Concepts for interpersonal system:** Interaction, communication, transaction, role and stress.
  - **Concepts for social system:** Organization, authority, power, status and decision-making.

Propositions Made in the Theory of Goal Attainment

The following propositions are made in the Theory of Goal Attainment (Fig. 7.9):

- If perceptual interaction accuracy is present in nurse-patient interactions, transaction will occur.
- If the nurse and patient make transaction, the goal or goals will be achieved.
- If the goal or goals are achieved, satisfaction will occur.
- If transactions are made in nurse-patient interactions, growth and development will be enhanced.
- If role expectations and role performance are perceived by the nurse and patient are congruent, transaction will occur.
- If role conflict is experienced by either the nurse or the patient (or both), stress in the nurse-patient interaction will occur.
- If a nurse with special knowledge communicates appropriate information to the patient, mutual goal setting and goal achievement will occur.
- The focus of nursing is the care of the human being (patient).

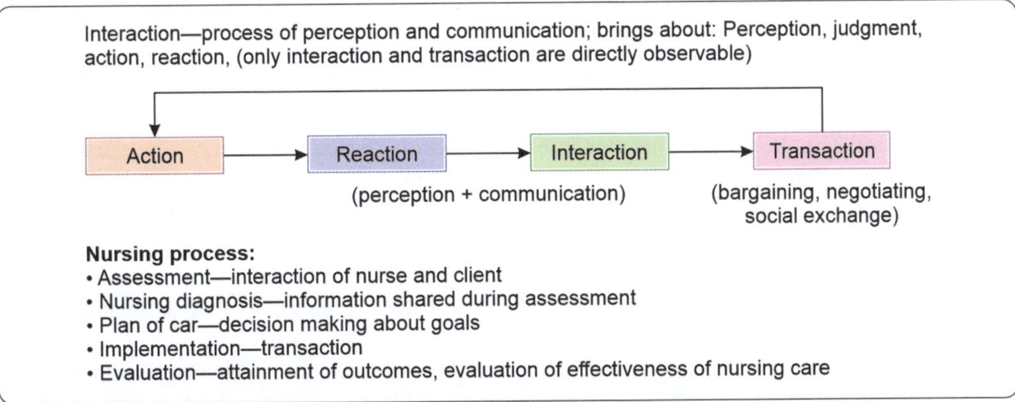

Figure 7.9: Propositions—theory of goal attainment

Assumptions Made in the Theory of Goal Attainment

The assumptions made in the model are as follows:

- The goal of nursing is the healthcare of both individuals and groups.
- Human beings are open systems interacting with their environments constantly.
- The nurse and patient communicate information, set goals mutually and then act to achieve those goals. This is also the basic assumption of the nursing process.
- Patients perceive the world as a complete person making transactions with individuals and things in the environment. Transaction represents a life situation in which the perceiver and the thing being perceived are encountered. It also represents a life situation in which a person enters the situation as an active participant. Each is changed in the process of these experiences.

Concepts of Theory of Goal Attainment

According to King, a human being refers to a social being who is rational and sentient. He/she has the ability to perceive, think, feel, choose, set goals, select means to achieve goals and make decisions. He/she has three fundamental needs:

1. The need for health information when it is needed and can be used.
2. The need for care that seeks to prevent illness.
3. The need for care when he/she is unable to help himself/herself.

Health involves dynamic life experiences of a human being, which implies continuous adjustment to stressors in the internal and external environment through optimum use of resources to achieve maximum potential for daily living. Environment is the background for human interaction. It involves the internal and external environments.

- The internal environment transforms energy to enable a person to adjust to continuous external environment changes.
- The external environment involves formal and informal organizations. In this model, the nurse is part of the patient's environment.

The Theory of Goal Attainment defines nursing as "a process of action, reaction and interaction by which nurse and client share information about their perception in a nursing situation" and "a process of human interactions between nurse and client whereby each perceives the other and the situation, and through communication, they set goals, explore means, and agree on means to achieve goals." The function of a professional nurse is "to interpret information in the nursing process to plan, implement, and evaluate nursing care."

King gives detailed information about the nursing process in her model of nursing. The steps of the nursing process are—assessment, nursing diagnosis, planning, implementations and evaluation.

1. **Assessment:** The theory explains that assessment occurs during interaction. The nurse brings special knowledge and skills whereas the patient brings knowledge of himself/herself as well as the perception of problems of concern to the interaction. During the assessment, the nurse collects data regarding the patient including his/her growth and development, the perception of self, and current health status. Perception is the base for the collection and interpretation of data. Communication is required to verify the accuracy of the perception as well as for interaction and translation.
2. **Nursing diagnosis:** The nursing diagnosis is developed using the data collected in the assessment. In the process of attaining goals, the nurse identifies problems, concerns and disturbances about which the patient is seeking help.

3. **Planning:** After the diagnosis, the nurse and other healthcare team members create a care plan of interventions to solve the problems identified. The planning is represented by setting goals and making decisions about the means to achieve those goals. This part of transaction and the patient's participation is encouraged in making decisions on the means to achieve the goals.
4. **Implementation:** The implementation phase of the nursing process is the actual activities done to achieve the goal. In this model of nursing, it is the continuation of transaction.
5. **Evaluation:** Evaluation involves determining whether or not goals were achieved. The explanation of evaluation in King's theory addresses meeting goals and the effectiveness of nursing care.

FURTHER READINGS

- Alligood MR. Nursing Theorists and Their Work (E-Book), 9th Edition. St. Louis: Elsevier Health Sciences; 2017.
- Colley S. Nursing theory: Its importance to practice. Nurs Stand. 2003;17(46):33-7.
- George JB. Nursing Theories: The Base for Professional Nursing Practice, 4th edition. Norwalk, Conn.: Appleton & Lange; 1995.
- Nightingale F. Notes on Nursing, 1st American edition. New York: D Appleton and Company; 1860.
- Peplau H. The art and science of nursing: similarities, differences, and relations. Nurs Sci Q. 1988;1(1):8-15.
- Rogers ME. An Introduction to the Theoretical Basis of Nursing. Philadelphia: FA Davis; 1970

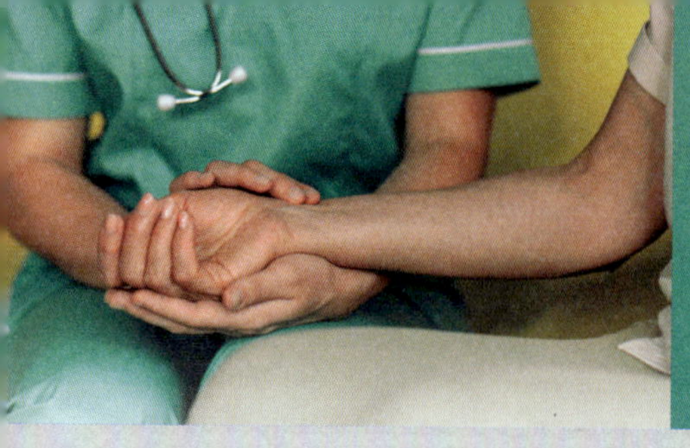

LONG ANSWER QUESTIONS

1. Discuss the environment theory given by Florence Nightingale.
2. Who gave the theory of goal attainment? Discuss the theory in detail.

SHORT ANSWER QUESTIONS

1. Write in brief about adaptive model.
2. Write in brief about interpersonal relations model.

MULTIPLE CHOICE QUESTIONS

1. **Which of the following is not considered metaparadigm of nursing?**
   a. Person
   b. Environment
   c. Health
   d. Diagnosis
   e. Nursing

2. **In 1958, which nurse believed the environment played a crucial role in patient care?**
   a. Sister Callista Roy, created by society, includes values and expectations
   b. Dorothea Orem, society's view on values and expectations
   c. Dorothea Orem, the direct influence on the health of a person
   d. Dorothea Orem, created by society, includes values and expectations
   e. Dorothea Orem, the environment was external influence on the person

3. **Dorothea Orem's theory states:**
   a. Human is willing to take care of themselves
   b. Basic human needs are met through self-care activities
   c. The self-care activities consist of fourteen detailed components
   d. The basic foundation to caring for oneself
   e. Basic humans need to be supported or educated on their limitations

4. **What was Betty Neuman's theory on a person?**
   a. A whole being that consists of spiritual, intellectual, and physiological components
   b. An integrated being constantly changing because of environmental influences
   c. An integrated whole being constantly seeking spiritual guidance
   d. Being whole and integrated into a variable state of change
   e. An integrated whole in a constant state of change because of the dynamic interrelationship of many variables

5. **Florence Nightingale believed the environment to be:**
   a. Either a negative or positive influence on the person
   b. Those aspects outside the person that affect health
   c. An external force that affects the person's health
   d. All of the above
   e. None of the above

6. **In 1964, which nurse believed the environment consisted of all internal and external influences that affect the human being?**
   a. Betty Neuman
   b. Florence Nightingale
   c. Virginia Henderson
   d. Dorothea Orem
   e. Sister Callista Roy

7. **Who proposed the self-care deficit theory?**
   a. Betty Neuman
   b. Virginia Henderson
   c. Dorothea Orem
   d. None of the above

ANSWER KEY

1. d   **2.** e   **3.** a   **4.** a   **5.** d   **6.** d   **7.** c

---

Note

8

Nursing Process

LEARNING OBJECTIVES

After the completion of the chapter, the readers will be able to:
- Discuss nursing process and practices.
- Know the components of nursing process—assessment, nursing diagnosis, planning, implementation and evaluation.
- Familiarize with documentation of nursing process.

CHAPTER OUTLINE

- Nursing Process
- Nursing Process—Cornerstone of the Nursing Profession
- Documentation of Nursing Process

KEY TERMS

Collaboration: A working practice whereby individuals work together for a common purpose to achieve business benefit.

Evaluation: Determination of the value, nature, character or quality.

Process: A series of actions done for a particular purpose.

NURSING PROCESS

The nursing process is a systematic method that directs both nurse and patient, as together they accomplish the following:

- Assess the patient to determine the need for nursing care
- Determine nursing diagnosis
- Identify expected outcome and plan care
- Implement the care
- Evaluate the results

Definitions

- Nursing process is a specific method of organizing and delivering nursing care or action.
- The nursing process is used by nurses every day to help patients improve their health and assist doctors in treating patients.
- It is a form of problem-solving approach. The nursing process is made-up of a series of stages that are used to achieve the objectives. Nursing knowledge is used throughout the process to formulate changes in approach to the patient's changing condition.
- Nursing process is a systematic problem-solving approach used to identify, prevent and treat actual or potential health problems and promote wellness.
- It is a systematic way to plan, implement and evaluate care for individuals, families, groups and communities.

Purposes

- To identify the client's health needs.
- To determine priorities of care goals and expected outcomes.
- To establish a nursing care plan to meet client-centered needs.
- To provide nursing intervention designed to meet these needs.
- Evaluate the effectiveness of the nursing care in achieving client goal.

Characteristics

The characteristics of a nursing process are as follows:

- Systematic
- Dynamic
- Client-centered
- Planned interpersonal and collaborative
- Universally applicable focus on problems or strengths
- Open and flexible
- Improves patient satisfaction
- Saves time and energy
- Provides guide for all staff members
- Humanistic and individualized
- Cyclical
- Outcome focused
- Emphasizes on feedback and validation.
- Promotes quality patient care
- Improves patient safety

Nursing process is a deliberate, rational, systematic, goal-directed method of planning and providing nursing care as shown in Figure 8.1.

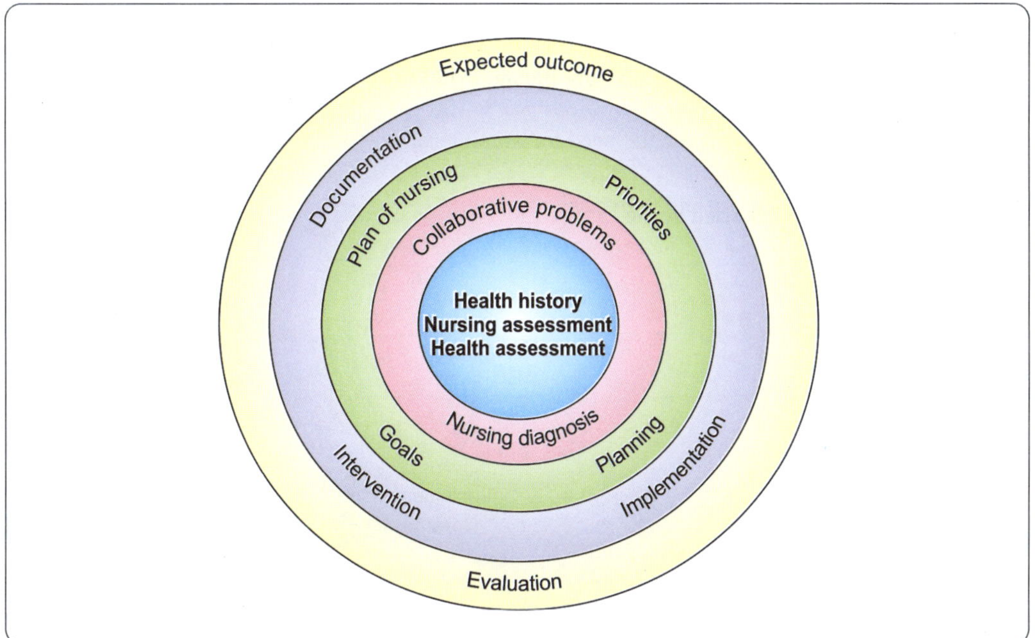

Figure 8.1: Nursing process model

Benefits of Using the Nursing Process

- Ensures continuity of care
- Prevents duplication
- Provides individualized care

- Maintains standards of care
- Increases client participation
- Encourages collaboration of care

NURSING PROCESS—CORNERSTONE OF THE NURSING PROFESSION

The nursing process is the base of a nursing theory developed by Ida Jean Orlando. She developed this theory in late 1950s. Ms Orlando proposed four steps in nursing process but through practical application over the past 40 years one step evolved and now there are total five steps.

Practical Advantages of Nursing Process

- The nursing process provides a framework for meeting the individual needs of patients, their families and community.
- The steps of the nursing process focus on the nurse's attention on the individual or human responses of a patient or group, about a given health situation, resulting in a holistic plan of care addressing their specific problem or needs.
- The use of nursing process promotes active involvement of the patient in his own healthcare.
- The use of nursing process enables a nurse to have more control over practice.
- The use of nursing process provides a common language for practice, unifying the nursing profession.

- It provides a means of assessing nurse's economic contribution to patient care.
- It provides an organized systematic method of problem-solving, which may minimize dangerous errors or omissions in caregiving and avoid time consuming repetition in care and documentation.

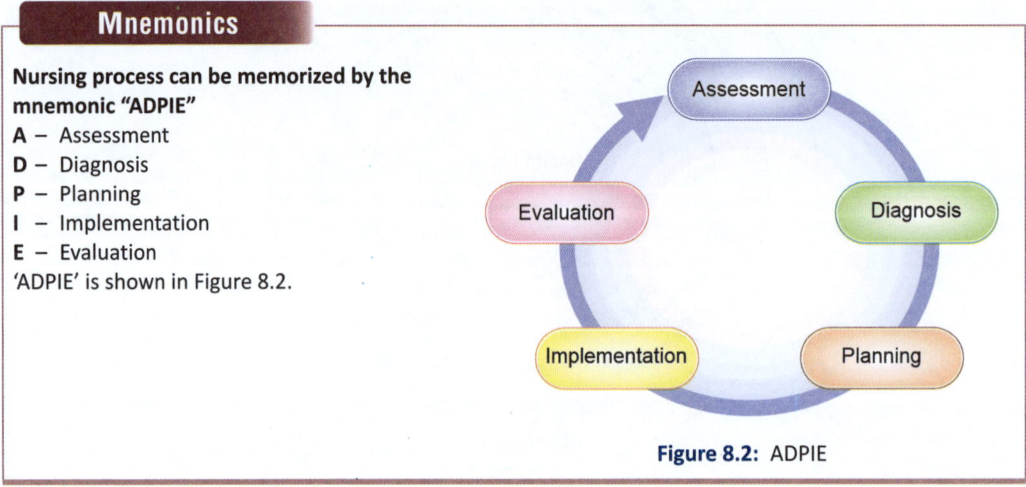

Mnemonics

Nursing process can be memorized by the mnemonic "ADPIE"
A – Assessment
D – Diagnosis
P – Planning
I – Implementation
E – Evaluation
'ADPIE' is shown in Figure 8.2.

Figure 8.2: ADPIE

Components of Nursing Process

The components of nursing process are shown in Figure 8.3.

Assessment

Assessment is the dynamic and continuous process of collecting, verifying and organizing information about a person or other entity. Assessment is obtaining information about a patient's response to health concerns/illness and their ability to manage these healthcare issues.

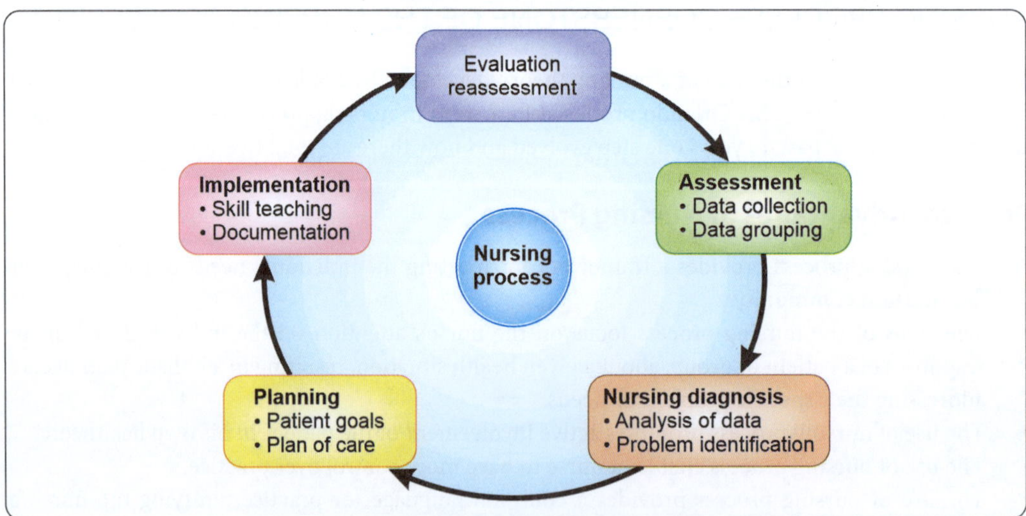

Figure 8.3: Components of nursing process

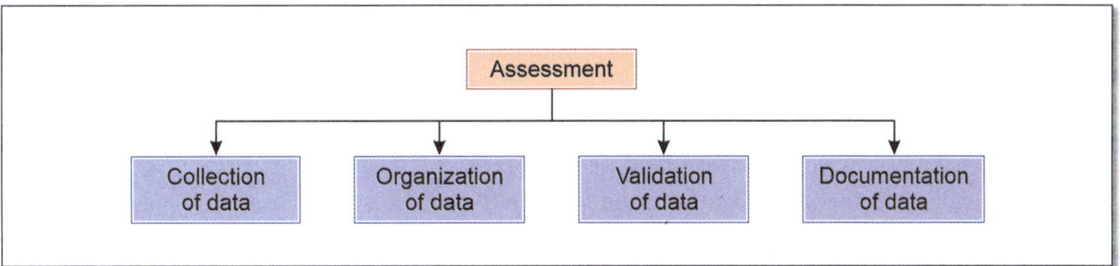

Figure 8.4: Components of assessment

Components of Assessment

The components of assessment are shown in Figure 8.4.

Assessing is a continuous process carried out during all phases of nursing process. All phases depend on the accurate and complete collection of data.

Assessment in nursing process involves:

- Collection of data
- Organization of data
- Validation of data
- Documentation of data

Purpose of Assessment

To establish a database about the client's level of wellness health practices, past illness and related experiences and healthcare goals. Assessment is a deliberate and systematic collection of data to determine a client's current and past health status and to determine the clients present and past coping patterns.

Types of Assessment

- **Initial assessment:** Performed within specified time after admission to a healthcare agency, e.g., nursing admission assessment.
- **Problem-focused assessment:** Ongoing process is integrated with nursing care to determine specific problem identified in an earlier assessment and to identify new or overlooked problems. For example, assessment of patient's ability to perform self-care while assisting client to take bath.
- **Emergency assessment:** It is done during psychiatric and physiological crisis of the client to identify life-threatening problems. For example, rapid assessment of ABC during cardiac arrest.
- **Time-lapsed assessment:** It is done several months after initial assessment to compare the client's status to baseline data previously obtained.

Data Collection

- Data collection is the process of gathering information about a client's health status. It includes, nursing health history, physical examination, result of laboratory and diagnostic test and information from healthcare team members and the client's family.
- Data collected during assessment should be describable, concise, complete and should not include interpretative statement.
- Several nursing models may be used to guide data collection. Using a nursing model as a framework for data collection rather than a body system approach or the commonly known

head-to-toe approach has the advantage of identifying and validating nursing diagnoses as opposed to medical diagnoses.

Types of Data

- Objective data (symptoms, covert data).
- Subjective data is client's perception about his health problems.

Objective data (signs, covert data)

These are observations and measurements made by data collectors. Objective data can be measured or tested against an accepted standard. They can be seen, heard, felt or smelled and they are obtained by observation or physical examination. Examples of objective data include blood pressure data, skin color, assessment of client's wound, etc.

Subjective data (client's perception)

Only client can provide this kind of information. Subjective data is the information obtained directly from the patient, the patient's family or from other healthcare providers who have observed changes or symptoms in the patient. Examples of subjective data include feeling of anxiety, physical discomfort or mental stress, pain, itching, etc.

Sources of Data

Sources of data are mentioned in Figure 8.5.

There are two kinds of sources of data:

1. **Primary (direct) source of data by client**
2. **Secondary source of data by family members**
    - Clients' records
    - Medical records
    - Records of therapies
    - Laboratory records
    - Team members

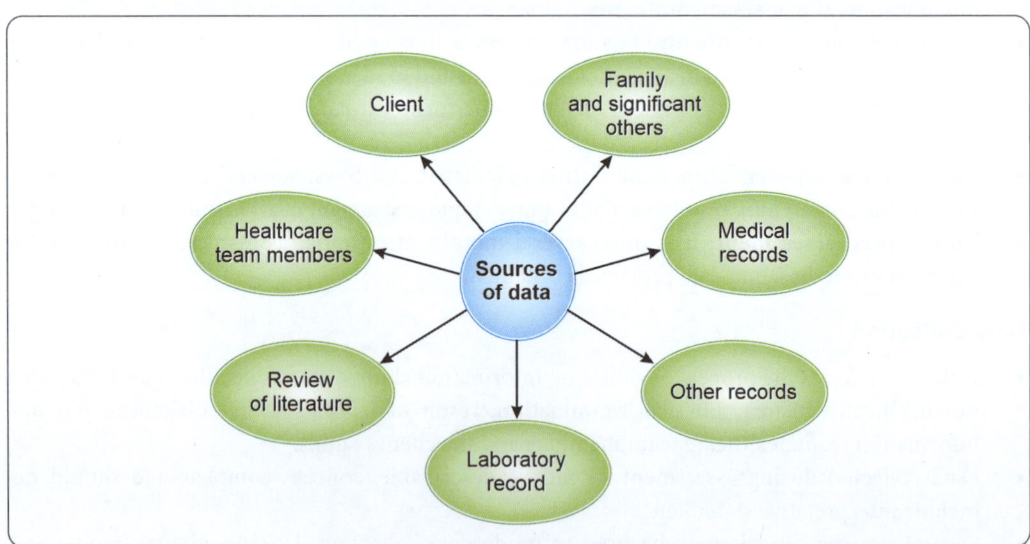

Figure 8.5: Sources of data

Methods of Data Collection

Data is collected in four ways which include interview process, nursing health history, physical examination and diagnostic and laboratory data.

Interview process: The interview process may involve problem-solving technique, or open ended questions.

- Problem seeking behavior—Problem-solving technique
- Direct questions—Open ended questions

Nursing health history it depends on following:

- Biological information—Reason for seeking healthcare
- Present illness—Past health history
- Family history—Environmental history
- Psychological history—Spiritual health
- Review of systems—Client expectations

Physical examination: The physical examination is performed systemically in a manner similar to the review of system in the health history. Physical examination includes various techniques like:

- Inspection
- Percussion
- Palpation
- Auscultation

Diagnostic and laboratory data: The results of diagnostic and laboratory tests can identify or verify alterations questioned or identified during the nursing health history and physical examination.

Interview Process

Information of the client database is obtained primarily from the client and then from family members/significant others, through conversation and observation during a structured interview. The nursing interview may take place over several contact sessions, but each contact should yield information. A well-conducted interview can be the first step in establishing a beneficial nurse–client relationship and the rapport needed for good communication.

The various phases of nursing interview process are mentioned in the Figure 8.6.

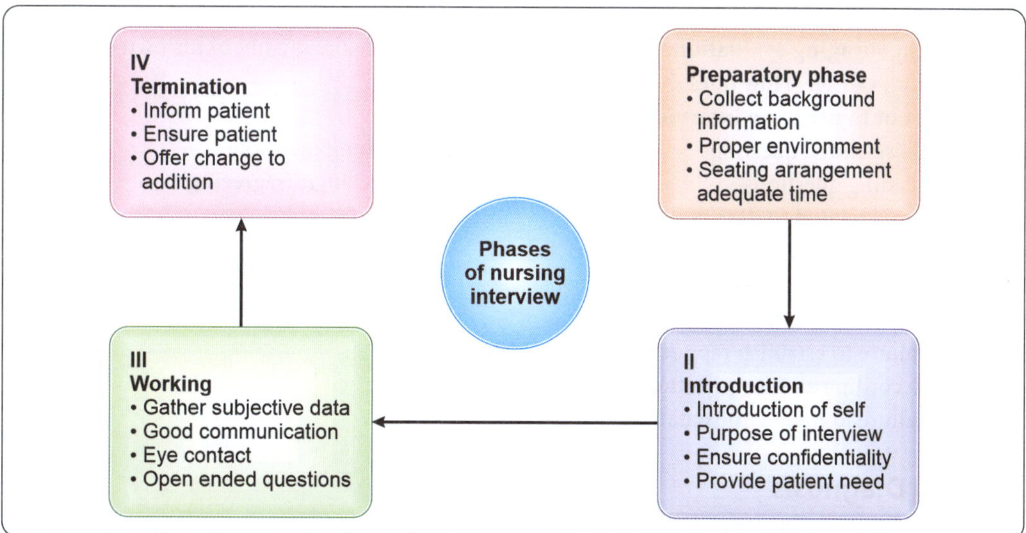

Figure 8.6: Phases of nursing interview process

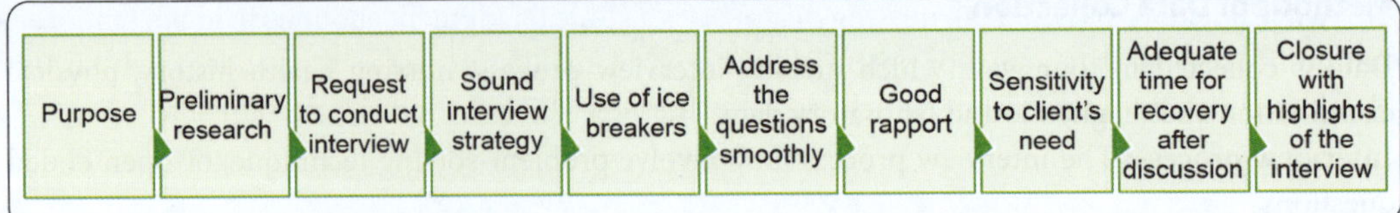

Figure 8.7: Elements of a successful interview

- **Elements of successful interview:** The elements of a successful interview are shown in Figure 8.7.
- **Techniques of data collection in an interview**
    - **Open ended questions:** These allow the client with maximum freedom to respond in his/her own way. For example: How do you feel?
    - **Hypothetical questions:** These types of questions pose a situation and ask the client how it might be handled. For example: What would you do if you feel lethargic?
    - **Reflecting or mirroring responses:** These are useful techniques in getting underlying meanings that might not be verbalized clearly. For example: You feel angry about having to use the nebulizer.
    - **Focusing:** This technique shows the client that you are attending to what is being said and consists of eye contact, body posture and verbal responses. For example: Tell me more about that.
    - **Giving broad openings:** This technique encourages the client to take the initiative about what is to be talked about. For example: Where would you like to begin?
    - **Offering general leads:** It encourages the client to continue.
    - **Exploring:** This technique pursues a topic in more detail. For example: Would you describe it completely?
    - **Verbalizing the implied:** This expresses what has been suggested? For example, if an interviewer mentions that taking a certain drug is no longer beneficial, a nurse might respond by acknowledging the concern that the drug doesn't seem to be making a difference for the person.
    - **Encouraging evaluation:** It helps the client to consider the quality of his own experience. For example: How does that seem to you?
- **What not to use in an interview?**
    - Close ended questions
    - Leading questions
    - Probing questions
    - Agreeing/disagreeing
- **Problems related to data collection:**
    - Inappropriate organization of the data base
    - Omission of pertinent data
    - Inclusion of irrelevant data
    - Failure to establish rapport and partnership
    - Recording an interpretation of data
    - Failure to update the database

Nursing Diagnosis

Definitions: As per Gebbie, Levin 1975, nursing diagnosis is the judgment or conclusion that occurs as a result of nursing assessment.

According to NANDA 1990, nursing diagnosis is a clinical judgment about individual, family or community responses to actual or potential health problems/life processes. It provides the basis for selection of nursing interventions to achieve outcomes for which the nurse is accountable.

Nursing diagnosis is:

- A statement of a client's potential or actual health problems resulting from analysis of data.
- A statement of client's potential or actual alteration in the health status.
- A problem statement that the nurse makes regarding a client condition which he/she uses to communicate professionally.
- A term used to classify health problems within the domain of nursing. Diagnosis means "to know" or "to distinguish".
- Diagnosing = Data analysis + Problem identification + Formulation of nursing diagnosis.

Purposes of Nursing Diagnosis

- To identify healthcare needs.
- To analyze assessment information and derive meaning from this analysis.
- To provide direction for nursing care plan.
- To identify how an individual, group, or community responses to actual or potential health and life process.
- Identify factors that contribute to or cause healths problems.
- Identify resources or strengths the individual, group or community can draw on to prevent or resolve a problem.

Importance

- Nursing diagnosis provides nurses with a common frame of reference and standardizes language that improves communication among nurses, helps organize research and is useful in educating new practitioners.
- Nursing diagnosis provides a classification system to describe the scientific foundation of nursing practices.
- Nursing diagnosis provides nomenclature for the reimbursement of nursing activities.

Steps of Nursing Diagnosis

The diagnostic process includes the decision-making steps and the nurse uses these steps to develop a diagnostic statement.

1. **Data clustering:** Data gathered in an interview, in physical examination and from other records, are organized and recorded in a concise systematic way and clustered into similar categories.
   - Cluster is a set of signs and symptoms that are grouped together in a logical order.
   - Clustering of data helps to focus on identification of the correct problem.
2. **Reviewing and validating findings:** Validation is an ongoing process that occurs during the data collection phase and on its completion when the data is reviewed and compared. Validation is important particularly when the data is conflicting and when the source of data is not reliable. Data that is grossly abnormal is rechecked. Objective and subjective data are compared for congruencies and inconsistencies.
3. **Interpretation of data:** The analysis involves recognizing patterns and trends, comparing these patterns with normal health patterns, and drawing conclusions about the client's response.

When a relationship among these patterns is identified, a list of client centered problems or needs begin to emerge. When looking for a pattern or trend, the nurse examines clusters of data that are a set of signs or symptoms grouped together in a logical order.

4. **Identification of client's needs:** Before formulating the nursing diagnosis, the nurse identifies the client's general health, needs or problems. To identify the client's needs, the nurse first determines what the client's health problems are and whether they are actual or potential problems.

- **An actual health problem:** It is one that is perceived or experienced by the client. For example, sleep pattern disturbance related to noisy environment.
- **A potential health problem:** It is one for which the client is at risk. For example, an overweight smoker at risk for in effective airway clearance related to incisional pain.

This step brings the nurse close to forming nursing diagnosis and making general analysis of clustered data.

5. **Formulation of nursing diagnosis:** Once clusters of data, containing defined characteristics are sorted, client's needs or problems are identified, the nurse is ready to formulate nursing diagnosis. Nursing diagnosis is based on the identification of client's needs.

The actual diagnosis is a statement of conclusion. It should be concise, precise and highly personalized to apply to the individual client. The diagnostic label should include the problem and its etiology.

NANDA has identified four types of nursing diagnoses:

1. Actual nursing diagnosis (describes human response to health conditions)
2. Risk nursing diagnosis (refers to human responses to health conditions)
3. Wellness nursing diagnosis (focuses more on opportunities than needs)
4. Resolved diagnosis (no longer requires intervention)

Another author has given following steps involved in formulating nursing diagnosis; these are:

1. **Problem sensing:** Rule out process
2. **Synthesizing the data:** Evaluating hypothesis
3. **List the client's needs:** Re-evaluate the problems list

Potential Errors in Choosing a Nursing Diagnosis

- Overlooking cues
- Making a diagnosis with an insufficient database
- Stereotyping

Characteristics of Nursing Diagnosis

- It states a clear and concise health problem.
- It is derived from existing evidences about the client.
- It is potentially amenable to nursing therapy.
- It is the basis for planning and carrying out nursing care.

Types of nursing diagnoses: Types of the nursing diagnoses with examples are tabulated in Table 8.1.

Steps in nursing diagnosis formulation: The steps of formulating nursing diagnosis are shown in Figure 8.8.

Mnemonics

Components of nursing diagnosis
The components of nursing diagnosis can be remembered with mnemonic **PES.**
- **P:** Problem statement
- **E:** Etiology/causes
- **S:** Defining characteristics/Signs/ Symptoms

TABLE 8.1:	Types of nursing diagnoses with examples
Type of nursing diagnoses	**Examples**
Actual nursing diagnosis	Imbalanced nutrition related to nausea, disturbed sleep pattern related to cough and pain
Potential nursing diagnosis	Possible nutrition deficit leads to possible low self-esteem (related to job)
Risk nursing diagnosis	Risk for impaired skin integrity related to decreased peripheral circulation, risk for infection related to compromised immune system
Wellness diagnosis	Appropriate family coping
Syndrome (nursing) diagnosis	Rape, trauma syndrome, post trauma syndrome

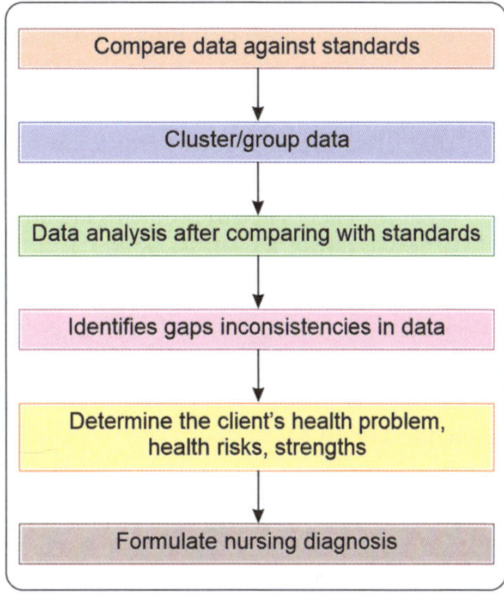

Figure 8.8: Steps in formulation of nursing diagnosis

Must Know

Tri Focal model for client assessment [Kelly, Frisch, Avant 1995]

Illness	Risk of Illness	Wellness
Actual nursing diagnosis	Risk nursing diagnosis	Wellness nursing diagnosis

Nursing Diagnosis Guidelines

- Phrase the nursing diagnosis as a patient problem or alteration in health's state rather than as a patient need.
- Patient's problem must precede the etiology and that the two are linked by the phrase "related to".
- Defining characteristics when included in the nursing diagnosis, should follow the etiology and be linked by the phrase "as manifested by" or "as evidenced by."
- Write in legally advisable terms
- Use non judgmental language
- Avoid using medical diagnosis
- Problem statement indicates what is unhealthy about the patient

Planning

Once the etiology, signs and symptoms previously identified are incorporated into a client's diagnostic statement, nurse can proceed to the planning step of the nursing process. Here, the focus is on determining the most appropriate actions to effectively address the patient's problems or needs.

The nurse begins to set priorities, establishes goals, identifies desired outcomes and determines specific nursing interventions. These actions are documented as a plan of care. It is a priority that the client and significant others be included in the planning process so that they may participate and take responsibility for their care.

Process of Nursing Planning

Setting Priorities for Client Care

The starting point for planning care is to rank the patient's problems or needs, so that the nurse's attention and subsequent actions are properly focused. The process helps a nurse attend to the client's most important needs and it assists the nurse in organizing ongoing care. Although there are many ways of prioritizing client's needs, a useful framework is developed by Abraham Maslow as shown in Figure 8.9.

Maslow's hierarchy

According to Maslow, physiological needs are generally considered baseline survival needs because they must be met in order, for life to continue.

This hierarchy can help nurse to identify and prioritize client's needs more and to plan desired outcomes and the associated nursing interventions. After determination of priority of care, the client care needs can also be ranked according to a system that can help in identifying basic to higher level actions/interventions. By ranking the client's needs, nurse can proceed in a logical way to facilitate his/her client's recovery.

Kalish's expanded hierarchy

Richard Kalish (1983) expanded and further subdivided the structure of Maslow's hierarchy as shown in Figure 8.10.

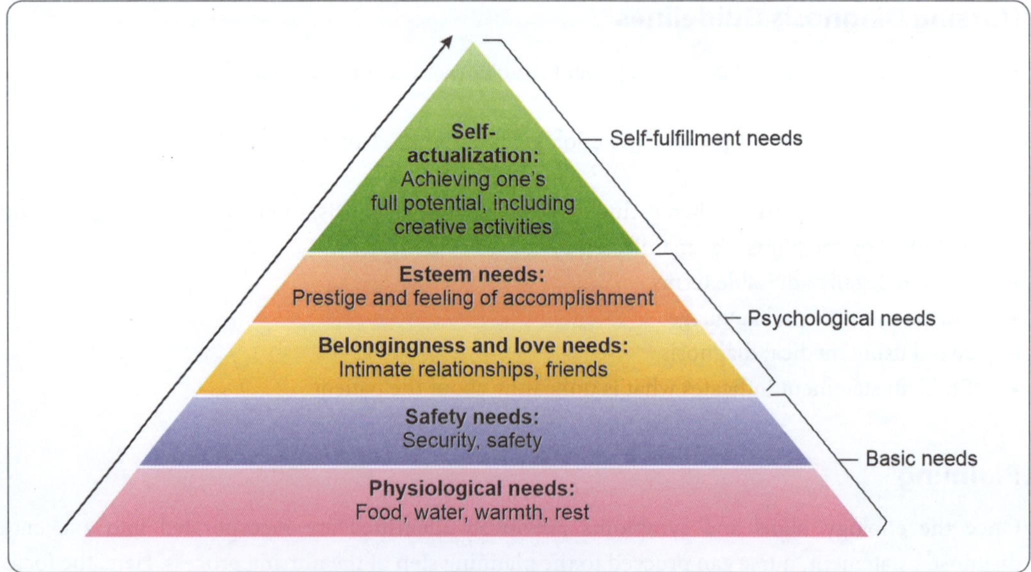

Figure 8.9: Maslow's hierarchy of needs

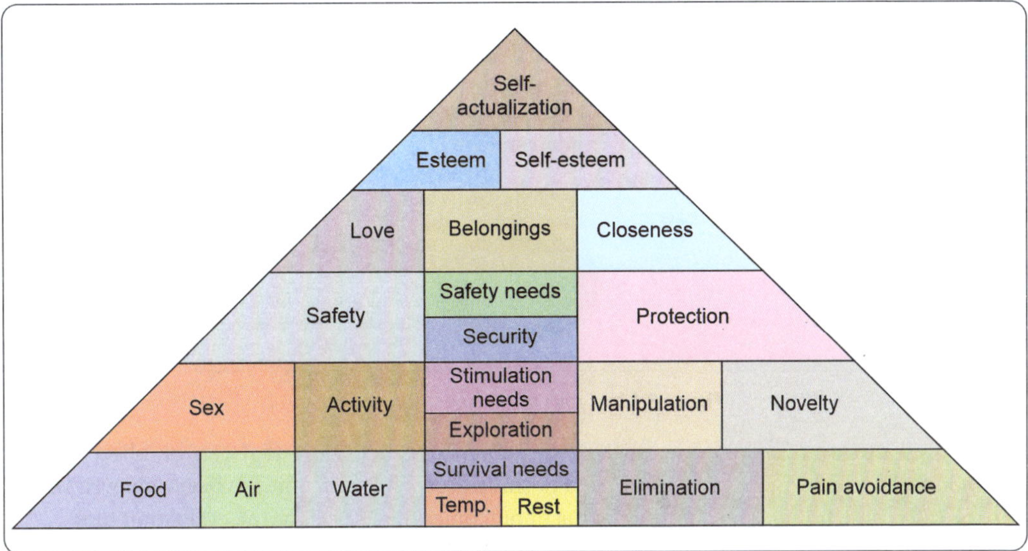

Figure 8.10: Kalish (1983) expanded structure of hierarchy

Establishing Goals and Expected Outcomes

Goals are broad guidelines indicating the overall direction of movement as a result of the intervention of the healthcare team.

Goals are specific statements of client's behavior or physiological response that a nurse sets to achieve as a problem resolution. The goals and outcomes provide a clear focus for the type of intervention necessary to care of the client.

Goals may either be long-term or short-term:

- **Long-term goals:** These indicate the overall direction or end result of care. For example: "Maintains control of blood glucose level".
- **Short-term goals:** These are more specific guides for care and must usually be met before discharge. Short-term goal may be evaluated within a few hours or over the period of several therapeutic sessions.

Identifying Expected Outcomes

- **Features of outcomes:** Because they must be measurable, outcome statements need to:
  - Be specific
  - Be realistic
  - Consider patient circumstances and desires
  - Indicate a definite time frame
  - Provide measurable evaluation criteria for determining success or failure.
- **Expected outcome:** It is a specific measurable change in a client's status, expected to occur in response to nursing care.
- **Planned outcomes:** These are the desired results of actions taken to achieve the broader goal. They are the measurable steps toward achieving the treatment/discharge criteria that were established earlier.

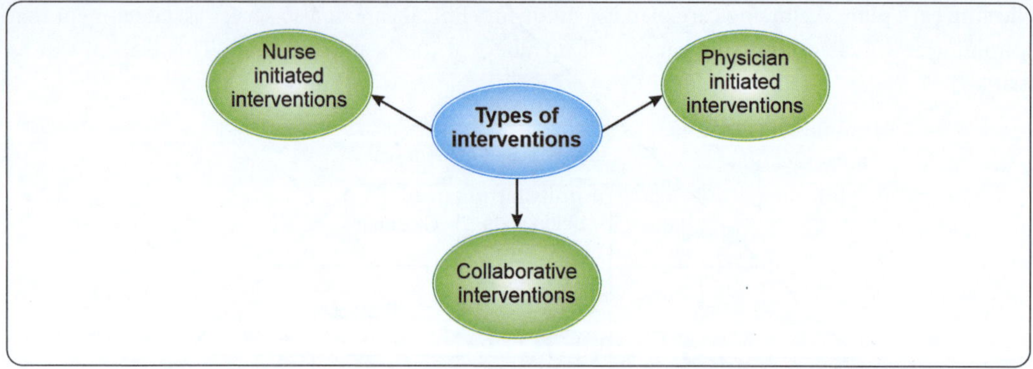

Figure 8.11: Types of nursing interventions

- **Desired outcomes:** These are written by listing items/behaviors that can be observed and monitored to determine whether or not a positive/acceptable outcome has been achieved within the rated time frame. The itemized listing of outcomes then serves as the evaluation tool.

Selecting Appropriate Nursing Interventions

Nursing interventions as shown in Figure 8.11, are prescriptions for behaviors, treatments, activities or actions that assist the client in achieving the expected outcome. The Nursing Interventions Classification (NIC) contains a list of 486 intervention labels such as infant care, organ procurement, mood, products, administration, and code management. Nursing interventions relate directly to all parts of the nursing diagnosis and are therapeutically effective and safe.

Factors that help in choosing intervention: When choosing intervention, a nurse keeps in mind the following important factors:

- Characteristics of nursing diagnosis
- Expected outcomes
- Research base for the interventions
- Feasibility of the interventions
- Acceptability of the client
- Competencies of the nurse

- Nursing standards and agency's policy must also be considered while selecting specific intervention.

The interventions must be deliberate and purposeful, they must include information on independent nursing activities, as well as any collaborative activities necessary for the nurse to carry-out orders from other healthcare providers.

Necessities of an intervention plan of care: The following items must be included when one is creating and documenting the intervention in the client's plan of care.

- The data when the intervention is written
- Activity to be performed
- Qualifiers of how, when, where and amount
- Signature or initials of originating nurse

Plan of Care

Planning care can save valuable time when the goals of care, client outcomes and nursing interventions to achieve them are clearly identified and then recorded. The documentation of the planning process is provided in the client's plan.

Nursing care plan: A nursing care plan is a guide for clinical care. It also serves as a document that communicates a client's nursing care to all members of the healthcare team. This plan of care is written to:

- Provide continuity of care
- Enhance communication
- Assist with determination of agency or unit staffing needs
- Document the nursing process
- Serve as a teaching tool
- Coordinate provision of care among disciplines.

> **Must Know**
>
> The term healthcare is not synonymous with medicine or nursing but includes many professional disciplines, each of these has its own definite characteristic and independent but overlapping functions. The fields of nursing and medicine are closely related. The relationship includes the exchange of data, the sharing of ideas and the development of a plan of care. The plan of care may be recorded on a single page or in a multiple page format.

Review the plan of care: Before the plan of care is implemented, it should be reviewed to ensure that:

- It is based on accepted nursing practice, reflecting knowledge of scientific principles, nursing standards of care and agency policies.
- It provides for the safety of the client.
- The client diagnostic statements are supported by the client data.
- It demonstrates individualized client care.

Types of Nursing Care Plans

In nursing, care plans are essential tools that outline the individualized care or treatment that a patient needs. Here are some common types of care plans:

- **Initial nursing assessment care plan:** Created based on the initial assessment of the patient's health status, identifying immediate needs and priorities.
- **Comprehensive care plan:** Provides a detailed outline of the patient's overall care needs, including medical, nursing, and other healthcare disciplines involved.
- **Long-term care plan:** Focuses on ongoing care needs for patients with chronic illnesses or long-term health conditions, outlining interventions and goals over an extended period.
- **Discharge care plan:** Developed to ensure a smooth transition from hospital or healthcare facility to home or another setting, addressing follow-up care, medications, and patient education.
- **Critical care plan:** Specifically tailored for patients in critical or intensive care settings, focusing on immediate interventions, monitoring, and management of complex conditions.
- **Palliative care plan:** Emphasizes comfort and quality of life for patients with serious illnesses, addressing pain management, emotional support, and end-of-life care preferences.
- **Rehabilitation care plan:** Designed for patients recovering from injuries, surgeries, or debilitating conditions, outlining therapies, exercises, and goals for restoring function and independence.

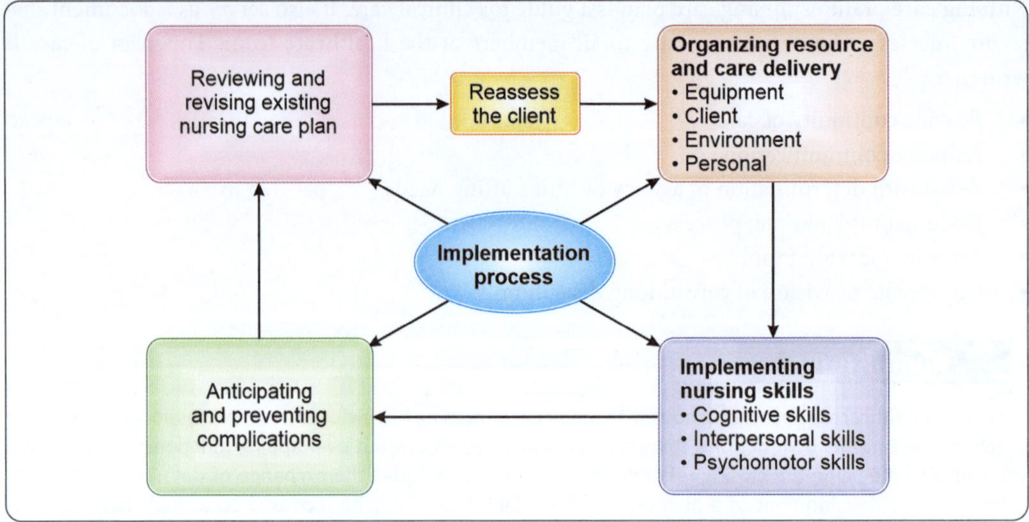

Figure 8.12: Process of implementation phase

Implementation

Implementation is the step of the nursing process where nurse provides care to patient. The nurse initiates and completes the nursing actions and interventions necessary for achieving the goals and expected outcomes of the nursing care.

Process

Preparation for implementation ensures efficient, safe and effective nursing care. Implementation is a continuous process that interacts with all steps of the nursing process. For the implementation to be effective, the nurse must be knowledgeable about the implementation process, implementation skills and specific direct and indirect care interventions as shown in Figure 8.12.

Legal and ethical concerns related to the interventions also need to be considered. Interventions may be composed of many activities ranging from simple task to complex procedure. These activities may require direct care or they may merely require the assistance of healthcare provider to the client.

Types of Interventions to be Implemented

Direct care: Direct care interventions are treatments and performed interactions with the client (Fig. 8.13). All direct care measures require competent and safe practice. This ensures an individualized approach (medication, counseling).

Indirect care: These interventions are performed away from client but on behalf of the client or group of clients (Fig. 8.14). These are measures/actions that support the effectiveness of direct care interventions. For example, managing client's environment, documentation, etc.

Evaluation

Evaluation is the final step of the nursing process. Evaluation is crucial after application of the nursing process, to determine the client's condition or well-being improvement. It is an ongoing process during the care process.

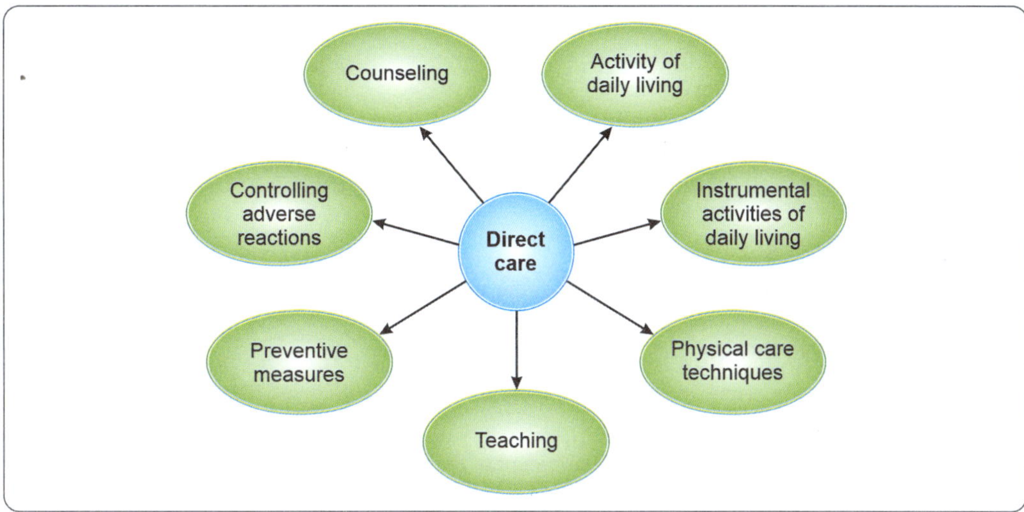

Figure 8.13: Measures of direct care

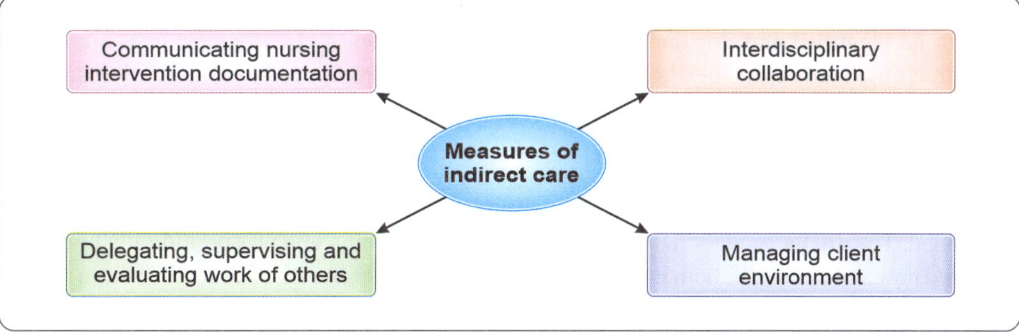

Figure 8.14: Measures of indirect care

This phase of the nursing process is used for making clinical judgment. Evaluation which is an ongoing process is necessary for determining how well the plan of care is working. It is an interactive continuous process.

Components of Evaluation

Evaluation step has three main components:

1. Reassessment
2. Modification of the plan of care
3. Termination of services; Termination includes completion of discharge planning.

Reassessment

Reassessment is a constant "measuring and monitoring" of the client's status. The evaluation process is ongoing, it does not occur only when an outcome is to be reviewed or a determination of the client's readiness for discharge is to be made.

Evaluation of the data determines:

- The appropriateness of the nursing actions.
- The need to revise the interventions.
- The development of new client needs.
- The need for referral to other resources.
- The need to rearrange priorities to meet the changing demands of care.

Nursing Considerations

While evaluating the patient's response to care, the nurse should note progress toward the specified outcomes.

Outcomes may be evaluated by:
- Direct observation
- Interview
- Review of records

An important aspect of this process is the involvement of the client.

Modification of the Plan of Care

At this step, a change in treatment approach is indicated and the plan of care must be modified to reflect these changes. When the desired outcomes are evaluated and found to be unmet, the reasons need to be identified and documented, the outcomes are then revised or new ones are written. When revising client's outcomes, keep in mind that they may simply need to be restated or their time frames lengthened so that the client can successfully achieve them.

Termination of Services

When the desired outcomes have been achieved and the broader goals are met, termination of care is planned. The discharge plan that began at the time of admission and was periodically updated, is finalized now and put into action. It must be verified that the client or significant others have received written and verbal instructions regarding treatments, medications and activities to be followed when referred to home.

Components of Evaluation Process

The evaluation process can also be more broadly applied at an institutional level to measure the overall quality of care. The evaluation level step needs to be viewed positively as an opportunity for growth for both individual and the profession as a whole.

Evaluation process (Fig. 8.15) which determines the effectiveness of nursing includes:

- Identifying evaluative criteria and standards.
- Collecting data to determine whether the criteria/standards are met.
- Interpreting and summarizing findings.
- Documenting findings and any clinical judgments.
- Terminating, continuing or revising the care plan.

Types of Evaluation

Types of evaluation in the nursing process include:

- **Formative evaluation:** Ongoing assessment and feedback during the care process to monitor progress and make adjustments as needed.

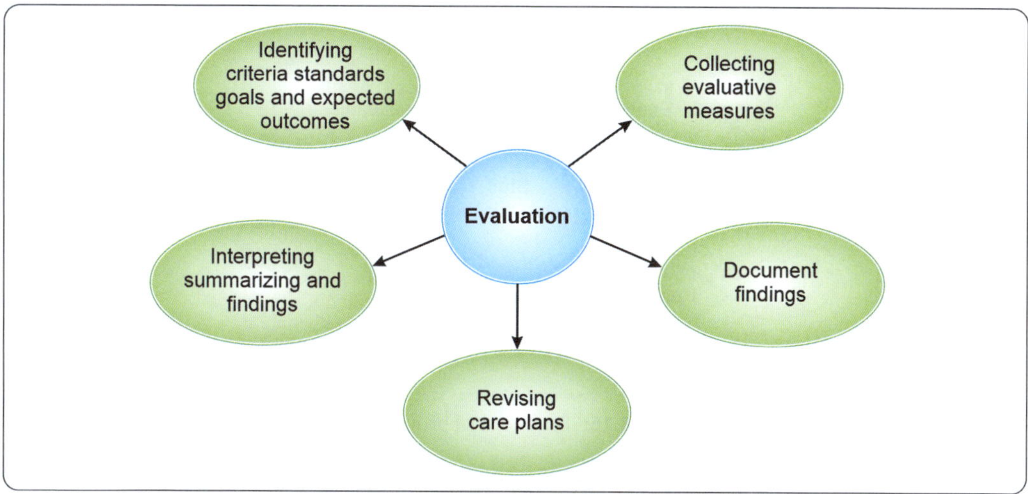

Figure 8.15: Components of evaluation process

- **Summative evaluation:** Assessing the outcomes of care interventions at the end of a specific period to determine their effectiveness.
- **Process evaluation:** Examining the steps and procedures followed during care delivery to ensure they align with standards and best practices.
- **Outcome evaluation:** Assessing the achievement of desired patient outcomes and goals to determine the overall success of the care provided.

DOCUMENTATION OF NURSING PROCESS

Documentation is not only a requirement for accreditation, it is also a legal requirement in any healthcare setting. Documentation provides a record of the use of the nursing process for the delivery of individualized client care.

The initial assessment is recorded in the client's history or database. The identification of client's needs and the planning of client care are recorded in the plan of care.

The implementation of the plan is recorded in the progress notes. The evaluation of care may be documented in the progress notes and plan of care.

Goals of Documentation

The goals of documentation are to:
- Facilitate the delivery of quality client care.
- Ensure documentation of progress.
- Facilitate interdisciplinary consistency and the communication of treatment goals and progress.

Types of Documentations

Progress Notes

These are an integral part of the overall medical record and should include all significant events that occur during the client's hospitalization (treatment program). The notes should be written in a clear

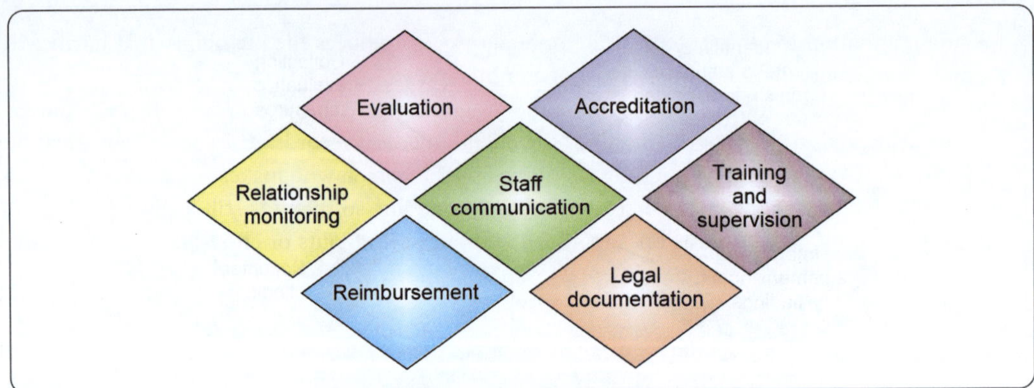

Figure 8.16: Functions of progress note

and objective fashion or in a manner that reflects progress toward desired measurable outcomes with the use of planned staff interventions.

Functions of Progress Notes

The functions of progress notes are shown in Figure 8.16.

Staff communication: Colleague to colleague communication is the most obvious function of the progress notes. Nursing staff members are in the unique position of being in contact with the client for extended periods and in a variety of situations.

Evaluation: To periodically review the client's progress and the effectiveness of the treatment plan performed by the nurse or the team. An evaluation of the client's progress may be documented on the plan of care or in the progress notes. For the purpose of review, the medical record should be written to facilitate an assessment of the care given to the client. The records serve as a method of tracking the client's response to treatment and as a means for evaluating the quality of care provided.

Relationship monitoring: The nurse/client relationship is the tool used by the nurse to help the client make the most of his/her own abilities. Monitoring the client's relationship is essential along with notes detailing the observations of these relationships.

The client's relationship with significant others can have an impact on general well-being progress toward recovery, independence in self-care and a successful transition to the home setting. So, observation and monitoring of interactions are useful components of nursing care.

Reimbursement: Third-party payers are insistent about why, when, where, how, what and who of the services, to be documented.

An absence of such documentation may result in termination of funding for an individual client and therefore termination of treatment. The record is a primary site for maintaining information about the client's treatment and associated revenues as it provides proof of services. Therefore, progress notes must document any significant observations about what is happening to the client during illness, treatment and recovery. Data about medications, details about equipment used and any other pertinent information must be recorded as well.

Legal documentation: Nurses have a legal and moral duty to do no harm to clients. Harm can result from nurse's action or inaction.

- Careful attention to all the steps of the nursing process reduces the possibility that harm will result from errors of omission or errors of commission.
- Both the implementation of interventions and progress toward the measurable outcomes should be documented in the progress notes of the client's medical records. These notations must be specific about date and time and must be signed by the person who makes the entry.
- Errors in the document must be crossed out with one line so that it is still legible. They must be identified by the author as on "error". The initiated white outs or cross outs that make the information unreadable are not acceptable because they could be construed to mean that the individual or facility is trying to alter the facts.

Accreditation: One of the essential requirements for healthcare facilities is maintenance of a medical record. Nursing care data related to patient assessment, nursing diagnosis, nursing intervention and patient outcomes are permanently integrated into the medical record.

Note Writing

Note writing is important for training and supervision purposes. An experienced nurse's description of how a complicated situation was handled, a supervisor's analysis of the problem presented by a new admission and a description of patterns noted in a particular client's response to care are all examples of notes that provide models for the remainder of the staff. Supervisors also gain insight into an employee's abilities by regarding his/her progress notes and may be able to isolate areas in which additional supervision or training/education would be beneficial.

Techniques of Note Writing

Following are the guidelines for writing observation-based notes to compare and contrast the judgmental and descriptive language.

- **Judgmental language:** Judgmental statements include phrases that:
    - Make a reference to undefined periods of time
    - Refer to undefined quantities
    - Refer to unsupported qualities
    - Fail to specify the objective basis for the judgment made.
      Examples are:
      - He is noncooperative today.
      - He asks for pain medication too often.
        Use of these and similar phrases without clarification may leave the statement unclear and judgmental.
- **Descriptive language:** Descriptive language includes observations only and avoids statements that are evaluative or judgmental, unless observational evidence can be presented to back-up the judgment. Descriptive statements contain measurable periods of time and quantity statements, in which nurse notes that the client "seemed" or "appeared" to be exhibiting a certain physical/emotional state which are inferential statements.

Nursing Consideration

Content should be as specific and accurate as possible. It is important to record in the progress notes any information that is of importance to oncoming shifts, as well as observation significant for other healthcare providers. When applying restraints, nurse need to document the exact time the procedure was initiated, whether any injuries resulted and henceforth.

Formats for Documentation

Several charting formats have been used for documentation. These include:

- Block notes (single entry covering entire shift)
- Narrative time notes (particular time, e.g., ate the breakfast at 7 am)
- Problem oriented medical record system (POMR)
- Focus charting: A system format created by nurses for documentation of frequent repetitive care is focus charting. It was designed to encourage looking at the client from a positive rather than a negative perspective by using precise documentation to record the nursing process.
- Documentation of patient care information, communication and reflection of the individualization of care nurse provided.

Benefits of Documentation

- Documentation promotes continuity of patient care among the varied healthcare providers and serves as a basis for evaluation of the care provided.
- The documentation process continuously reinforces accountability and responsibility to implement and evaluate the nursing process.

FURTHER READINGS

- Carpenito L J. Nursing Diagnosis. Lippincott, 8th edition. 2000.
- Potter P, Boxerman S, Wolf L, Marshall J, Grayson D, Sledge J, et al. Mapping the Nursing Process: A New Approach for Understanding the Work of Nursing. J Nurs Adm. 2004;34(2):101-9.

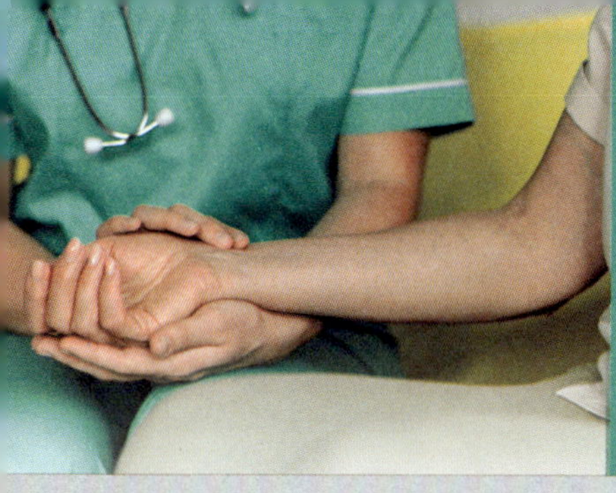

STUDENT ASSIGNMENT

LONG ANSWER QUESTIONS

1. What do you understand by the term nursing process? What are its components? What are the benefits of applying nursing process?
2. What is data collection? Discuss the types of data along with their sources.
3. What is documentation? Explain.

SHORT ANSWER QUESTIONS

1. Define nursing diagnosis.
2. Define progress notes?
3. Write about Maslow's Hierarchy.

MULTIPLE CHOICE QUESTIONS

1. **The systematic problem-solving approach toward providing individualized nursing care is known as ___________________.**
   a. Nursing care plan
   b. Nursing process
   c. Nurses practice act
   d. Nursing method

2. **What purpose does the nursing process serve?**
   a. Assisting family members in making important healthcare decisions.
   b. Providing nurses with a framework to aid them in delivering comprehensive care.
   c. Help other healthcare professionals know what is going on with the client.
   d. Organize information so the doctor knows what is wrong with the client.

3. **Once a nurse assesses a client's condition and identifies appropriate nursing diagnoses:**
   a. A plan is developed for nursing care.
   b. Physical assessment begins.
   c. List of priorities is determined.
   d. Review of the assessment is conducted with other team members.

4. **Planning is a category of nursing behavior in which:**
   a. The nurse determines the healthcare needed for the client.
   b. The physician determines the plan of care for the client.
   c. Client-centered goals and expected outcomes are established.
   d. The client determines the care needed.

5. **As goals, outcomes, and interventions are developed, the nurse must:**
   a. Be in charge of all care and planning for the client.
   b. Be aware of and committed to accepted standards of practice from nursing and other disciples.
   c. Not change the plan of care for the client.
   d. Be in control of all interventions for the client.

6. **When establishing realistic goals, the nurse:**
   a. Bases the goals on the nurse's personal knowledge.
   b. Knows the resources of the healthcare facility, family, and the client.
   c. Must have a client who is physically and emotionally stable.
   d. Must have the client's cooperation.

7. **To initiate an intervention the nurse must be competent in three areas, which include:**
   a. Knowledge, function, and specific skills.
   b. Experience, advanced education, and skills.
   c. Skills, finances, and leadership.
   d. Leadership, autonomy, and skills.

8. **A client-centered goal is a specific and measurable behavior or response that reflects a client's:**
   a. Highest possible level of wellness and independence in function.
   b. Response when compared to another client with a same problem.
   c. Physician's goal for the specific client.
   d. Desire for specific healthcare interventions.

ANSWER KEY

1. b   **2.** b   **3.** a   **4.** c   **5.** b   **6.** b   **7.** a   **8.** a

9

Quality Assurance in Nursing

LEARNING OBJECTIVES

After the completion of the chapter, the readers will be able to:
- Discuss quality assurance in nursing.
- Know nursing standards and nursing audit.
- Describe total quality management.

CHAPTER OUTLINE

- Quality Assurance
- Role of a Nurse in Developing Quality Nursing Care
- Nursing Standards
- Five Nursing Standards
- Standard Statements for Prevention of Infection
- Nursing Audit
- Total Quality Management

KEY TERMS

Approach: A way to deal with a problem or a situation, etc.

Assurance: A promise that something will certainly happen.

Criteria: The standard that you use when you decide or form an opinion about somebody/something.

Performance: The way a person performs.

QUALITY ASSURANCE

Definitions

Quality assurance is defined as follows:

- Quality is defined as the extent of resemblance between the purpose of healthcare and truly granted care.   **—Donabedian, 1986**
- Quality assurance is a program adopted by an institution that is designed to promote the best possible care.   **—DeLoughery**
- Quality assurance is the process of achieving excellence in the service rendered to every client.
- Quality assurance is defining of nursing practice through well written nursing standards and the use of those standards as a basis for evaluation on improvement of client care.   **—Maker, 1998**
- Quality assurance is defined as a process designed to monitor objectively and systematically, and evaluate the quality and appropriateness of patient care, pursue the opportunities to improve patient care and resolve identified problems.   **—Joint commission, 1971**
- Quality assurance originated in manufacturing industry. The idea was "to ensure that the product consistently achieved customer satisfaction".
- Quality assurance is a dynamic process through which nurses assume accountability for quality of care they provide. It is a guarantee to the society that services provided by nurses are being regulated by members of profession.

Objectives

The objectives of quality assurance are as follows:

- To ensure the delivery of quality client care.
- To demonstrate the efforts of the healthcare providers.
- To provide technical assistance in correcting systemic deficiencies.
- To refine existing methods for ensuring optional quality healthcare.
- To provide the best possible results.

Principles

Quality assurance:
- Is oriented towards meeting the needs and expectations of clients
- Focuses on systems and processes
- Uses data to analyze service delivery
- Encourages the use of teams in problem solving and quality improvement
- Uses effective communication to improve service delivery.

Components

There are four essential components of quality assurance:

1. Setting program objectives
2. Promoting quality
3. Activity monitoring quality control
   - Quality supervision

4. Performance assessment quality review
    - Quality evaluation
    - Quality approval

Approaches

The two approaches of quality assurance are as follows:

1. General approach:
    - Credentialing
    - Licensure
    - Accreditation
    - Certification
2. Specific approach:
    - Peer review
    - Utilization review
    - Evaluation study
    - Audit
    - Client satisfaction
    - Incident review
    - Standards

General Approach

It involves a large governing official body's evaluation of a person's or agency's ability to meet established criteria or standards at a given time.

Credentialing

Credentialing is a formal recognition of professional or technical competence and attainment of minimum standards by a person or agency.

Functional Components

Credentialing process has four functional components which are as follows:

1. To produce a quality product
2. To confer a unique identity
3. To protect provider and public
4. To control the profession

Principles of Credentialing

The principles of credentialing are as follows:

- Credentialing benefits both the credentialed individuals and the public.
- The legitimate interests of the involved occupation or institution and of the general public should be reflected in each credentialing mechanism.
- Accountability should be an essential component of any credentialing process.
- A system of checks and balances within the credentialing system assures equitable treatment for all parties involved.
- Periodic assessments with the potential for sanction are essential components of an effective credentialing mechanism.
- Standard objectives, set criteria and person's competencies are essential for the credentialing process.
- Professional identity and responsibility should evolve from the credentialing process.
- Coordination of credentialing mechanisms should lead to efficiency and cost-effectiveness and avoid duplication.

Licensure

Individual licensure is a contract between the profession and the state in which the profession is granted control over entry and exit from the profession and control over the quality of professional practice. Licensures of nurses have been mandates by law since 1903.

Accreditation

Accreditation is the establishment of the status, legitimacy or appropriateness of an institution program or module of study. Accreditation is usually for a limited duration at which time reaccreditation procedures come into operation. Accreditation process is primarily evaluated based on agency's physical structure, organizational structure and personal qualifications.

Certification

Certification is usually a voluntary process within the profession. Personal educational achievements, experiences and performances in examinations are used to determine the person's qualifications for functioning in an identified specialty area.

Specific Approach

Peer Review

To maintain high standards, peer review has been initiated to carefully review the quality of practice demonstrated by members of a professional group. Peer review is divided into:
- Recipients of health services
- Health professionals

Utilization Review

Utilization review activities are directed toward assuring that care is actually needed and that the cost appropriate for the level of care is provided. Three types of utilization reviews are:
1. **Prospective:** It is an assessment of the necessity of care before giving service.
2. **Concurrent:** A review of necessity of care while the care is being given.
3. **Retrospective:** A review of necessity of care after the care has been given.

Evaluation Studies

Three models have been used to evaluate quality. These are:
1. **Donabedian's structure process model:** It includes:
   - Structural evaluation
   - Outcome evaluation
   - Process evaluation
2. **The tracer method:** This is a measure of both process and outcome of care. This method provides nurses with data to show the differences in outcomes as a result of nursing care standards.
3. **The sentinel method:** It is an outcome measure for examining specific instances of client care.

Audit

Audit is a detailed review and evaluation of selected clinical records in order to evaluate the quality of nursing care performance by comparing it with accepted standards.

Client Satisfaction

Client satisfaction can be assessed using in-person or telephonic interviews, and mailed questionnaire. Data from client satisfaction surveys are used to measure structure, process and outcome of care given.

Incident Review

During a patient's hospitalization, several incidents may occur which have a bearing on the treatment and patient's final recovery. The critical incidents may be:

- Delayed attendance
- Incorrect medications
- Lack of cleanliness
- Lack of asepsis

Standards

Standards are the predetermined baseline conditions or levels of excellence that comprise a model to be followed and practiced or used to do a service.

For example, The American Nurses Association Standards of Practice include:

Standard 1: Data collection

Standard 2: Nursing diagnosis

Standard 3: Goals

Standard 4: Priorities and prescribed nursing approach

Standard 5: Nursing action (health maintenance)

Standard 6: Nursing action (maximize health capabilities)

Standard 7: Evaluation

Factors Affecting Quality Assurance in Nursing Care

A list of various factors affecting the quality assurance are as follows:

- **Lack of resources:** Insufficient resources, infrastructure, equipment, money for recurring expenses and staff, make it impossible for output of a certain quality.
- **Personnel problem:** Lack of trained, skilled and motivated employees, disciplined staff, etc. affects the quality of care.
- **Unreasonable patients and attendants:** Illness, anxiety, absence of immediate response to treatment, unreasonable and noncooperative attitude which in turn affects the quality care.
- **Improper maintenance:** Building as well as equipment require proper maintenance for efficient use. Bad quality of equipment will definitely hamper the quality of care.
- **Absence of well-informed population:** To improve quality nursing care, it is necessary that the people become knowledgeable and assert their rights to quality care.
- **Absence of accreditation laws:** There is no organization which is strictly empowered with legislation to lay down standards for nursing and medical care so as to regulate the quality of care.
- **Basic requirements in a hospital are not met:** Enquire into major incidents of negligence and act against health professionals involved in malpractices.
- **Lack of incident review procedures:** During a patient's hospitalization, several incidents may occur which have a bearing on the treatment and the patient's final recovery.

- **Delayed attendance by physician/nurse:** Incorrect medication, burns arising out of faulty procedures, death in a corridor with no nurse/physician accompanying the patient care.
- **Lack of good hospital information system:** A good management information system is essential for the appraisal of quality care.
- **Absence of conducting patient satisfaction surveys:** Surveys must be carried out through questionnaires, interviews, etc. by social worker, hospital management trainees and consultant groups.
- **Lack of nursing care records:** Nurses should use the problem-oriented record system or use nursing process while recording the care given.
- **Miscellaneous:** Lack of good supervision, absence of knowledge about the philosophy of nursing care, lack of policy and administrative manual, lack of procedure manual, substandard education and training, inadequate quality and number of professionals, lack of evaluation techniques, lack of coordination between and within departments, lack of written job descriptions and job specifications, lack of in-service and continuing educational programs.

ROLE OF A NURSE IN DEVELOPING QUALITY NURSING CARE

A nursing administrator has to develop a formalized quality program, which includes:
- Reviewing organizational and personal environment.
- Focusing on standards of nursing care and methods of delivering nursing care.
- Focusing on the outcome of nursing care.

NURSING STANDARDS

Definition: Standard is a statement of expected level of quality.

Professional standards describe the competent level of care in each phase of the nursing process. They reflect a desired and achievable level of performance against which a nurse's actual performance can be compared. The main purpose of professional standards is to direct and maintain safe and clinically competent nursing practice. Professional standards assist us, our management team, and our healthcare organization to develop safe staffing practices, delegate tasks to licensed and unlicensed personnel, ensure adequate documentation, and even create policies for new technology such as social media.

Definitions of Nursing Standards

Various definitions of nursing standards are as follows:
- Standards are professionally developed expressions of the range of acceptable variations from a norm or criterion.
  —**Avedis Donabedian**
- It means the minimal professional practice expectations for any registered nurse in any setting or role, approved by nursing council.
- Benchmark of achievement which is based on a desired level of excellence.
- A desired and achievable level of performance against which actual performance can be compared.
- A statement, reached through consensus, which clearly identifies the desired outcome.

Purposes of Nursing Standards

The purposes of nursing standards are as follows:

- To promote, guide, direct and regulate professional nursing practice.
- To set out the legal and professional basis for nursing practice.
- To describe the desirable and achievable level of performance.
- To serve as a guide to the professional knowledge, skill, and judgment needed to practice nursing safely.

Functions of Nursing Standards

Standards are always applied to all registered nurses in Registered Nurse practice roles, including nurse practitioners. Standards range from the unwritten but inherent requirements of a profession, to these broad profession-wide standards established by the college, and onto detailed standards for client care. As standards progress from profession-wide expectations to specific levels of nursing care, the focus changes accordingly. Standards are measured by clients, employers, colleagues, themselves and others.

The standards:

- Provide guidance to assist registered nurses in decision-making and self-assessment as part of continuing competence.
- Are the foundation for the development of specific standards to various contexts of practice.
- May be used in conjunction with other resources to guide nursing practice.
- May be used to develop position descriptions, and performance appraisal and quality improvement tools.
- Support registered nurses by outlining practice expectations of the profession.
- Inform the public and others about what they can expect from practicing registered nurses.
- Reflect the values of the nursing profession.
- Clarify what the profession expects of nurses.
- Represent the criteria against which nurse practice.

Principles of Nursing Standards

The principles of nursing standards are as follows:

- The standards apply at all times to all registered nurses in practice roles.
- They provide guidance to assist registered nurses in decision-making and self-assessment as part of continuing competence.
- Standards are the foundation for the development of standards specific to various contexts of practice.
- Standards may be used to develop position descriptions, and performance appraisal and quality improvement tools.
- Standards support registered nurses by outlining practice expectations of the profession.
- Standards inform the public and others about what they can expect from practicing registered nurses.
- Standards are used as a legal reference for reasonable and prudent practice.

Importance of Nursing Standards

The importance of nursing standards are as follows:

- They promote and guide clinical practice.
- They provide an evaluation tool for nurses and their colleagues to ensure clinical proficiency and safety.
- They are used to provide a framework for developing clinical competency checklists.
- They are used as a comparison tool to evaluate care provided by nurse.
- They ensure that nurses are accountable for clinical decisions and actions, and for maintaining competence during career.
- They encourage nurses to persistently enhance knowledge base through experience, continuing education, and the latest guidelines.
- They utilize professional standards to identify areas for improvement in clinical practice and work areas, as well as to improve patient and workplace safety.

Approaches of Nursing Standards

There are various approaches that can be used to develop and implement the standards. The most common approaches are mentioned in Table 9.1.

- **Structure:** This approach involves the setup of the organization, philosophy, goals and objectives, structure of the organization, facilities, equipment and qualification of employees.
- **Process:** The process approach involves the activities concerned with the delivery of patient care. They measure nursing interventions or their shortcomings.
- **Outcome:** The outcome approach reflects the effectiveness and the results rather than the process of giving care.

Characteristics of Nursing Standards

Standards are directed toward an ideal which are:

- Based on current knowledge
- Realistic
- Made in positive terms
- Attainable
- Measurable
- Acceptable
- Expertise
- Understandable

Areas of Application of Nursing Standards

The nursing standards are applied in the following areas:

- Nursing education
- Administration
- Research
- Nursing practice

TABLE 9.1: Approaches of nursing standards			
Parameters	**Structure**	**Process**	**Outcome**
Resource	Need	Work	Achievement
Evaluation of	Physical environment, building policies, rules and regulations, staff, equipment schedules	Assessment techniques procedures nursing care, patient education, documentation	Recovery rate, mortality rate, patient's satisfaction, behavior, knowledge, self-care

Types of Nursing Standards

There are two types of standards mentioned below:

1. **Standard of practice:** It is an authoritative statement that describes assessment, diagnosis, planning, implementation and evaluation. These standards emphasize the nurse's practice in caring for the client.
2. **Standards of professional performance:** It describes a competent level of behavior in the professional role, including activities related to quality of care, performance appraisal, education, collegiality ethics, collaboration and research.

Uses of Nursing Standards

For nurses:

- To understand their professional obligations.
- To support their own continuing competence and professional development.
- To explain what nursing is and what nurses do.
- To advocate for changes to policies and practices.
- To define and to resolve professional practice problems.
- To include in nursing education courses/programs.

For society: To understand the expectations of professional nursing practice.

For employers: Employers can use the professional standards to develop systems that support nurses:

- To develop job descriptions that identify expectations for practice.
- To develop orientation programs.
- To create performance appraisal tools.

FIVE NURSING STANDARDS

Standard 1: Responsibility and Accountability

Registered nurses are responsible and accountable to practice safely, compassionately, competently and ethically in accordance with their legislated and individual scopes of practice.

Indicators

Each registered nurse:

- Is responsible and accountable for her/his own actions and decisions.
- Is accountable to evaluate her/his own practice.
- Exercises reasonable judgment and makes timely decisions.
- Seeks assistance appropriately.
- Demonstrates behaviors that uphold the public trust in the profession.
- Takes appropriate action in situations where client safety and well-being are potentially or actually compromised.
- Contributes to safe, supportive and professional practice environments.
- Promotes practice environments that support professional accountability.
- Promotes quality practice environments that support best practices and the ability of registered nurses to practice safely, effectively and ethically.

- Makes appropriate decisions about the distribution of resources under her/his control.
- Promotes a learning environment that supports professional accountability.
- Provides appropriate supervision of learners that supports their ability.
- Promotes research environments that support professional accountability.

Standard 2: Knowledge-Based Practice and Competence

Registered nurses continuously attain, maintain and demonstrate competence relevant to their individual scope of practice.

Indicators

Each registered nurse:

- Has appropriate competencies to practice safely and provide patient-centered care.
- Applies a theoretical and/or evidence-informed rationale for decisions.
- Establishes, maintains and evaluates the nursing component of a plan of care.
- Monitors the effectiveness of a plan of care and revises the plan appropriately in collaboration with the healthcare team.
- Completes documentation in a manner that is clear, timely, accurate and comprehensive.
- Uses appropriate and effective communication skills.
- Demonstrates continuing professional development.
- Promotes practice environments that encourage learning and evidence-informed practice.
- Utilizes and integrates current research findings in his/her practice.
- Encourages and supports the integration of research, evidence-informed theory.
- Encourages, supports and promotes practice environments that facilitate engagement in continuous professional development.
- Promotes learning environment.
- Encourages and supports learners to engage in continuous learning and professional development.
- Integrates research findings into educational activities.
- Promotes research environment that support and facilitate research utilization.
- Communicates best practices and research findings to others.

Standard 3: Client-Focused Care

Registered nurses establish professional, therapeutic relationships and advocate for clients in their relationships with the healthcare system.

Indicators

Each registered nurse:

- Establishes, maintains and appropriately ends professional, therapeutic relationships with clients.
- Maintains appropriate boundaries between professional, therapeutic relationships and non-professional and personal relationships.
- Demonstrates a professional presence with clients.
- Respects clients' cultural diversity.
- Provides relevant information to clients regarding their health.
- Respects and promotes clients' rights to informed decision-making and informed consent.

- Protects the privacy and dignity of clients.
- Maintains the confidentiality of client and health information.
- Coordinates resources to promote quality care.
- Participates in and supports the development and implementation of policies.
- Advocates for systems of care and services that assist nurses to advocate for clients.
- Promotes practice environments that support client advocacy and enable nurses to fulfill their advocacy role.
- Implements educational activities to assist learners to develop, maintain and enhance therapeutic relationships.
- Maintains appropriate professional relationships with learners, recognizing potential authority imbalances between learner and educator.
- Assists learners to recognize potential and actual boundary crossings and/or violations.
- Promotes learning environments that support client advocacy.
- Promotes research environments that support the enhancement of client relationships.

Standard 4: Professional Relationships and Leadership

Registered nurses establish professional relationships with healthcare team members and demonstrate leadership to deliver quality nursing and healthcare services.

Indicators

Each registered nurse:
- Demonstrates leadership in developing strategies to improve client care outcomes.
- Coordinates client care and/or health services throughout the continuum of care.
- Shares relevant information and knowledge with the healthcare team.
- Practices independently and collaboratively as a member of the healthcare team.
- Develops and sustains collaborative relationships with members of the healthcare team.
- Demonstrates professional judgment and accountability.
- Supports and participates in developing, implementing and evaluating quality initiatives.
- Acts as a role model, resource, preceptor, coach and/or mentor to clients, learners, nursing peers, students and colleagues.
- Seeks continuing education opportunities to facilitate growth in leadership skills.
- Promotes healthy violence-free workplace environments.
- Promotes practice environments.
- Facilitates learning environments that encourage learners.
- Advances nursing leadership through communicating research and best practice findings.

Standard 5: Individual Self-Regulation

Registered nurses are accountable to regulate themselves.

Indicators

Each registered nurse:
- Maintains current registration.
- Follows all regulations and legislations.

- Follows policies relevant to profession.
- Practices within their own level of competence.
- Regularly assess their practices.
- Ensures their fitness to practices.
- Attempts to resolve professional practice issues.

STANDARD STATEMENTS FOR PREVENTION OF INFECTION

Application of Infection Control Measures

Nurses understand and apply control measures to prevent and control transmission of microorganisms that are likely to cause infection.

Indicators

The nurse:
- Adheres to appropriate hand hygiene protocols.
- Uses a systematic approach to care based on current infection control principles and research.
- Knows his/her personal immunization status relevant to the practice setting.
- Knows a client's immunization status and takes appropriate action to ensure protection of clients, others and self.
- Takes all measures necessary to prevent the transmission of infection from the nurse to client or other healthcare providers.
- Maintains competence in infection control practices by accessing appropriate resources.
- Advocates for an environment and equipment that reduce the risk for disease transmission.

Risk Reduction for Infection

Nurses reduce the risk to self and others by appropriately handling, cleaning and disposing of materials and equipment.

Indicators

The nurse meets the standard by:
- Participating in education on the use of safer medical devices and work practices relevant to the practice setting.
- Adhering to best practices or manufacturer's guidelines on the cleaning, disinfecting and disposal of wastes or hazardous material.
- Using safety devices when available.
- Following established guidelines when disposing of biomedical waste.
- Identifying hazards and the potential for injury.
- Reporting a break in infection control technique and acting to limit damage.
- Advocating for safety devices.

Communication

Nurses use appropriate and timely communication strategies with clients and their significant others.

Indicators

The nurse meets the standard by:

- Inculcating the psychosocial needs of clients into the plan of care.
- Using appropriate teaching strategies to communicate health information to clients.
- Developing creative or innovative communication strategies.
- Maintaining open communication with the healthcare team, including support staff.

NURSING AUDIT

Definition

- Nursing audit refers to assessment of the quality of clinical nursing. **—Elison**
- Nursing audit is an exercise to find-out whether good nursing practices are followed.
  —Goster Welfer
- Nursing audit is defined as a part of the cycle of quality assurance. It incorporates the systematic and critical analysis by nurses, midwives and health visitors, in conjunction with other staff, of the planning, delivery and evaluation of nursing and midwifery care, in terms of their use of resources and the outcomes for patients/clients, and introduces appropriate change in response to that analysis. **—NHS ME, Framework for Audit for Nursing Services, 1991**

In other words, nursing audit is the systematic evaluation of nursing which results in an improvement in the quality of patient care. The word 'audit' is concerned with the control to improve the quality of patient care.

The following functions of professional nursing are used as the framework for an audit:

- Nurse care of the patient
- Care given by other professionals
- Observation of clinical features and complication, side effects
- Application of nursing procedures
- Health promotion
- Recording and reporting
- Implementation of physician's prescriptions.

Purposes of Nursing Audit

The purposes of nursing audit are as follows:

- It evaluates the nursing care given by nurses.
- It stimulates better recording.
- It evaluates the care given according to the set standards.

Goals of Nursing Audit

The various goals of nursing audit are as follows:

- Improve quality of healthcare.
- Promote improved communication among nurses and other health team members.
- Improve quality of nursing care.

- Detect and analyze problems and errors.
- Ensure that nurses are accountable or answerable for the care.
- Contribute to research.
- For the purpose of reimbursement.

Steps in Audit Process

There are some steps to conduct an audit as mentioned in Figure 9.1.

1. **Selection of a topic:** Before the auditing is done one needs to identify the aspect of care which is to be audited. It may be related to current situation or direct patient needs.
2. **Development of a criteria:** The criteria for assessing the quality care have to be developed. Any type of audit needs to have particular criteria on the basis of which auditing is done. An audit criterion is a statement of what should be happening. Ensure that the criterion is measurable.
3. **Review of records:** In a retrospective type of auditing, the auditor needs to decide at what particular time he/she reviews the charts.
4. **Data collection:** After setting the criteria/standards for the audit, collect the audit data. Data can be collected from questionnaires, computers and paper records and data collection sheets.
5. **Analysis of variation:** Analysis involves calculating percentages to determine whether the standards have been achieved. Audit data should also be analyzed to identify particular trends/problems.
6. **Development of solutions to correct problem**
7. **Implementation of change:** This stage of the audit cycle is one of the most crucial and difficult. After analyzing the data, the audit team need to decide what changes should be implemented. A detailed action plan should be made. All members of the team should be informed of the proposed change.
8. **Evaluation and reaudit:** The final phase of the audit cycle is to undertake a reaudit to ensure that any remedial action undertaken in response to the first audit has been affective.

Complete audit cycle is shown in Figure 9.2.

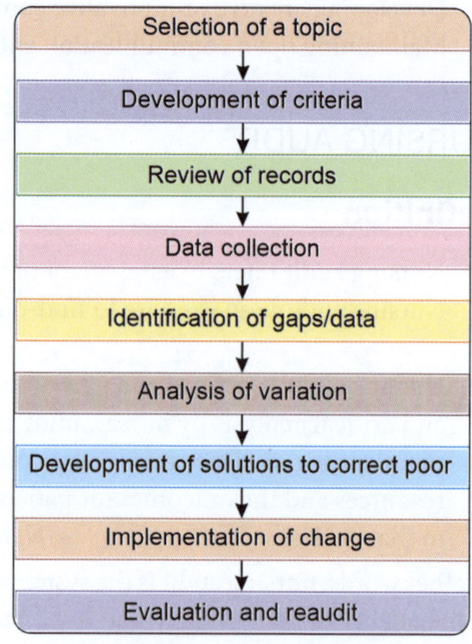

Figure 9.1: Steps in audit process

Types of Audit

An audit can be:

- **Retrospective audit:** A retrospective nursing audit will identify the specific nurse who is responsible for patient care at various times during hospitalization. Deficiencies in performance or charting will be reported back to the nurse.

- **Concurrent audit:** It reviews and evaluates records while persons are receiving care. The advantage is providing opportunities for making changes in the ongoing care program.
- **Prospective audit:** It identifies how future performance will be affected by current interventions. Most frequently used quality controls are process audit, structure audit and outcome audit.
  - **Process audit:** Process audits are used to measure the process of care or how the care was carried out. Process audit is task oriented and focuses on whether or not practice standards of nursing practice are being met.
  - **Structure audit:** These audits assume there is a relationship between setting, quality care, and appropriate structure.
  - **Outcome audits:** They are end results of care. They determine what results occurred as a result of specific intervention by nurses for clients.

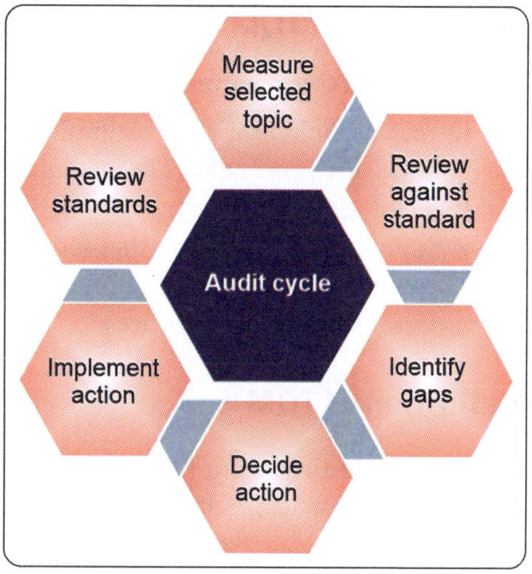

Figure 9.2: Audit cycle

Advantages of Nursing Audit

Some of the advantages of nursing audit are as follows:

- A biographical index of quality of nursing.
- A patient is assured of good services.
- It will give a valuable and pertinent information for the staff.
- It will lead to cooperation and communication among the nurse and health team.
- It will help each professional nurse for her self-evaluation.
- It helps the administration as better planning.
- It will reduce the incidence of medico legal complication.
- It will broaden and strengthen nursing service.

TOTAL QUALITY MANAGEMENT

The total quality management (TQM) requires a total paradigm shift in healthcare management, meaning that the organization must commit to total participatory involvement, collective responsibility, continuous improvement and flexible objective and plans. TQM demands that change based on the needs of the customer and not the values of the providers. It requires the meaningful participation of all personnel and a rapid and thoughtful response from top management to suggestions made by participating personnel. The customers in TQM include patient's families, medical staff, referring physicians, government, accrediting bodies, employers and nurses.

Philosophy of TQM

Philosophy of TQM revolves around customer driven management.

- Its major emphasis is on determining customer need or expectation from the product.
- Total quality is the culture of the organization.
- It is attitude of people how they perform their assigned work with aims to provide customers with products and services that satisfy their needs.
- The culture change means all members of the organization participate in the improvement of process, products, and services.

Definition of TQM

Total Quality Management (TQM) involves quality and leadership commitment, which provide the energy and rationale for implementing TQM processes within the organization's comprehensive quality strategy.

Hospitals and other healthcare organizations across the globe have been progressively implementing TQM to reduce costs, improve efficiency and provide high quality patient care. TQM, which places on improved customer satisfaction, offers the prospect of great market share and profitability. TQM can be an important part of hospital's competitive strategy in quality of healthcare system.

TQM Principles in Nursing

The TQM principles in nursing are shown in Figure 9.3.

Mnemonics
Fours "Ps" of TQM in nursing
P1 – People commitment
P2 – Patient need satisfaction
P3 – Process improvement
P4 – Product in time

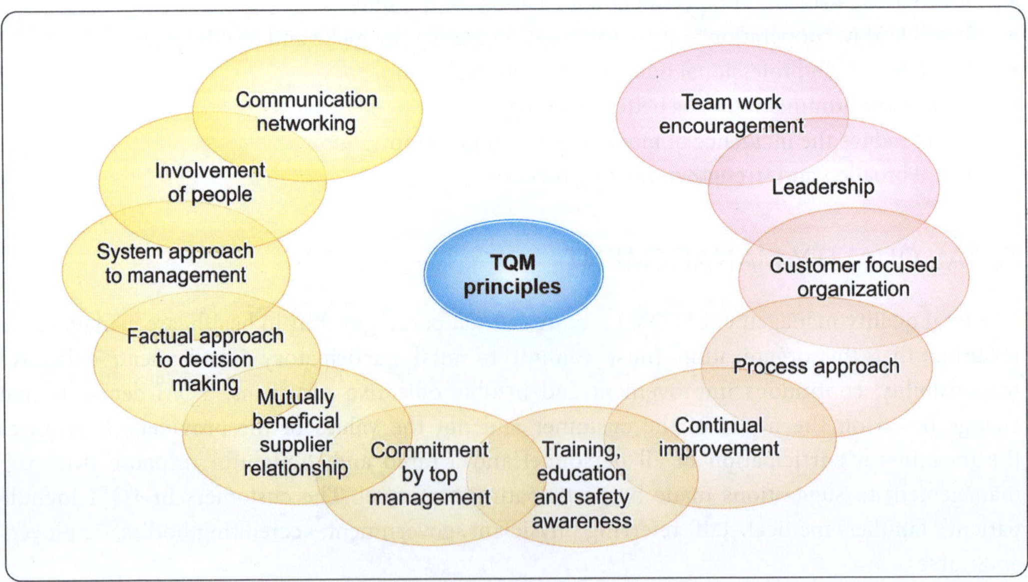

Figure 9.3: TQM principles in nursing

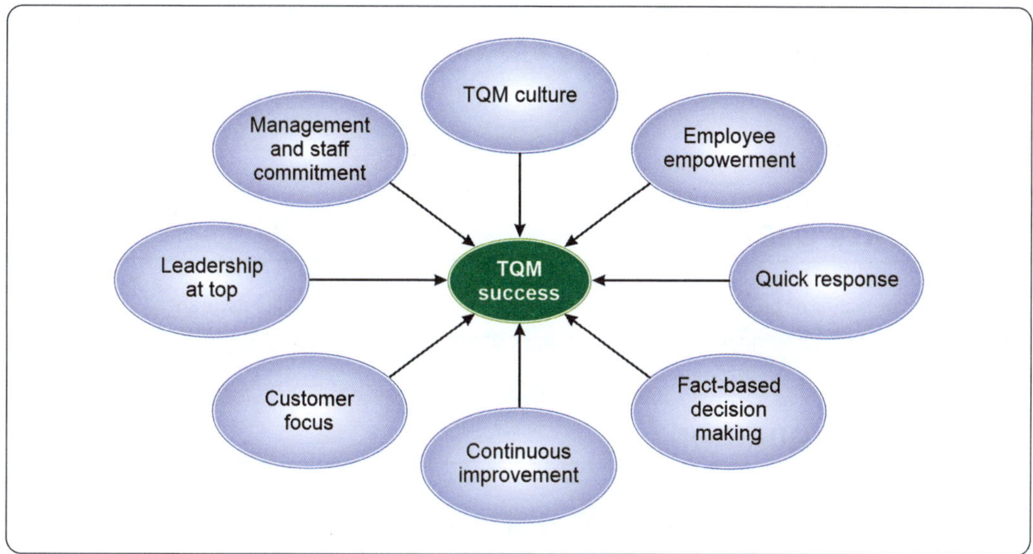

Figure 9.4: Factors responsible for the success of TQM

Success of TQM

Success of TQM depends on factors shown in Figure 9.4.

TQM Activities

Some of the TQM activities are as follows:
- Reducing processing time and cost
- Meeting customer needs
- Finishing task in predetermined time
- Bringing customer satisfaction
- Improving plan of care
- Empowering employees
- Providing recognition and awards
- Setting new targets

FURTHER READINGS

- Alzoubi MM, Hayati KS, Rosliza AM, Ahmad AA, Al-Hamdan ZM. Total Quality Management in the Healthcare Context: Integrating the Literature and Directing Future Research. Risk Manag Healthc Policy. 2019;12:167-77.
- Morey W. Total Quality Management and Nursing: A Shared Vision. Contemp Nurse. 1996;5(3):112-6.

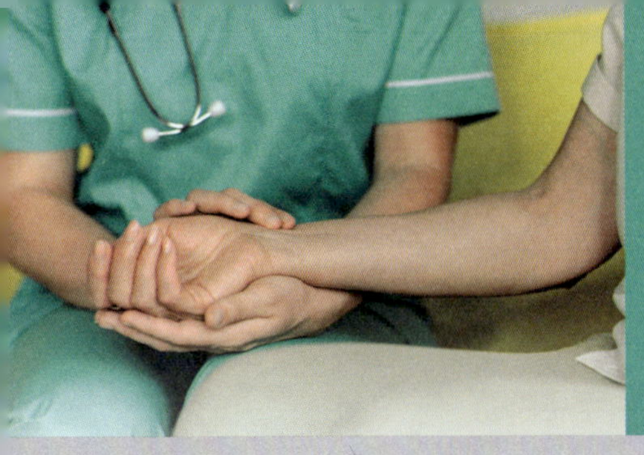

STUDENT ASSIGNMENT

LONG ANSWER QUESTIONS

1. Discuss approaches of quality assurance. What are the factors affecting quality assurance?
2. What are the nursing standards? What is their importance and uses?

SHORT ANSWER QUESTION

1. Write about:
   a. TQM
   b. Types of audits
   c. Approaches of standards

MULTIPLE CHOICE QUESTIONS

1. **When documenting an assigned client's record during and at the end of the shift, the nurse must keep in mind which of the following facts?**
   a. In order to get the care done for all assigned clients, the charting must be as brief as possible.
   b. The proper format, such as SOAP or PIE, as chosen by the hospital, must be adhered to.
   c. The chart is a legal document and may be all a nurse has to support care that was given if called to court.
   d. Clients need to be assessed and the care documented at least once every hour during the shift.

2. **According to the nursing code of ethics, when working as a nurse and a conflict comes up between your client's needs and what the family and/or the physician wants, and/or the hospital policies, your first loyalty is to the:**
   a. Hospital
   b. Client
   c. Family
   d. Physician

3. **Which of the following strategies can most help you as a nurse to enhance your ethical practice and client advocacy?**
   a. Reading a book on religions of the world
   b. Examining and clarifying your own values
   c. Talking with peers about their beliefs and values
   d. Buying a nursing book on ethical decisions

4. **__________ is a part of quality management focused on providing confidence that quality requirements will be fulfilled.**
   a. Quality management
   b. Quality
   c. Quality assurance
   d. Updating

5. **Quality Council of India sponsored accreditation system for hospitals and healthcare provider:**
   a. NABH
   b. Joint Commission International
   c. NIS
   d. NABET

ANSWER KEY

1. c   **2.** b   **3.** b   **4.** c   **5.** a

10

Professional Bodies in Nursing

LEARNING OBJECTIVES

After the completion of the chapter, the readers will be able to:
- Know the professional bodies in nursing.
- Discuss the roles of professional bodies in nursing.

CHAPTER OUTLINE

- Nursing Profession
- Professional Organizations in Nursing
- Nursing as a Profession
- Various Professional Bodies and their Functions
- Roles of Regulatory Bodies in Nursing

KEY TERMS

Advisor: A person who gives advice to a company, government, etc.

Authority: The powers and rights to give orders and make others obey.

Autonomy: The quality or state of being self-governing.

Legislation: The processes or result of enrolling, enacting or promulgating laws.

Self-regulation: The ability to control one's behavior, emotions, and thoughts in the pursuit of long-term goals.

NURSING PROFESSION

Nursing is a profession within the healthcare sector focused on the care of individuals, families and communities. So, they may attain, maintain or recover optimal health and quality of life. Professions are those occupations possessing a particular combination of characteristics generally considered to be the expertise, autonomy, commitment and responsibility.

Definitions of profession:

Various definitions of profession are as follows:

- A paid occupation, especially one that involves prolonged training and a formal qualification.
- A vocation requiring advanced training and usually involving mental rather than manual work.
- A profession is an occupation based on specialized intellectual study and training, the purpose of which is to supply skilled services with ethical components and others.

PROFESSIONAL ORGANIZATIONS IN NURSING

Professionals create organizations to work collectively on behalf of issues that improve their work and their involvement in communities, ensure continued learning and competence, and use political action to influence policy makers to support mission of organization. Professional organizations offer a supportive way to learn leadership skills, to test ideas, and to follow these ideas to completion. Nursing has national organizations open to all graduate nurses—Indian Nursing Council (INC) and Trained Nurses' Association of India (TNAI).

Objectives

- To understand the role of professional organizations in empowering nurses in their emerging professionalism.
- To discuss the functions of each professional organization.
- To discuss importance of self-assertiveness in safeguarding our profession.
- To study the vast scope of collective bargaining in nursing profession.

Various Vital Components of a Profession

- Education takes place in a college or university.
- Education is prolonged.
- Work involves mental creativity.
- Decision making is based largely on science or theories.
- Values, beliefs and ethics are an integral part of preparation.
- Commitment dominates material reward.
- Accountability rests with Individual.

Criteria of a Profession

The various criteria of a profession are as follows:

- **Based on systematic theory:** A distinct way of viewing phenomena surrounding the knowledge base of the profession.
- Specialized competencies and practitioners who are effective in practicing the professional role.
- Dedication to raise the standards of the profession's education and practice.

- Availability of professional education as a life-long process and mechanisms to advance the education of professionals established by the profession.
- The presence within the profession of individuals with varied identities and values forming groupings and coalitions that coalesce into unified segments—known as specialties with specific missions.
- Authority recognized by society and the clientele of the profession.
- Approval of the authority sanctioned by a broader community or society.
- A code of ethics to regulate the relationships between professionals and clients.
- Self-regulation that protects practitioners and supports disciplinary criteria and actions to censure, suspend or remove code violators.
- A professional culture sustained by formal professional associations, such that the membership may develop a biased perspective through their profession's lenses.

NURSING AS A PROFESSION

The nursing pathway to professionalism has not been smooth. For decades, an ongoing subject for discussion in nursing circles has been the question—"Is nursing a profession?" Sociologists do not agree that nursing is a profession. They believe it is an emerging profession. Nursing is rather considered by everyone as a profession now. Nursing complies with all criteria of a profession. It has greatly changed now as:

- There is a body of knowledge that is uniquely nursing's own.
- Nursing is no longer based on trial and error but increasingly relies on theory, development and research as a basis for practice. We call it evidence-based practice.
- Nursing is now engaged in an ongoing effort to identify and standardize nursing diagnoses, interventions and outcomes—all of which are parts of nursing process.
- Individual accountability has become a part of nursing practice. Now society holds nurses individually responsible for their actions.
- Majority of programs offering basic nursing education are now associate degree and baccalaureate programs available in colleges and universities.

VARIOUS PROFESSIONAL BODIES AND THEIR FUNCTIONS

International Council of Nurses

ICN is a federation of over 130 national nurses' associations (NNAs), representing the millions of nurses worldwide. We work directly with these member associations on issues of importance to the nursing profession. In addition, we grant affiliate status to a number of international specialist nursing organizations, which allows them certain privileges and benefits. ICN's mission is to represent nursing worldwide, advance the nursing profession, promote the well-being of nurses, and advocate for health in all policies. Our vision is that the global community recognizes, supports, and invests in nurses and nursing to lead and deliver health for all.

In alignment with the ICN mission of advancing the nursing profession, promoting the well-being of nurses, and advocating for the health of all, ICN works within policy advocacy, global health partnerships, leadership development, expanding networks, forming congresses and more.

ICN advances nursing, nurses and health through its policies, partnerships, advocacy, leadership development, networks, campaigns, congresses and special projects.

Functions of ICN

To provide policy direction to fulfil the objectives of ICN.

- To establish categories of membership and determine their rights and obligations as well as dues.
- To act upon recommendations of the Board of Directors relating to admission and readmission of member associations into ICN.
- To receive and consider information from the Board regarding ICN activities since the last CNR.
- To receive nominees for the Board and to elect the Board.
- To act upon proposed amendments to the ICN Constitution.
- To act upon recommendations of the Board of Directors for the amount of NNA dues.
- To act through mail, written, or electronic communication on ICN business that requires immediate attention by the CNR between meetings.
- To act upon recommendations for the dissolution of the ICN.

ICN's Strategic Plan 2019-2023 had four goals under which nurses' work was presented:

- **Goal 1. Global impact:** ICN aim is to inform and influence the design and implementation of health, social, educational and economic policies at a global and regional level to promote health for all.
- **Goal 2. Membership empowerment:** ICN aim is to strengthen NNAs across the three pillars of ICN to enable them to address key challenges at regional and national levels.
- **Goal 3. Strategic leadership:** ICN aim is to provide strategic leadership to advance the nursing profession to meet current and future needs of the population, health systems (including health and social care) and nurses.
- **Goal 4. Innovative growth:** ICN aim is to identify, secure and diversify business and revenue.

Recent Updates

ICN has set five goals as a strategic Plan 2024–2028.

Goal 1. Global voice, influence and impact: Provide strategic leadership to inform and influence the design and implementation of global and regional health, social, educational, regulatory and economic policies that promote health for all and advance the nursing profession.

Goal 2. Workforce solutions and nurse empowerment: Create sustainable change and influence to build and retain the nursing workforce for the future.

Goal 3. Member vitality: Strengthen National Nursing Associations to grow membership, advance the nursing profession in their country, and address key health system challenges at regional and national levels.

Goal 4. Leadership to transform nursing practice at all levels: Lead the formulation of future-focused policies that enhance and elevate the nursing profession and strengthen health systems.

Goal 5. Diversifying and growing revenue for sustainability: Expand and grow revenue generating opportunities to support ICN goals, diversify business and promote sustainability.

Indian Nursing Council

The Indian Nursing Council is an autonomous body under the Government of India, Ministry of Health and Family Welfare was constituted by the Central Government under section 3(1) of the Indian Nursing Council Act, 1947 of parliament in order to establish a uniform standard of training for nurses, midwives and health visitors.

Functions

- To establish and monitor uniform standards of nursing for nurse midwifes, auxiliary nurse midwifes and health visitors' education by doing inspection of the institutions.
- To recognize the qualification(s) under section 10(2)(4) of the Indian Nursing Council Act, 1947 for the purpose of registration and employment in India and abroad.
- To prescribe minimum standards of education and training in various nursing programs and prescribe the syllabus and regulations for nursing programs under section 16 of the Indian Nursing Council Act, 1947.
- Power to withdraw the recognition of qualification under Section 14 of the Indian Nursing Council Act, 1947 in case the institution fails to maintain its standards under Section 14(1)(b) of the Act when an institution recognised by a State Council for the training of nurses midwives, Auxiliary Nurse Midwives or health visitors does not satisfy the requirements of the Council.
- To recognise Degree/Diploma/Certificate awarded by Foreign Universities.
- To give approval for registration of Indian and Foreign Nurses possessing foreign qualification under Section 11(2)(a) of the Indian Nursing Council Act, 1947.
- To maintain Indian Nurses Register for registration of nursing personnel.
- To advise the State Nursing Councils, Examining Boards, State Governments and Central Government in various important items regarding nursing education in the country.
- To promote research in nursing.
- To prescribe code of ethics and professional conduct.
- To regulate the policies of training of nursing programs in the field of nursing to improve the quality of nursing education.

Services

- To attend all matters relating to recognition of nursing qualification awarded by different university w.r.t INC Act 1947 and regulation there under. The Council stripes to deal such matters on priority basis so that the decision in these matters are taken at the earliest and conveyed to the concerned.
- To deal with all matters relating to accord suitability and annual renewal of suitability of a large number of nursing educational institutions all over India. The Council has made this work completely online without any personnel interaction which is a big boon to the institutions who can get the work done without need for any travel to INC office with bulky documents etc.
- A large number of candidates approach INC to verify the credential of their qualification which is also an online process done on priority basis.

Role of Indian Nursing Council

The Indian Nursing Council (INC) plays a pivotal role in regulating and advancing nursing education and practice in India (Fig. 10.1). Here are the key roles of the Indian Nursing Council:
- **Setting standards:** The INC establishes and maintains standards for nursing education and practice in India. This includes defining the curriculum, course content, and clinical training requirements for nursing programs to ensure that they meet the highest standards of quality and proficiency.

- **Regulatory oversight:** The INC regulates nursing education institutions and programs across the country. It approves nursing courses, conducts inspections of nursing schools and colleges, and ensures compliance with regulatory norms and guidelines.
- **Accreditation:** The INC accredits nursing institutions and programs that meet its prescribed standards. Accreditation serves as a mark of quality assurance, indicating that the institution or program has undergone rigorous evaluation and meets established benchmarks of excellence.
- **Licensing and registration:** The INC oversees the licensing and registration of nurses in India. It sets the criteria for eligibility, conducts examinations for registration, and maintains a registry of qualified nurses who are authorized to practice professionally.
- **Curriculum development:** The INC formulates comprehensive curriculum frameworks and guidelines for nursing education. It ensures that nursing programs cover essential topics and competencies required for effective nursing practice, including clinical skills, patient care, ethics, and professionalism.
- **Promotion of research and development:** The INC promotes research and development in the field of nursing. It encourages nursing institutions and professionals to engage in research activities aimed at advancing knowledge, improving patient outcomes, and enhancing nursing practice.
- **Advocacy and collaboration:** The INC advocates for the interests of the nursing profession and collaborates with government agencies, healthcare institutions, and professional nursing associations to address issues related to nursing education, practice, and policy.
- **Continuing education:** The INC promotes continuing education and professional development for nurses. It encourages nurses to pursue further education, training, and certification to enhance their skills, knowledge, and career opportunities.

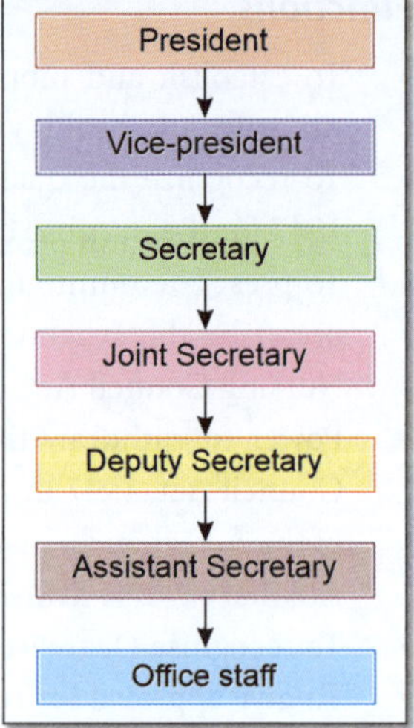

Figure 10.1: Hierarchy of INC

The Trained Nurses Association of India

The 117 glorious years of Trained Nurse's Association have passed and TNAI is still moving ahead with commitment and dedication.

Overview

The Trained Nurses' Association of India (TNAI) is a national organization of nurse professionals at different levels. It was established in 1908 and was initially known as Association of Nursing Superintendents. The Government of India has recognized TNAI as a service organization in 1950. A similar recognition by all the State Governments has been an asset to the promotion of its objectives.

Foundation stone for TNAI was laid by Late Dr S Radharishnan and the Headquarter was inaugurated by Late Smt. Indira Gandhi.

Objectives

Upholding in every way the:
- Dignity and honor of the nursing profession.
- Promoting a sense of espirit de corps among all nurses.
- To advance professional, educational, economic and general welfare of nurses.

Functions

- To enunciate standards of nursing education and implement these through appropriate channels.
- To establish standards and qualifications for nursing practice.
- To enunciate standards of nursing service and implement these through appropriate channels.
- To establish a code of ethical conduct for practitioners.
- To stimulate and promote research designed to enhance.
- To stimulate and promote research designed to enhance the knowledge for evidence-based nursing practice.
- To promote legislation and to speak for nurses in regard to legislative action.
- To promote and protect the economic welfare of Nurses.
- To provide professional counselling and placement service for nurses.
- To provide for the continuing professional development of practitioners.
- To represent nurses and serve as their spoke person with allied national and international organizations, governmental and other bodies and the public.
- To serve as the official representative of the Nurses of India as a member of the International Council of Nurses.
- To promote the general health and welfare of the public through the Association programs, relationships and activities, e.g., disaster management.
- To render care as per the changing needs of the society.

Membership

A life member is a person who is a registered Nurse and Midwife (equivalent of midwifery training in case of male nurse), trained from an institution recognised by the Indian Nursing Council/State Nursing Council and holds a certificate of training issued by a Nursing Registration Council or Board of Examinations recognised by the Indian Nursing Council.

Student Nurses' Association (SNAI)

The Student Nurses' Association of India (SNAI) is an affiliated association of the student nurses under the umbrella of TNAI. The main purpose behind the establishment of SNAI was to uphold the dignity and to promote a team spirit among students with professional ethics.

SNAI was established in 1929 during TNAI Annual Conference in Madras. Miss LN Jeans, Nursing Superintendent, Government General Hospital, Madras, was the first Honorary Organizing Secretary of SNAI. The pioneer unit of SNA was established in General Hospital, Madras. The first SNA Annual Conference was held in Delhi during November 1932. The first one-day SNA Conference was held in 1951, and the first Biennial SNA Conference was held at Nagpur in 1961.

Miss I. Dorabji was appointed as first SNAI Secretary followed by Miss M.Philip. In 1970 with the reorganization of TNAI the designation of the SNAI Secretary was changed to SNAI Advisor. Mrs. Narender Nagpal was appointed as the first SNA Advisor followed by Ms. D. K. Singh (1978-79). The office was re-designated as Assistant Secretary-cum-SNA Advisor. In 2005, again re-designated as Deputy Secretary General-cum-SNA Advisor.

Further the SNAI units are expanded gradually to many nursing institutions in India and started functioning. Now there are 900 SNAI units and 150000 SNAI members in the country.

Objectives

- To help the students to uphold the dignity of the profession.
- To promote team spirit among students for common goal.
- To help the students to develop professional ethics.
- To encourage students to gain positive attitude towards the nursing profession
- To encourage the students to develop leadership quality and effective communication skills for overall development.
- To encourage students to participate and compete in various events at state, regional and national conferences.

SNA Management

Affairs of SNA are managed at the Unit, State and at National level.

At the unit level, the unit executive committee manages SNA affairs. It comprises of President (Principal of the institution - TNAI member), SNA Advisor (any elected faculty - TNAI member), Vice President, Secretary, Treasurer and the conveners of various committees are student nurses elected by the students during their SNA General Body meeting.

At the State level, the State SNA Executive Committee comprises of the State TNAI President as ex-officio member, SNA Advisor, Student Vice President, student Secretary elected by all unit Vice president and Secretary of their state during state SNA conference/Meeting

At the National level, the SNA General Committee Comprises of TNAI President, Honorary Treasurer, Secretary-General, Dy. Secretary General-cum-SNA Advisor and State SNA Advisors and Student SNA Vice Presidents and Student Secretaries.

Activities of SNA

Number of activities are assigned to the SNAI members at all levels to achieve the objectives of the association. The professional, educational, social, cultural and recreational activities are arranged to strengthen their curricular and co-curricular components at the Unit, State and National level. Organizing conferences and meetings at all levels is one of the important activities which provide a forum for the members to discuss and find solutions for various problems faced by the students.

- **Organization of conferences and meetings:** At the TNAI Conference student representatives, i.e., Vice-President and the Secretary of the State Branch from each State are invited to attend the SNA General Committee meeting every year.
- **Maintenance of SNA dairy:** The SNA Diary was instituted in 1939. This is the biennial record book drawn up for the use of the unit secretaries. There are assessed by the State SNA Advisors annually and the 2 best diaries from each State are then sent to the National SNA Advisor for Biennial evaluation and awards. These diaries are assessed for professional, educational, extracurricular social, cultural and recreational activities.
- **Exhibition of posters:** All categories of student nurses are eligible to participate in exhibitions, both as groups and as an individual. They can prepare charts, posters on the topics announced in the TNAI Bulletin and NJI. The posters are competed at the state level, and after thorough scrutinization, only one best entry at the state level under each category and section is entertained at the national level.
- **Public speaking and writing:** Public speaking and writing is encouraged to increase self-confidence and to help them develop communication skills. In order to achieve this, the

competition on scientific paper presentations related to the theme of the conference is being organized. The Scientific Papers presented by many students are scrutinized at state level. Only one scientific paper on each sub-theme of the conference was sent to the national level for final evaluation. The best three scientific papers, one on each of the sub-themes are selected at the national level.

- **Project:** The students undertake community projects such as school health projects, health surveys, nutrition surveys, medical camps, immunization programs, health mela are also undertaken by the student nurses. In addition, fund raising activities are also recommended and encouraged.
- **Advocacy of nursing profession:** To acquaint the general public with the nursing profession, general public is invited to the celebrations and festive of professional and non professional nature, such as Nurses' week, WHO Day, Lamp Lighting, Graduation Ceremonies, Sports, Tournaments, TV Shows and Radio Talks which are organized by nurses.
- **Fund raising:** Fund raising is an important and necessary activity of SNA done by getting voluntary donations, sale of donation tickets and organizing variety entertainment activities to raise the fund.
- **Socio-cultural and recreational activities:** The association believes that the professional development remains incomplete without this component. Dynamism and energy of present youth who enters the nursing profession is channelized constructively into fine arts, dramas, and different varieties of dance, music, paintings, and other competitive activities. Sports and games are becoming extremely popular and competitions are held at unit level, state level and at the national level.

  In addition, there are numerous other activities in the shape of article writing, poetry writing, flower arrangement, cooking, sewing, interior decoration and gardening, etc. which are also encouraged. The personality contest Mr. SNA and Miss SNA was introduced for the first time in the SNA Platinum Jubilee and XXI Biennial Conference.
- **Program for ANM students:** Since 2006 a separate session has been organized for ANM students during SNA Biennial Conference and this provides an opportunity to discuss the problems and issues of ANM and ways to resolve them.

Proposed National Nursing and Midwifery Commission

The National Nursing and Midwifery Commission Bill, 2023 was introduced in Lok Sabha on July 24, 2023. It repeals the Indian Nursing Council Act, 1947. The Bill provides for the regulation and maintenance of standards of education and services for nursing and midwifery professionals. Key features of the Bill are:

Key Features of the Bill

- **National nursing and midwifery commission:** The Bill provides for the constitution of the National Nursing and Midwifery Commission. It will consist of 29 members. The chairperson should have a postgraduate degree in nursing and midwifery and have at least 20 years of field experience. Ex-officio members include representatives from the Department of Health and Family Welfare, National Medical Commission, Military Nursing Services, and the Directorate General of Health Services. Other members include nursing and midwifery professionals, and one representative from charitable institutions.

- **Functions of commission:** Functions of the commission include:
  - Framing policies and regulating standards for nursing and midwifery education
  - Providing a uniform process for admission into nursing and midwifery institutions
  - Regulating nursing and midwifery institutions, and
  - Providing standards for faculty in teaching institutions.
- **Autonomous boards:** The Bill provides for the constitution of three autonomous boards under the supervision of the National Commission. These are:
  - The Nursing and Midwifery Undergraduate and Postgraduate Education Board, to regulate education and examination at undergraduate and postgraduate levels
  - The Nursing and Midwifery Assessment and Rating Board, to provide the framework for assessing and rating nursing and midwifery institutions; and
  - The Nursing and Midwifery Ethics and Registration Board, to regulate professional conduct and promote ethics in the profession.
- **State nursing and midwifery commissions:** Every state government must constitute a State Nursing and Midwifery Commission where no such Commission exists under state law. It will consist of 10 members. The members will include representatives from the health department, from any nursing or midwifery college of the state, and nursing and midwifery professionals.
- **Functions of the state commission:**
  - Enforcing professional conduct, code of ethics and etiquette
  - Maintaining state registers for registered professionals
  - Issuing certificates of specialisation, and
  - Providing for skill-based examination. Appeals against decisions taken by state commissions may be filed with the Ethics and Registration Board. Decisions taken by the Board will be binding on the State Commission unless a second appeal is filed with the National Commission.
- **Establishment of nursing or midwifery institutions:** Permission of the Assessment and Rating Board would be needed to establish a new nursing and midwifery institution, increase the number of seats, or start any new postgraduate course. The Board must decide on the proposals within six months. In case of disapproval, an appeal can be made to the National Commission and a second appeal can be filed with the Central Government.
- **Practicing as a professional:** The Ethics and Registration Board will maintain an online Indian Nurses and Midwives' Register, containing the details and qualifications of professionals and associates. Individuals must be enrolled in the National or State Register to practice nursing or midwifery as qualified professional. Failure to comply may result in imprisonment of up to one year, a fine of up to five lakh rupees, or both.
- **Advisory council:** The central government will also establish the Nursing and Midwifery Advisory Council. The chairperson of the National Commission shall be the chairperson of the Council. Other members include representatives from each State and Union territory, Ministry of Ayush, the University Grants Commission, the National Assessment and Accreditation Council, the Indian Council of Medical Research, and nursing and midwifery professionals. The Council will provide advice and support to the National Commission in matters concerning nursing and midwifery education, services, training, and research.

Functions of Proposed National Nursing and Midwifery Commission

- Conducting a common national entrance examination for diploma, undergraduate and postgraduate nursing and midwifery courses and exit test for professional practice.

- Setting and maintaining the standards of nursing and midwifery education which will include curriculum, facilities, assessment, research, clinical affiliations and faculty quality and development and approval of institutes.
- Regulate nursing and midwifery institutions, researches, professionals and associates.
- Assessing nursing and midwifery requirements in healthcare and advising the government.
- Regulate professional code of conduct and promote nursing and midwifery ethics.
- Regulate the standards and scope of practice of registered nurses and midwives, nursing associates, midwifery associates and postgraduates of nursing and midwifery profession.
- Regulate the limited prescribing authority for nurse practitioners (NPs) who have obtained the requisite nursing and midwifery qualification criteria prescribed by the Post Graduate education board.
- Maintaining a national register of nursing and midwifery professionals and another register for associates and state commissions will have state registers.
- Ensuring rights and obligations of registered nursing and midwifery professionals and associates.
- Provide for mechanisms for receiving complaints and grievance redressal.

> **Recent Updates**
>
> The Ministry of Health and Family Welfare (MOFFW) has introduced the National Nursing and Midwifery Commission Rules, 2024. These rules aim to regulate and advance nursing and midwifery education in the country. These rules were published on March 13, 2024.

ROLES OF REGULATORY BODIES IN NURSING

A regulatory body is like a professional body but it is not a membership organization and its primary activity is to protect the public. Unlike professional bodies, it is established on the basis of legal mandate. A regulatory body for health professionals is mandated by the government to regulate professionals in the interests of the public. Its role is to protect the public by ensuring that the professionals it regulates provide safe, competent and ethical care. Self-regulation is a privilege granted by the government.

Functions of Regulatory Body

Regulatory bodies exercise regulatory functions, that are:

- Imposing requirements
- Putting restrictions and conditions
- Setting standards in relation to any activity
- Securing compliance or enforcement

Vital Role of Regulatory Bodies

Few of the important roles of regulatory bodies are as follows:

- To ensure quality healthcare service.
- To support and assist professional members.
- Set and enforce standards of nursing practice.

- Monitor and enforce standards for nursing education.
- Monitor and enforce standards of nursing practice.
- Set the requirements for the registration of nursing professionals.

Nursing regulatory bodies also called colleges or associations, are responsible for the licensing of nurses within their respective provinces' territory. The Nursing Regulatory Bodies receive their authority from legislation.

The professional body may have a number of functions such as:

- To set and assess professional examinations.
- To provide support for continuing professional development through learning opportunities and tools for recording and planning.
- To publish professional journals or magazines.
- To provide networks for professionals to meet and discuss their field of expertise.
- To issue a code of conduct to guide professional behavior.
- To deal with complaints against professionals and implement disciplinary procedures.
- To enable fairer access to the professions, so that people from all backgrounds can become professionals.
- To provide career support and opportunities for students, graduates and people already working.

FURTHER READINGS

- International Council of Nurses. (2023). The global voice of nursing. [online] Available from https://www.icn.ch/[Last accessed August, 2023].
- The Trained Nurses' Association of India. (2023). [online] Available from https://www.tnaionline.org/ [Last accessed August, 2023].
- World Health Organization. (2023). [online] Available from https://www.who.int/ [Last accessed August, 2023].
- https://Prsindia.org

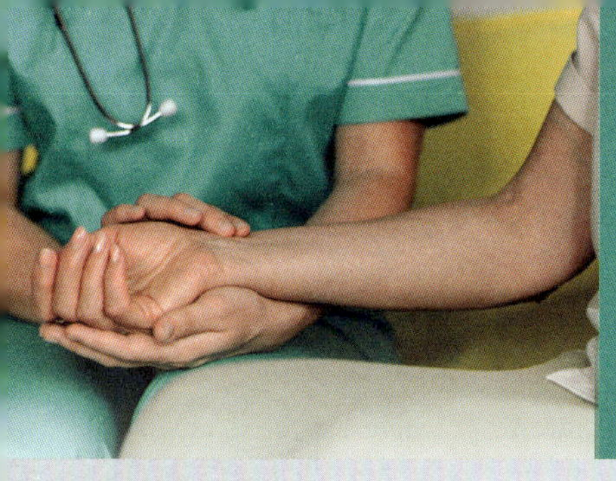

STUDENT ASSIGNMENT

LONG ANSWER QUESTIONS

1. What is a nursing profession? Define it. Discuss various nursing organizations.
2. Discuss the vital roles of nursing regulatory bodies.

SHORT ANSWER QUESTION

1. Write about:
   a. INC
   b. TNAI

MULTIPLE CHOICE QUESTIONS

1. **Criteria of a profession include; except:**
   a. A profession should be intellectual
   b. It should be self-governing
   c. In a profession there is no place for higher education
   d. A profession should be service oriented
2. **Which of the following are reasons to join a nursing professional organization? (Select all that apply)**
   a. It makes you look good
   b. Stay current in clinical specialty or role
   c. You get paid for joining
   d. Leadership development
3. **All professional organizations have their own mission statement.**
   a. True
   b. False

ANSWER KEY

1. c   **2.** b, d   **3.** a

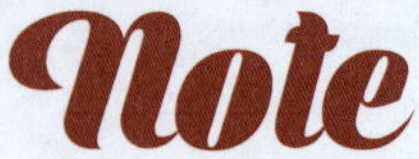

11

Nursing Care Systems

LEARNING OBJECTIVES

LEARNING OBJECTIVES

After the completion of the chapter, the readers will be able to:
- Describe various types of nursing such as holistic, community-based, progressive patient care, team nursing and functional nursing.

CHAPTER OUTLINE

- Nursing Care Systems
- Holistic Nursing
- Primary Nursing
- Family-Oriented Nursing Concept
- Progressive Patient Care
- Person-Centered Care
- Functional Nursing Method

KEY TERMS

Holistic nursing: A nursing practice that aims to heal the whole person, not just their physical body.

Person-centered care: A healthcare practice that involves patients working with their health professionals to actively participate in their own medical treatment.

Progressive patient care: The systematic grouping of patients according to their degree of illness and dependency on the nurse rather than by classification of disease and sex.

NURSING CARE SYSTEMS

Nursing care system can be defined as the organization and structure through which nursing care is delivered to the clients. These systems are designed to ensure that clients receive the quality care while using maximum use of available resources. Nursing care delivery system is actually a subsystem of the practice model that describes our approach to delivering patient care by:

- Detailing assignments, responsibilities and authority to accomplish patient care.
- Determining who is going to perform what task, who is responsible and who make decisions.
- Assigning nurses as per client care meets.

Characteristics of Nursing Care Delivery Systems

- **Coordination:** Ensuring interaction amongst various healthcare providers to provide comprehensive care.
- **Flexibility:** Modifying care plans as per the changing needs as the client.
- **Efficacy:** Striving for the optional health outcomes within available resources.
- **Continuity:** Assuring that the care provided is consistent and uninterrupted.

Components of Nursing Care Delivery System

- **Task allocation:** The process is determining who does what is crucial. This should consider the proficiency level of nursing staff, allowing their skills to be civilized as per client need.
- **Effective communication:** Communication is important to ensuring tasks are understood coordinates and executed efficiently.
- **Collaboration:** Working as one unit ensures all care aspects are covers from direct patient care to documentation.
- **Resource Utilization:** Optional utilization of available resource including nurses, medicines etc. is a key to efficient systems.

Selection of nursing care delivery model depend on following factors:

- Care setting
- Patient care needs
- Resource availability

The nursing care approach is shown in Figure 11.1.

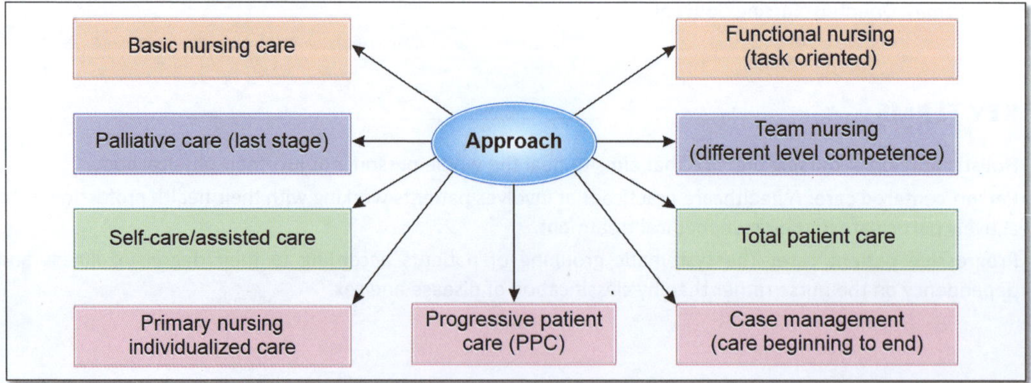

Figure 11.1: Nursing care approach in community-based nursing

- **Self-care:** It is taking care of self to keep healthy rather than neglecting health. It emphasizes to adopt a health-seeking behavior. Self-care is also seen in disease management. It empowers individuals to make informed healthcare decisions and is an essential component of self-care. The nurse plays a vital role in ensuring that the client's family is informed about self-care. Although community-based nursing affords the opportunity for direct interventions, it also requires self-care teaching for the client and family members.
- **Preventive healthcare:** Community-based nursing considers all three levels of preventive.

HOLISTIC NURSING

"Holism" in healthcare is a philosophy that emanated directly from Florence Nightingale, who believed in care that focused on unity, wellness, and the interrelationship of human beings, events, and environment. Holistic nursing focuses on promoting health and wellness, assisting healing, and preventing or alleviating suffering. Healing is the integration of the totality of humankind in body, mind, emotion, and spirit. Holism acknowledges and values the connectedness of the body, mind, and spirit; the inherent goodness of human beings; the ability to find meaning and purpose in our lives and experiences; the practitioner's support for each client so that the client may find comfort, peace and harmony; and the body's innate power to heal itself. With a holistic approach, the person is treated, rather than just the treatment of symptoms. Individuals are viewed as unique, therefore two people with the same disease may be treated very differently.

Holistic nursing integrates complementary modalities, relaxation, meditation, guided imagery, breathwork, biofeedback, reiki, journaling, etc., with traditional nursing interventions. It draws on nursing knowledge, theories of wholeness, expertise, caring and intuition, as nurses and clients become therapeutic partners in a mutually evolving process toward healing, balance, and wholeness. Holistic nurses conduct holistic assessments, select appropriate interventions, and assist the client in exploring self-awareness, spirituality, and personal transformation in healing. They work to alleviate clients' signs and symptoms, provide health counseling and education, and guide clients in making choices between conventional medicine and complimentary/alternative therapies. Holistic nursing is a practice of nursing that focuses on healing the whole person. It addresses the interconnectedness of the mind, body, spirit, social/cultural, emotions, relationships, context, and environment as shown in Figure 11.2.

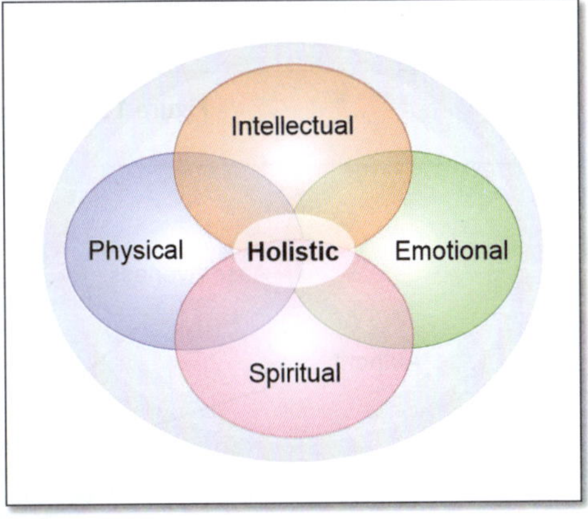

Figure 11.2: Holistic nursing care model

PRIMARY NURSING

Primary nursing was originally developed in the late 1960s/early 1970s in response to changes in nursing academic preparation. Primary nursing refers to comprehensive, individualized care provided by the same nurse throughout the period of care. The primary nursing framework is shown in Figure 11.3. Primary nursing is a method of nursing practice which emphasizes continuity of care by having one nurse provide complete care for a small group of patients within a nursing unit of a hospital (Fig. 11.3). Registered Nurse (RN) is responsible for a patient's care throughout the entire stay. This type of nursing care allows the nurse to give direct patient care. The primary nurse accepts total 24-hour responsibility for a patient's nursing care. Nursing care is directed toward meeting all of the individualized patient's needs. The primary nurse communicates with other members of the healthcare team regarding the patient's healthcare (Fig. 11.4).

Each registered nurse is a primary nurse to a small group of patients and an associate nurse to other patients that he/she helps to care for. The head/charge nurse also acts as a primary nurse with a slightly reduced patient load. The charge nurse assigns patients to the primary and associate nurses. The primary nurse plans 24-hour care for his/her primary patients and follows the plan while caring for other patients. Nurses care for their clients during their entire hospital stay and may even make home visits. As a whole primary nursing includes many factors as given in (Fig. 11.4).

Advantages of Primary Nursing

It promotes continuity of care and empowers nurses.

Disadvantages of Primary Nursing

It requires consistent alignment.

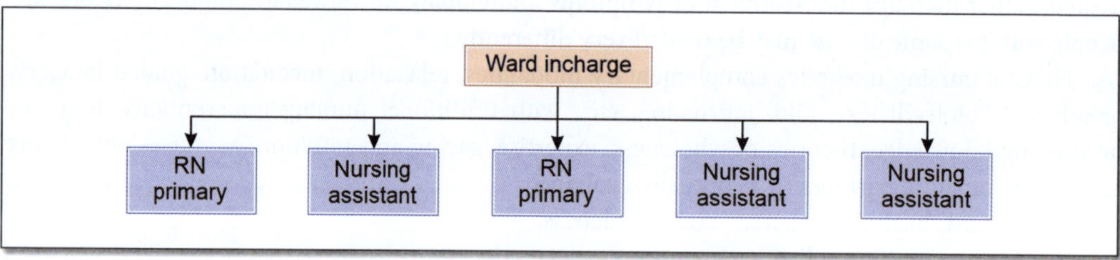

Figure 11.3: Framework for primary nursing

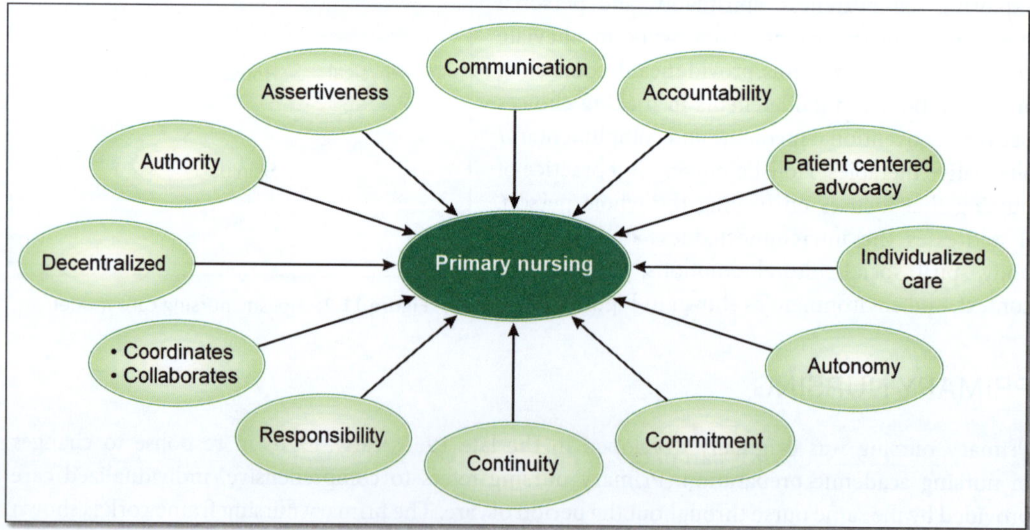

Figure 11.4: Primary nursing

FAMILY-ORIENTED NURSING CONCEPT

Family-oriented nursing can be defined as the process of providing healthcare needs of families within the scope of nursing practice. Family nursing is considered the community and cultural aspect of the family. Family health nursing is offered in a setting where the individuals live with physiological and psychological problems (Fig. 11.5).

It considers the relationship between and among family members. Family nurse manipulates the environment to increase the family interaction. It focuses on strength of individual family members.

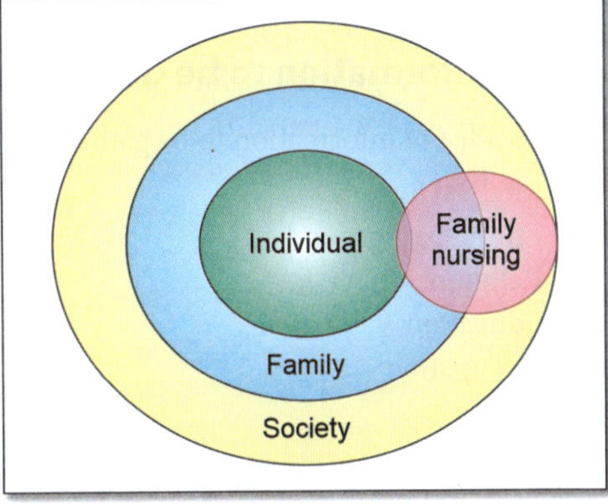

Figure 11.5: Model of family-oriented nursing concept

Setting for Family-Oriented Nursing

The setting for family-oriented nursing includes:

- Home
- Clinic
- School
- Job area

Objectives of Family-Oriented Nursing

The objectives of family-oriented nursing are as follows:

- To identify health and nursing needs and problems of each family.
- To ensure family's understanding and acceptance of those needs and problems.
- To plan and provide nursing services with active participation of family members.
- To help families develop abilities to deal with their health needs and health problems independently.

Approaches for Family Nursing

Various approaches of family nursing are as follows:

- Family as a context
- Family as a client
- Family as a system
- Family as a component of society
- To educate, counsel and guide family members.

Principles of Family-Oriented Nursing

Various principles of family-oriented nursing are as follows:

- Family nursing is family focused.
- Nurse must establish good relationship with the family.
- Family health nursing is part of family healthcare services.
- It should be realistic in terms of resources available.
- Family as a unit is responsible for their members health.
- Family should be related to the community where it lives.

- Health education, counseling, guidance and supervision are integral part of family nursing.
- Effective recording and reporting are essential.

Initial Information to be Gathered from a Family

Here is a list of information to be gathered from a family, initially:

- Medical history
- Ethnic background
- Religion
- Education
- Occupation
- Abuse if any
- Smoking and alcohol
- Income
- Location

PROGRESSIVE PATIENT CARE

Progressive patient care is one of the nursing care concepts. The concept began to take shape in the middle of 1950s, the overall aim of this concept was to organize hospital services in such way that the patient receives optimum care according to his/her medical and nursing needs.

Under progressive patient care system, the patient is classified and placed in different units of the hospital according to the needs and not according to the medical diagnosis. The patient may need intensive care or long-term care and accordingly he/she is admitted to the appropriate unit irrespective of the medical diagnosis.

Definitions

Various definitions of progressive patient care are as follows:

- Progressive patient care is described as the organization of the hospital facilities' services and staff around the changing medical and nursing needs of the patient.
- Progressive patient care is the area where the patient is nursed in different units according to the illness suffered.

Principle Elements of Progressive Patient Care

Various principle elements of progressive patient care (PPC) are shown in Figure 11.6.

- **Intensive care:** It is for critically ill patients who receive intensive care round the clock, who need constant attention, are being admitted to intensive care unit (ICU). The purpose of this unit is lifesaving.
- **Intermediate care:** When condition improves and vital functions are stabilized, the patient no longer needs the close attention by the nurses. Now the patient is transferred to the intermediate care unit.
- **Convalescent or self-care:** It is for the ambulatory patient who is mostly self-sufficient in terms and needs daily care requirement. Self-care patient requires minimal nursing care.
- **Long-term care:** It is for chronically ill patient or disabled patient who requires nursing care for a prolonged period. Rehabilitation is an occupational therapy although physical therapy may be needed for such patients. Patient teaching is emphasized with a view to help these patients learn how to adjust to their illness and disabilities.

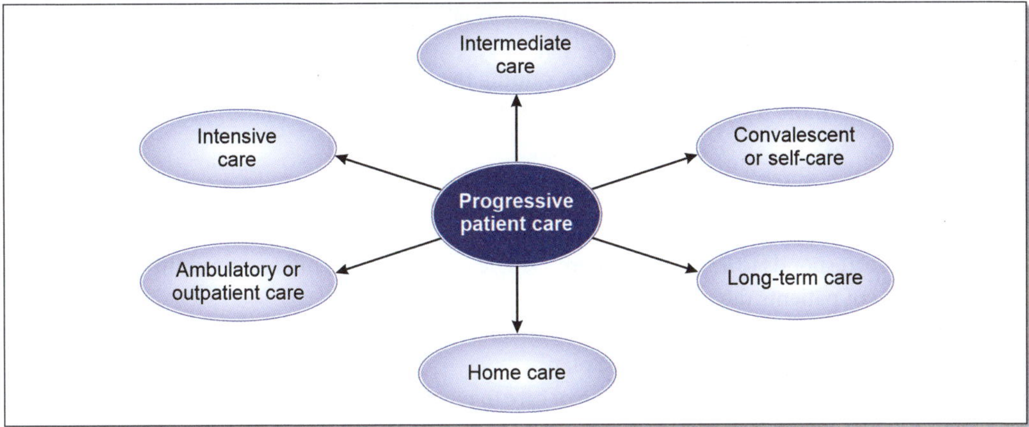

Figure 11.6: Elements of progressive patient care

- **Home care:** Home care is for patients who can be adequately cared for in the home through the extension of certain services. A hospital care-based care program provides staff equipment and supplies for the patient.
- **Ambulatory or outpatient care:** It is for the ambulatory patient requiring simple diagnostic, curative, preventive and rehabilitative services.

Advantages of Progressive Patient Care

The advantages of progressive patient care are as follows:

- Clients receive specialized attention when they need it.
- Assistance in making the adjustment to the hospital and later to home and community.
- Nurses can make effective use of special skills and capabilities.
- Placement can be made according to the skills and competencies of nursing staff.
- Team can include semi-skilled staff to extend the nursing services to low-risk patients, under the guidance of qualified registered nurses.
- Nurses can deliver increased and improved quality of nursing services.
- Hospitals can enhance the quality of patient care as a result of effective and efficient use of personnel.
- Hospitals can maintain continuity of care and coordinate home care services.

Disadvantages of Progressive Patient Care

Some of the disadvantages of progressive patient care are as follows:

- There may be discomfort to the client who is moved often.
- Long-term nurse-client relationships are difficult to manage.
- There is often difficulty in meeting the administrative needs of the organization's staffing, evaluation and accreditation.

PERSON-CENTERED CARE

In this method, care is delivered according to the scientific method, starting with the identification of the nursing care needs, the definition of priorities, planning, implementation, and evaluation of interventions and providing individualized and personalized care to the patient as an interconnected and integrated whole.

It is a part of the humanistic perspective, valuing the relationship and the concern for the other, where the whole is more than the sum of its parts. Thus, it comes closer to the systemic-contingency perspectives.

Individual Method—Case Method or Total Patient Care

This method corresponds to a situation where a single nurse assumes full responsibility for delivering care to a group of patients during the shift.

Although, care is not fragmented, its coordination does not prevail between shifts, and changes may occur in the established nursing care plan.

In this method, the overall organization of care to meet the needs identified by the nurse depends on the nurse's view of his/her role as a professional and may prioritize the patient or the performance of tasks. In addition, because the individual method limits the nurses' actions during a shift and the patient(s) to which he/she is allocated, outcome evaluation is based only on circumstantial objectives.

The coordination of the care delivered to all patients in the unit is under the responsibility of a single nurse, usually the head nurse, who supervises and evaluates the delivery of nursing care and makes the most significant decisions throughout the process. However, the delivery of care in the shift is delegated to the nurse allocated to that shift.

Advantages

Some of the advantages of individual method—case method or total patient care are as follows:

- The individualization of care, with satisfaction of patient's needs.
- Promotion of the nurse–patient relationship.
- The patient can identify the nurse who provides care in a given shift, resulting in a close, humanized, and personalized care.
- It also reinforces the confidence in the nurse and the patient's safety.

Team Nursing

Team nursing originated in the 1950s and 1960s. It involves use of a team leader and to provide various aspects of nursing care to a group of patients. Mostly team nursing was never practiced in the purest form but was instead a combination of team and functional structure.

It is a decentralized system in which the care of a patient is distributed among the members of a group working in coordinated manner. Team nursing is a care delivery model that assigns staff to teams (Fig. 11.7). A unit may be divided into teams and each team is led by a registered nurse.

In team nursing, medications might be given by one nurse while bath and physical care are given by a nursing assistant under the supervision of a nurse team leader. Skill mixes include experienced and specially qualified nurses to nursing orderlies (Fig. 11.8). The quality of patient care with this system is questionable, and fragmentation of care is of concern.

Small team requires less communication, better use of members' time for direct patient care activities. Team nursing is a care delivery model that assigns staff to teams who are then responsible for a group of patients. A unit may be divided into two teams, and each team is led by a registered nurse. The team leader supervises and coordinates all the care provided by those on his team.

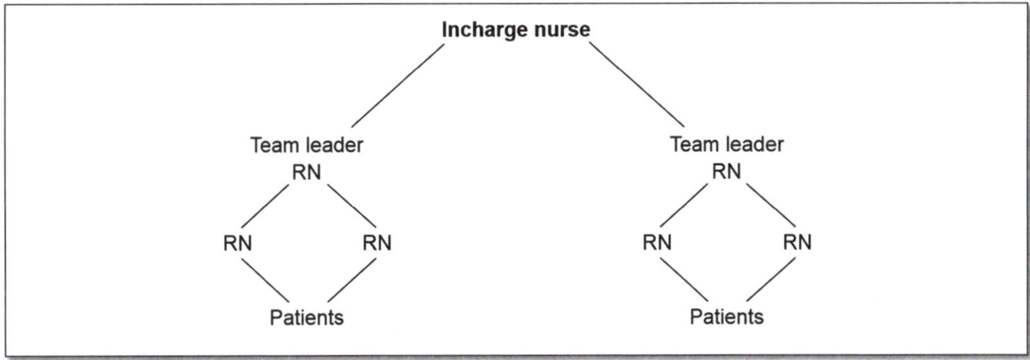

Figure 11.7: Team nursing model

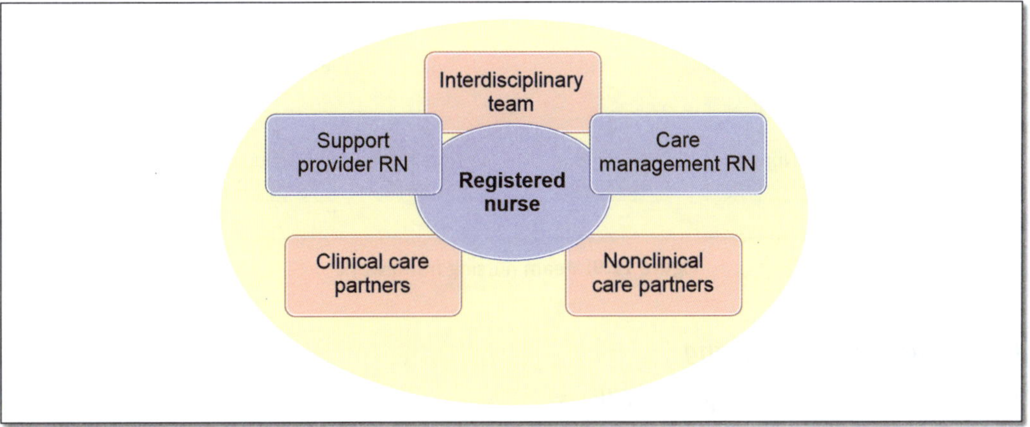

Figure 11.8: Team nursing

Abbreviation: RN, registered nurse

The nurse is responsible for condition and needs of all the patients assigned to him/her and for planning individual care.

Objective

To provide the best patient-centered care.

Team Nursing Framework

The team nursing framework is shown in Figure 11.9.

Responsibilities of Team Leader

The team leader's duties vary depending on the patient's needs and the work load. Duties of team leader are:

- To assist team members
- To provide direct care to patient
- To teach
- To coordinate patient activities
- To divide work
- To provide professional direction

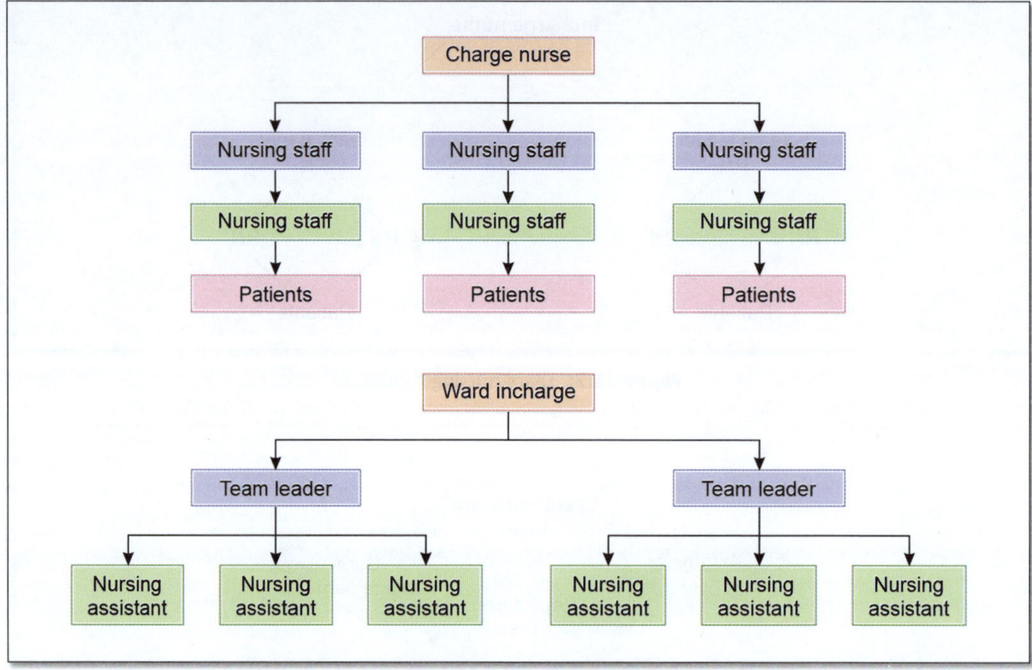

Figure 11.9: Team nursing framework

Advantages of Team Nursing

The advantages of team nursing are as follows:

- Team nursing allows members to contribute their own special expertise or skills.
- By recognition of individual worth of all employees and giving autonomy to team members, team nursing provides high job satisfaction.
- Nurses help one another more readily. Nurse is more eager to assist his/her peers without being asked. Every nurse knows something about all the patients.
- The team concept pairs expert nurses with novices, which helps boost retention rates.
- Less experienced nurses have gains significant self-confidence, patient care skills and efficiency.

Disadvantages of Team Nursing

Few of the disadvantages of team nursing are as follows:

- Improper implementation.
- Insufficient time for team care planning and communication. Communication barriers may cause some problems in rendering patient care.

Responsibilities of a Team Nurse

The various responsibilities of a team nurse are as follows:

- Coordinating the team members' actions with respect to implementing total patient care.
- Serving as a role model for each member.

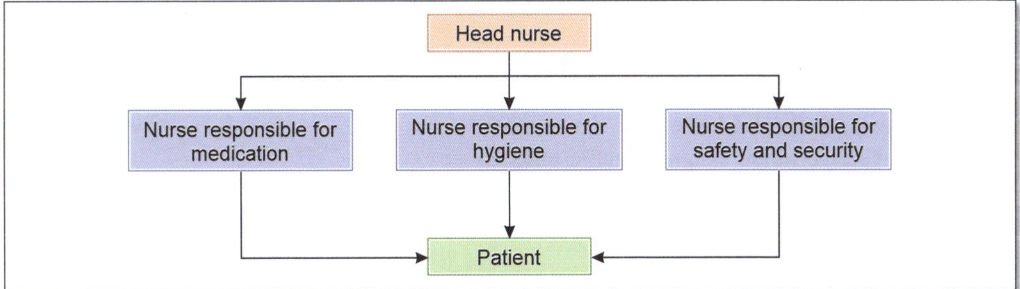

Figure 11.10: Structure of the functional nursing method

- Performing any delicate task to be done on the patient which is outside the scope of a team member's knowledge and capacity.
- Planning patient's care.
- Coordinating with team members.
- Filling in for any team member who is unavailable.
- Observing the implementation done by the members.

FUNCTIONAL NURSING METHOD

The functional nursing method became popular during World War II, given the need for nurses to care for many wounded people in hospital settings. The delivery of nursing care was based on the distribution of standardized tasks by the nurses, who achieved proficiency through the systematic repetition of techniques such as intravenous drug administration and monitoring of vital signs (Fig. 11.10).

Functional Nursing—Task Oriented

Functional nursing, also known as task nursing, focuses on the distribution of work based on the performance of tasks and procedures, where the target of the action is not the patient but rather the task. The work is thus broken down into tasks performed by different professionals, from a mechanistic perspective. Functional nursing was designed around an efficacy model that seeks to get many tasks accomplished in a short period. It is task-oriented in scope. Instead of one primary nurse performing many functions, several nurses are given one or two assignments. The focus of functional nursing is getting the job done. This method divides the work to be done with each person being responsible to the nurse in charge (Fig. 11.11). It is suitable for short term use.

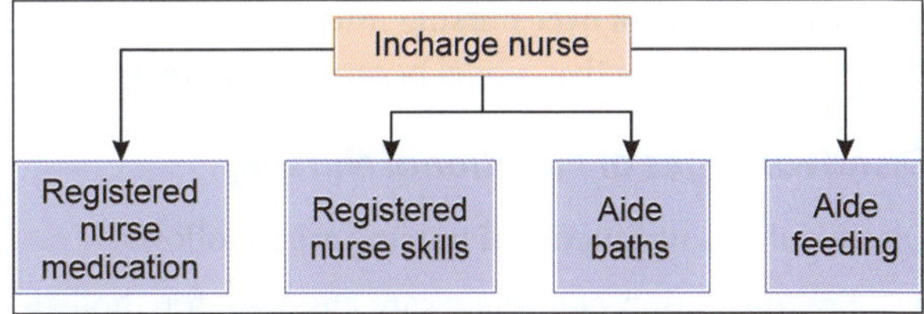

Figure 11.11: Model of functional nursing—task oriented

Assignment of Tasks

In functional nursing, separate tasks are assigned to each nurse based on:

- The difficulty of the task or skill to be performed.
- The ability and qualification of the nurse.

Division of Tasks

In this method, nursing care is divided into tasks like medication administration, dressing change and other treatments, baths and beds, vital signs and so on. Head or Charge nurse assigns specific tasks to each staff member (Fig. 11.12).

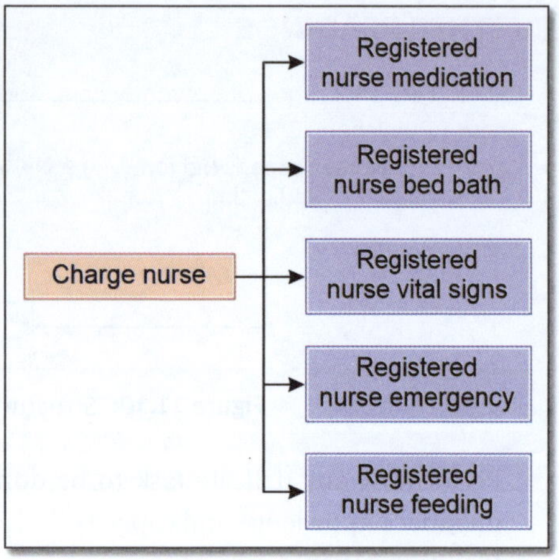

Impact of Functional Nursing

Impact of Functional Nursing on Unit

Some of the impacts of functional nursing on the unit are as follows:

- Things get done.
- There is an efficient use of staff.
- It is cost-effective.

Figure 11.12: Division of task

Impact of Functional Nursing on Staff

Following are the impacts of functional nursing on staff:

- Often boring to do only one thing all day.
- Little growth.
- Client gets fragmented care.
- Patient has no one who really knows all about his needs.

Advantages of Functional Nursing

Advantages of functional nursing are as follows:

- The repetitive nature of only doing one thing lends itself to the staff member acquiring the skill faster.
- It allows most work to be accomplished in short-time.
- Workers learn to work fast.
- Workers gain skills fast.
- Greater control over nursing interventions.
- It is a cost-effective model because fewer registered nurses are needed.

Disadvantages of Functional Nursing

Disadvantages of functional nursing are as follows:

- Fragmentation of nursing care and therefore holistic care is not achieved.
- Nurses' accountability and responsibility are diminished.
- Patients cannot identify who their "real nurse" is.
- Nurse–patient relationship is not fully developed.
- Evaluation of nursing care is poor and outcomes are rarely documented.
- It is difficult to find specific person who can answer the patient's relatives' questions.
- Holistic care is not achieved.
- Staff feels boredom to do same work.
- Staff performs task only without responsibility.

FURTHER READINGS

- Park K. Park's Textbook of Preventive and Social Medicine, 25th edition. Jabalpur, India: Banarsidas Bhanot Publishers; 2019.
- Parreira P, Santos-Costa P, Neri M, Marques A, Queiros P, Salgueiro-Oliveira A. Work Methods for Nursing Care Delivery. Int J Environ Res Public Health. 2021;18(4):2088.
- Wessel S L, Manthey M, Smith R. Primary Nursing: Person-Centered Care Delivery System Design, 1st edition. Minneapolis, MN: Creative Healthcare Management; 2015.

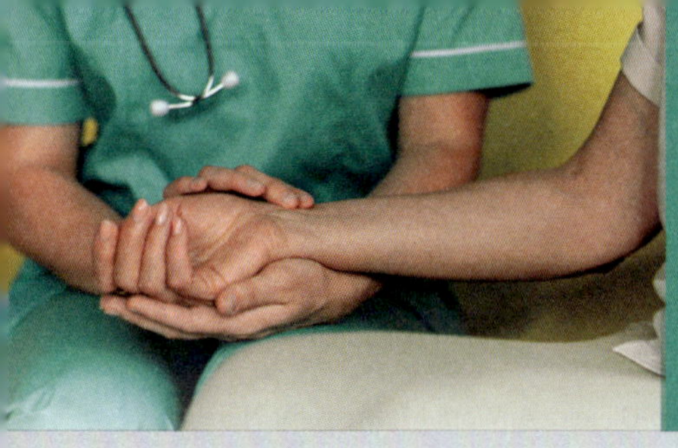

STUDENT ASSIGNMENT

LONG ANSWER QUESTIONS

1. What are the principles and characteristics of primary healthcare?
2. Discuss the advantages and disadvantages of functional nursing.
3. What is team nursing? Discuss the various advantages of team nursing.
4. What is family-oriented nursing? Discuss the various objectives of the same.

SHORT ANSWER QUESTION

1. Write about:
   a. Functional nursing
   b. Team nursing
   c. Holistic nursing

MULTIPLE CHOICE QUESTIONS

1. **As well as taking a holistic approach, nurses ensure the care they provide is ______.**
   a. Of a quality acceptable to the nurse
   b. Of a quality acceptable to the patient
   c. Of the highest quality
   d. Of a good quality
2. **Nurses work ______.**
   a. Independently
   b. As part of a multidisciplinary team
   c. In partnership with patients
   d. All of the above
3. **Patients value nurses who ______.**
   a. Care for them as individuals
   b. Make them feel more comfortable
   c. Make them feel less afraid
   d. All of the above
4. **Nurses on a unit provide personal hygiene, administer medications, educate the patient and family about treatments, and provide emotional support. These nurses provide patient care based on which nursing delivery system?**
   a. Total patient care
   b. Partnership nursing
   c. Team nursing
   d. Functional nursing

5. **The nurse manager is planning staffing levels and realizes that the first step is to:**
   a. Know the intensity of care needed by patients according to physical and psychosocial factors.
   b. Examine the educational level of the staff.
   c. Assess the skill level of the staff.
   d. Review the budget to determine the financial consequences of past staffing patterns.

6. **A nursing unit is comparing team nursing to the partnership model and finds that:**
   a. With the partnership model, the RN does not have to be a part of the mix.
   b. Leadership abilities of the RN is a major determinant of effectiveness of care for both models.
   c. The RN teaches the LPN/LVN or unlicensed assistive personnel (UAP) how to apply the nursing process in team nursing.
   d. With team nursing the RN cares for the patient while the team members work with the family or significant others.

ANSWER KEY

1. c   **2.** d   **3.** d   **4.** a   **5.** a   **6.** b

Note

12

Communication

LEARNING OBJECTIVES

After the completion of the chapter, the readers will be able to:
- Discuss communication, its forms and barriers.
- Understand the principles of communication.

CHAPTER OUTLINE

- Communication
- Principles of Communication
- Levels of Communication
- Models of Communication
- Types of Communication
- Organizational Communication
- Communication Network Pattern
- Barriers to Communication
- Precautions While Communicating

KEY TERMS

Credibility: The quality that somebody has that makes people believe or trust him/her.

Formal: Appear serious or official in situations in which you do not know the other people very well.

Probability: A measure of the likelihood of an event to occur.

COMMUNICATION

The word communication has been derived from the Latin word 'communis' which means common. Communication therefore refers to the sharing of ideas, opinion, information and understanding.

Definitions

The various definitions of communication are as follows:

- Communication is the process of passing information and understanding from one person to another. It is essentially a bridge of meaning between people. By using this bridge of meaning a person can safely cross the river of misunderstanding that separates all people. —**Prof. Dasgupta**
- Sending, giving or exchanging ideas and information, which it often expressed nonverbally or verbally.   —**Webster**
- The act or process of transmitting information.
- Communication is the process whereby speech, signs, actions transmit information from one person to another.
- The art and technique of using words effectively to import information or ideas.
- Communication is the process of transmitting thoughts, feelings, facts and other information including verbal and nonverbal behavior.
- The importing or exchanging of information or news.
- Passage or an opportunity or means of passage.

Objectives of Communication

The various objectives of communication are as follows:

- To develop information and understanding.
- To foster an attitude necessary for motivation, cooperation and job satisfaction.
- To discourage the spread of misinformation, rumors, gossip and to release the emotional tensions of workers.
- To encourage ideas and suggestions from subordinates for an improvement in the product and work conditions.
- To improve relationships.
- To ensure free exchange of information and ideas.
- To maintain social relations among human beings.

Process of Communication

The process of communication (Fig. 12.1) consists of the following steps or stages:
- **Message:** This is the background step to the process of communication; which, by forming the subject matter of communication necessitates the start of a communication process. The message might be a factor, an idea, or a request, or a suggestion, or an order, or a grievance.
- **Sender:** The actual process of communication is initiated by the sender; who takes steps to send the message to the recipient.
- **Encoding:** Encoding means giving a form and meaning to the message through expressing it into—words, symbols, gestures, graphs, drawings, etc.

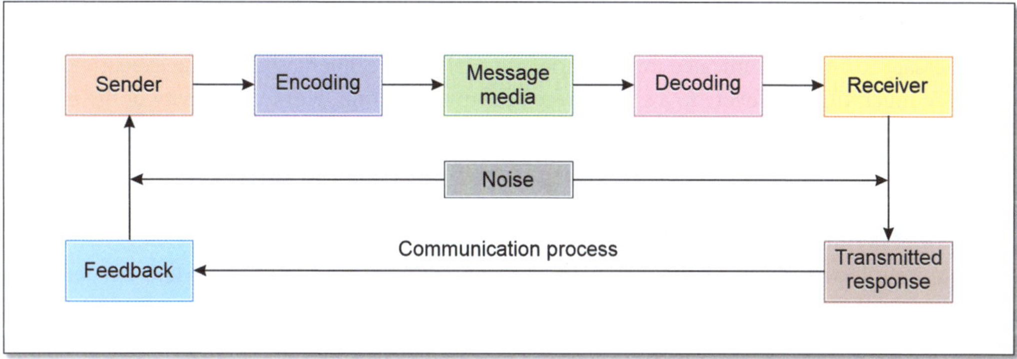

Figure 12.1: Communication process

- **Medium:** It refers to the method or channel through which the message is to be conveyed to the recipient. For example, an oral communication might be made through a peon or over the telephone, etc. while a written communication might be routed through a letter or a notice displayed on the notice board, etc.
- **Recipient (or the Receiver):** Technically, a communication is complete, only when it comes to the knowledge of the intended person, i.e., the recipient or the receiver.
- **Decoding:** Decoding means the interpretation of the message by the recipient with a view to get the meaning of the message, as per the intentions of the sender.
- **Feedback:** To complete the communication process, sending feedback to communication by the recipient to the sender is imperative. 'Feedback' implies the reaction or response of the recipient to the message, comprised in the communication.
- **Interpersonal variables:** These are the factors within both the sender and receiver that influence communication. For example, perception, educational and development levels.
- **Environment:** It is the setting for sender-receiver interaction. For effective communication the environment should meet participant's needs for physical and emotional comfort and safety.

PRINCIPLES OF COMMUNICATION

Principle of Understanding

Communication must be such, which transmits understanding of the communication message to the recipient, as per the intentions of the sender. Practical application of the principle is that the message must be clearly expressed whether made orally or in writing. Further, the message must be complete – leaving no scope for any doubts likely to confuse the recipient and compel him towards a misinterpretation of the message.

Principle of Attention

Communication must be made in such a manner that in invites the attention of the recipient to it. Practical application of the principle, is imperative. Not only the message must be expressed in a pleasant and sound manner but also the purpose of the sender in making communication must be absolutely clarified.

Principle of Brevity

The message to be communicated must be brief as usually the recipient, specially an executive, would not have much time to devote to a single piece of communication. However, brevity of the message must not be sought at the cost of clarity or completeness of the message. The sender must strike a balance among these three factors—brevity, clarity and completeness.

Principle of Timeliness

The communication must be timely, i.e., it must be made at the high time, when needed to be communicated to the recipient. An advance communication carries with it the danger of 'forgetting', on the part of the recipient, while a delayed communication loses its purpose and charm, and becomes meaningless, when the right time for action on it has expired.

Principle of Appropriateness (Or Rationality)

The communication must be appropriate or rational, in the context of the realization of organizational objectives. Communication must be neither impracticable to act upon; nor irrational, making no contribution to common objectives.

Principle of Feedback

Communication must be a two-way process. The feedback (or reaction or response) of the recipient to the message, must be as easily transferable to the sender, as the original communication made by the sender. The idea behind emphasizing on the feedback aspect of communication is that it helps the sender to modify his subsequent communications in view of the reactions of the recipient–making for better and improved human relations.

Principle of the Constructive and Strategic use of Informal Groups

The management must not hesitate in making a constructive and strategic use of informal groups, for ensuring and facilitating speedier communication in emergency situations. Such a use of informal groups would also help to develop good human relations by upgrading the status of informal groups and their leaders.

Principle of Clarity

The idea or message to be communicated should be clearly spelt out. It should be worded in such a way that the receiver understands the same thing which the sender wants to convey. There should be no ambiguity in the message. It should be kept in mind that the words do not speak themselves but the speaker gives them the meaning. A clear message will evoke the same response from the other party. It is also essential that the receiver is conversant with the language, inherent assumptions, and the mechanics of communication.

Principle of Informality

Formal communication is generally used for transmitting messages and other information. Sometimes formal communication may not achieve the desired results, informal communication may prove effective in such situations. Management should use informal communication for assessing the reaction of employees towards various policies. Senior management may informally convey certain decisions to the employees for getting their feedbacks. So this principle states that informal communication is as important as formal communication.

Principle of Consistency

This principle states that communication should always be consistent with the policies, plans, programs and objectives of the organization and not in conflict with them. If the messages and communications are in conflict with the policies and programs then there will be confusion in the minds of subordinates and they may not implement them properly. Such a situation will be detrimental to the interests of the organization.

LEVELS OF COMMUNICATION

Various levels of communication are as follows:

- Interpersonal
- Therapeutic
- Social
- Transpersonal
- Structured
- Organizational

MODELS OF COMMUNICATION

Communication model is a pictorial representation of the communication process, ideas, thoughts or concepts through diagram.

Communication models help (Fig. 12.2) in understanding the potential barriers to effective communication, roles of different elements involved and the importance of feedback for successful communication.

Types of Communication Models

A communication model is a pictorial representation of the communication process, ideas, thoughts, or concepts through diagrams, etc. Communication models help in understanding the potential barriers to effective communication, roles of different elements involved, and the importance of feedback for successful communication. By applying the models of communication, individuals and organizations can enhance their communication skills and improve the interaction quality.

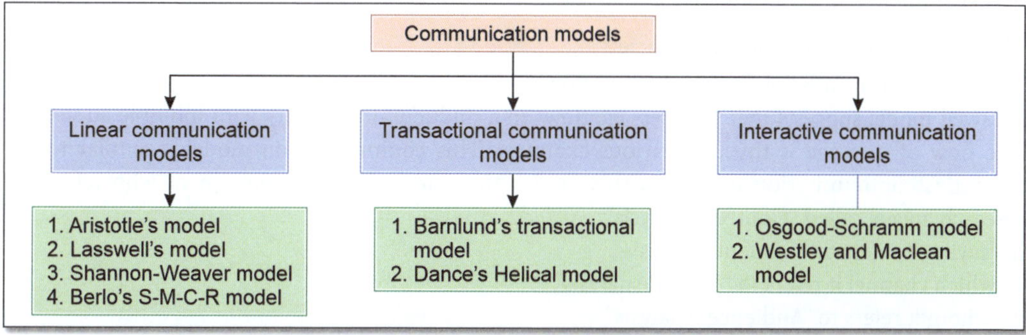

Figure 12.2: Types of communication models

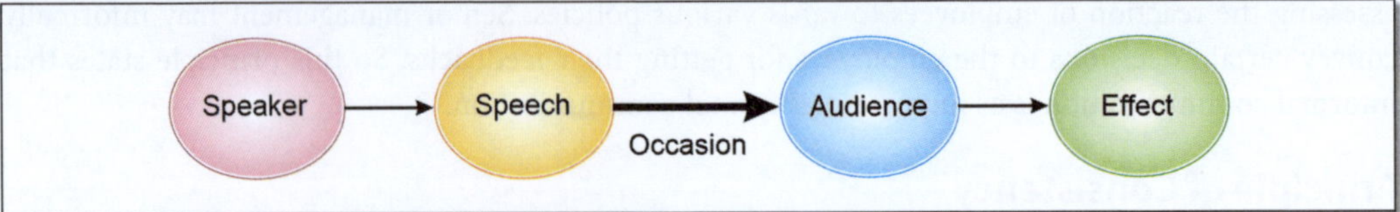

Figure 12.3: Aristotle model of communication

Linear Communication Model

Linear model of communication depicts one-way communication and are used to communicate with the masses. Linear model of communication are models where the sender sends the message and the receiver only receives the message. There is no concept of feedback involved. Linear model of communication is of four types. The introduction of noise may affect clear communication in these four types of communication models.

1. Aristotle Model of Communication

Aristotle, a great philosopher initiated the earliest mass communication model called "Aristotle's Model of Communication" (Fig. 12.3). He proposed model before 300 B.C. He found the importance of audience's role in communication chain in his communication model. This model is more focused on public speaking than interpersonal communication.

Aristotle's model of communication is formed with five basic elements:

(i) Speaker, (ii) Speech, (iii) Occasion, (iv) Audience and (v) Effect.

Aristotle advises speakers to build speech for different audience at different time (occasion), for different effects.

2. Lasswell's Model of Communication

Harold Dwight Lasswell, the American political scientist states that a convenient way to describe an act of communication is to answer the following questions.

- Who
- Says What
- In Which Channel
- To Whom
- With what effect?

This model (Fig. 12.4) is about process of communication and its functions to the society. According to Lasswell there are three functions for communication are:

1. Surveillance of the environment
2. Correlation of components of society
3. Cultural transmission between generation

Lasswell model suggests that the message flows in a multicultural society with multiple audiences. The flow of message is through various channels. This communication model is similar to the Aristotle's communication model. In this model, the communication component who refers the research area is called "Control Analysis",

Says what it refers to "Content Analysis",

In which channel it refers to "Media Analysis",

To whom it refers to "Audience Analysis",

With what effect it refers to "Effect Analysis"

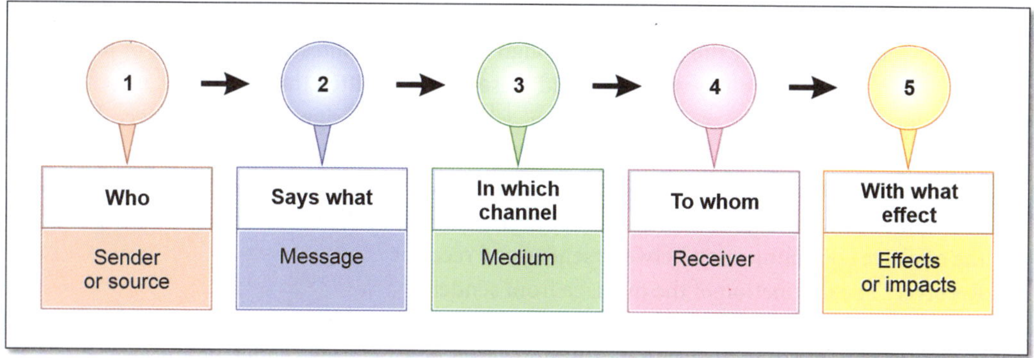

Figure 12.4: Lasswell's communication model

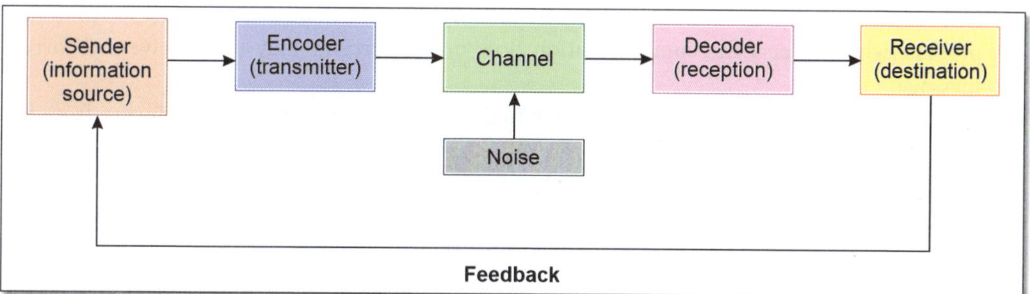

Figure 12.5: The Shannon-Weaver model of communication

3. Shannon and Weaver Model of Communication

In 1948,Claude Shannon an American mathematician, electronic engineer at Bell Telephone Company and Weaver an American scientist joined together to write an article in "Bell System Technical Journal" called "A Mathematical Theory of Communication" and also called as "Shannon-Weaver model of communication" (Fig. 12.5).

As the Shannon-Weaver model suggests, a message begins at a source, is then relayed through a transmitter where it is sent using a signal towards a receiver. This message travels from sender to receiver while encountering all kinds of noise (sources of interference). The last step is for the receiver of the message to let the source know if the message was understood. This is referred as "Feedback" and is a repeat of the communication process described here but for the "Receiver" back to the "Sender".

This model is specially designed to develop the effective communication between sender and receiver. Also they found factors which affect the communication process called "Noise". At first the model was developed to improve the technical communication. Later it was widely applied in the field of communication.

The model deals with various concepts like information source, transmitter, noise, channel, message, receiver, channel, information destination, encode and decode.

- **Sender:** The originator of message or the information source, selects desired message
- **Encoder:** The transmitter which converts the message into signals

Note: The sender's messages converted into signals like waves or binary data which is compactable to transmit the messages through cables or satellites. For example, in telephone, the voice is converted into wave signals and these are transmitted through cables

- **Decoder:** The reception place of the signal which converts signals into message. A reverse process of encode
  Note: The receiver converts those binary data or waves into message which is comfortable and understandable for receiver. Otherwise receiver can't receive the exact message and it will affect the effective communication between sender and receiver
- **Receiver:** The destination of the message from sender
  Note: Based on the decoded message the receiver gives their feedback to sender. If the message distracted by noise, it will affect the communication flow between sender and receiver
- **Noise:** The messages are transferred from encoder to decoder through channel. During this process, the messages may get distracted or affected by physical noise like horn sounds, thunder and crowd noise or encoded signals may be distracted in the channel during the transmission process, which affects the communication flow or the receiver may not receive the correct message.
- **Feedback:** It is information that is sent back to the source. It can come in many forms, from the "receiver falling asleep to a verbal message". Feedback tells the sender how accurately you have decoded the message, and how you have decided to respond to it. Communication is a flowing process that moves from a sender to receiver and back again. Communication does not start and stop or move from one direction to another. It is a flowing process.

4. Berlo's SMCR Model of Communication

David Berlo's SMCR Model of Communication represents the process of communication in its simplest form. The acronym SMCR stands for Sender, Message, Channel, and Receiver.

Berlo's SMCR Model of Communication (1960) describes the different components that form the basic process of communication. Because this communication tool also emphasises the coding and decoding of the message, it can be used for more efficient communication Figure 12.6.

Berlo's SMCR Model of Communication includes four components that describe the communication process. The different components in the model are influenced by various factors.

Sender

The sender of the message is the source who creates and sends the message to the receiver. The source is the start of the communication process and is the person who encodes the message.

Factors that may influence the sender are also applicable to the receiver. Consider how the message is interpreted Berlo's SMCR Model of Communication identifies the following factors that affect the source:

- **Communication skills:** Communication skills include: Reading, listening, speaking etc.
- **Attitude:** One's attitude in relationship to the audience, receiver and subject changes the meaning and consequence of the message.
- **Knowledge:** Familiarity with the subject of the message makes communication more effective.
- **Social systems:** Values, beliefs, religion and rules influence the way in which the sender communicates the message, alongside location and circumstances.
- **Culture:** Cultural differences may result in the message being interpreted differently.

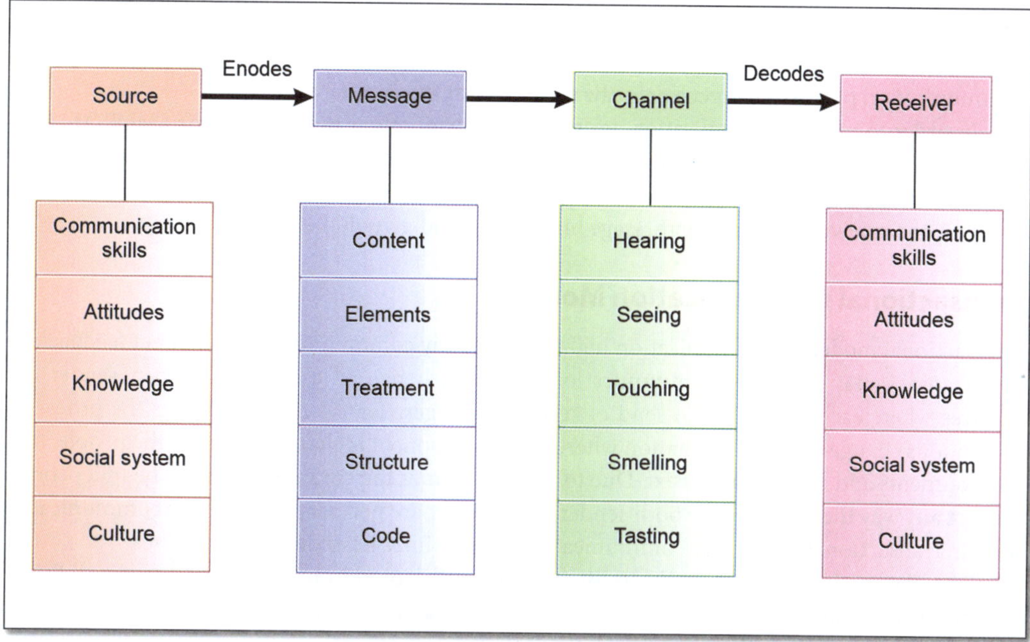

Figure 12.6: Berlo's SMCR model of communication

Message

The message is the package of information or meaning that is sent from sender to receiver. The message can be sent in various forms, such as audio, speech, text, video or other media.

The sender of the messages always wants the receiver to interpret the message in a certain way. The source's intention is therefore translated into a coded message. The receiver should understand the message with reasonable accuracy. The message is influenced by:

- **Content:** The content of the message from beginning to end.
- **Elements:** Elements are (non) verbal aspects, such as gestures and signs, that may influence the message.
- **Treatment:** Treatment refers to the way in which the message is sent, the message's packaging.
- **Structure:** As the word suggests, the structure of the message refers to the way in which it is structured.
- **Code:** The code of the message is the form in which the message is sent. This may include text, language, video, gestures, music, etc.

Channel

The channel is the medium used to send the message. The medium must be able to be picked up by the sensory system of the receiver and may therefore involve vision, sound, smell, taste or touch. Humans have the following senses:

- Hearing
- Touching
- Tasting
- Seeing
- Smelling

Mass communication always involves technical tools, such as phones, the Internet and television. In these cases, the transmitted information is assimilated via vision and sound.

Receiver

The receiver is the person who receives and subsequently decodes the coded message. In a linear communication process, the receiver is always located at the end.

In order to make communication as effective and smooth as possible, Berlo's SMCR Model of Communication assumes the receiver's thinking pattern must be in accordance with that of the sender. The same factors therefore influence this component in Berlo's SMCR Model of Communication. After all, the receiver decodes the message him/herself and gives it their own meaning.

Transactional Communication Model

Transactional model of communication highlight two-way communication with direct feedback.

Transactional model of communication is the exchange of messages between sender and receiver where each take turns to send or receive messages. Transactional model is the process of continuous change and transformation where every component is changing such as the people, their environments and the medium used. Due to this, it assumes the communicators to be independent and act any way they want. Since both sender and receiver are necessary to keep the communication alive in transactional model, the communicators are also interdependent to each other.

The transactional model is the most general model of communication. Everyday talk and interactions are also a form of transactional model communication. It is more efficient for communicators with similar environment and individual aspects. For instance, communication between people who know each other is more efficient as they share same social system.

In transactional model, efficiency and reliability of communicated message also depends on the medium used. For example, the same message might not be perceived by a person the same way when it is sent through a phone and when it is provided face to face. It is because of possible loss of message on a phone call or absence of gestures.

1. Barnlund Transactional Model of Communication

Dean Barnlund proposed a transactional model of communication in 1970 for basic interpersonal communication which articulates that sending and receiving of messages happens simultaneously between people which is popularly known as Barnlund's Transactional Model of Communication.

Barnlund's Transactional Model is a multi-layered feedback system. This is a continuous process where sender and receiver interchange their places and both are equally important. The passing of message passing takes place with a constant feedback being provided by both parties. A feedback for one is the message for the other.

Components of Barnlund's Model

Cues refers to the signs for doing something. As per Barnlund there are:
- Public cues
- Private cues and
- Behavioral cues.
  In the model diagram shown in Figure 12.7, spiral lines give graphic representation to the assumptions like public cues and private cues.
- **Public cues (Cpu)** are physical, environmental or artificial and natural or man-made.
- **Private cues (Cpr)** are also known as private objects of orientation which include senses of a person. Both these cues can be verbal as well as non-verbal. Another set of cues are behavioral cues.

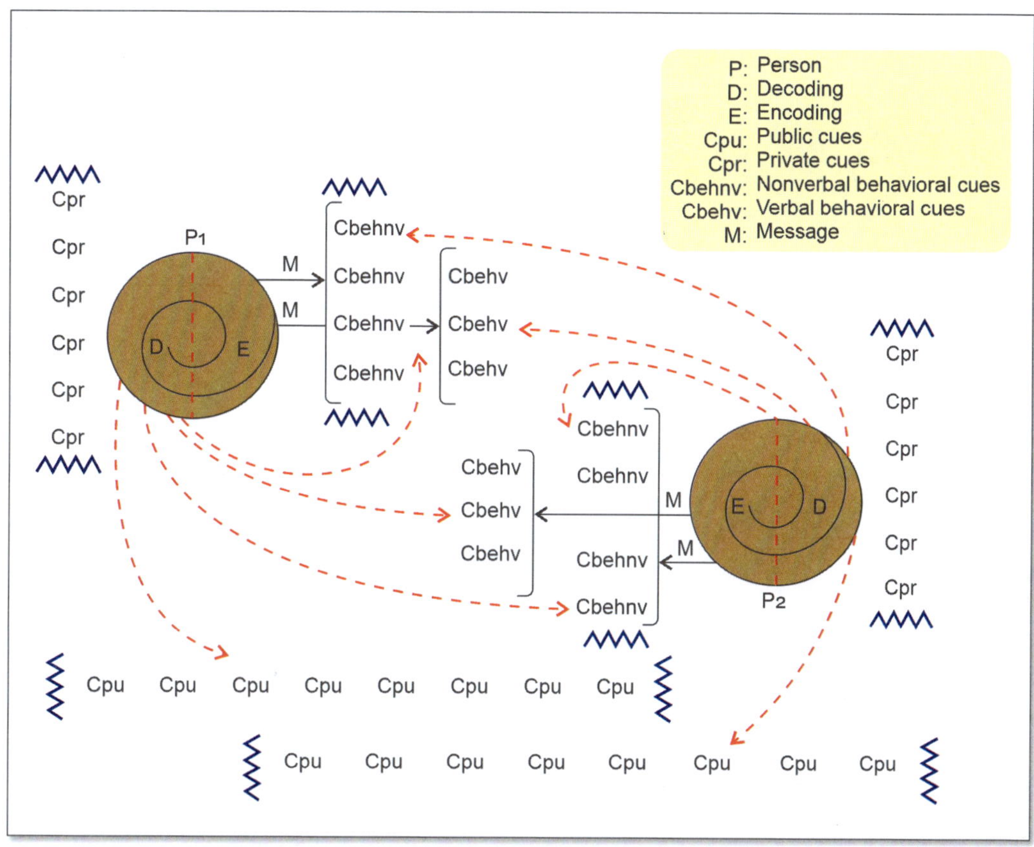

Figure 12.7: Barnlund transactional model of communication

- **Behavioral cues can be verbal (Cbehv)** as well as non-verbal (Cbehnv).
- The arrows and their directions show that the message is intentionally sent and actively taken where the receiver plays a key role of giving feedback. Arrows also show the process of production of technical encoding, interpretation and decoding.
- The **jagged lines** show that the availability of cues can be unlimited and are denoted as **VVVV**.
- The **valence signs**, +,0 and – are also attached to these types of cues which illustrates the amount/ degree/strength of attractiveness of the cues in the message.
- **Speech act** refers to a particular instance of communication in the model.
- **Filters** are the realities of people engaged in communication. Here the senders' and receivers' personal filters might differ according to cultures, traditions, content of the message, etc.
- **Noise** is the problem that arises in communication flow and disturbs the message flow.

2. Helical Model of Communication

In 1967, Frank Dance has proposed the communication model called Dance's Helix Model for a better communication process. The name helical comes from "Helix" which means an object having a three-dimensional shape like that of a wire wound uniformly around a cylinder or cone. He shows communication as a dynamic and non-linear process Figure 12.8.

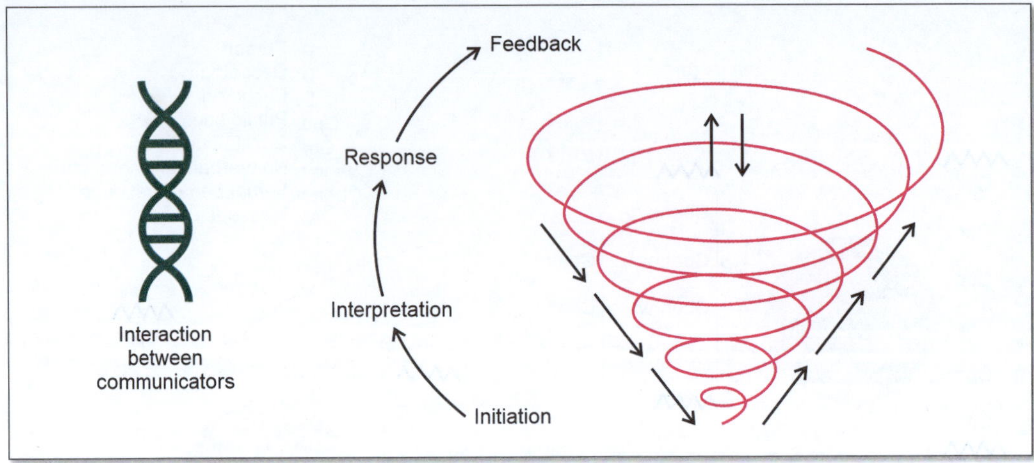

Figure 12.8: Dance's helical model

Explanation

Dance's model emphasized the difficulty of communication. Frank Dance uses the form of a helix to describe the communication process. He developed this theory based on a simple helix which gets bigger and bigger as it moves or grows. The main characteristics of a helical model of communication is that it is evolutionary.

Frank Dance explains the communication process based on this Helix structure and compares it with communication. In the helix structure, the bottom or starting is very small then it gradually moves upward in a back and forth circular motion which forms the bigger circle in the top and it is still moves further. The whole process takes some time to reach. As like helix, the communication process starts very slowly and defined small circle only. The communicators shared information only with a small portion of themselves to their relationships. Its gradually develops into next level but which will take some time to reach and expanding its boundaries to the next level. Later the communicators commit more and shared more portions by themselves.

The helical model of communication is largely dependent on its past. A child learns to pronounce a word in his elementary classes and throughout his life he uses that word in the same way he learnt. Just like that, we used to react to certain things in a certain way in our childhood and such reactions and habits lasts with us forever. The communication evolves in the beginning in some simple forms then the same process of communication functions and develops based on past activities. Thus, his way of communication or his reactions may also different from the past behavior and experiences. It develops further with modifications according to the situations.

Therefore the model concludes that the process of communication is like a continuous curve with some changes or flexibilities. The base of the helical curve (lower level) can be affected and/or altered at any time according the experience of an individual.

Interactive Communication Models

Interactional model of communication highlight a two-way communication with indirect feedback. The interactive communication models highlight that the feedback may get delayed when the messages are exchanged between the sender and receiver.

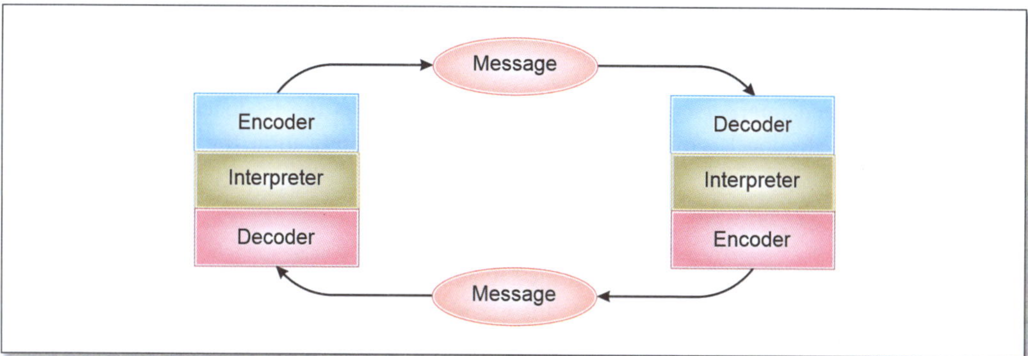

Figure 12.9: Osgood-Schramm/Circular model of communication

1. Osgood-Schramm Model of Communication

In 1954 Charles E. Osgood presented the theory of meaning. Wilbur Schramm changed this theory of meaning into a model and after this model became the Circular Model of communication or the Osgood-Schramm model of communication (Figure 12.9).

Charles E. Osgood was an American psychologist who developed the technique of measuring the 'connotative meaning' of the concept, known as semantic differential. Osgood was born in Somerville, Massachusetts and did his PhD from Yale University.

Wilbur Schramm was a scholar and also known as the authoritarian of mass communication. He was a great influencer of mass communication and was the one who established the departments of mass communication studies across the universities of the United States. He was the first person who called himself a communication scholar. Schramm did a pilot project called Mass Communication Program for his PhD in Lowa University.

The Osgood and Schramme model is about two way of communication between Sender and Receiver. Osgood popularized the statement that communication is circular rather linear, which requires sender and receiver for sharing their information.

It is a circular model, means that communication is something circular in nature

- **Encoder:** Who does encoding or Sends the message (message originates)
- **Decoder:** Who receives the message.
- **Interpreter:** Person trying to understand (analyses, perceive) or interpret

This model breaks the sender and receiver model and it seems communication in a practical way. It is not a traditional model. It can happen within, where, or between two people, where each person acts as both sender and receiver and hence uses interpretation. It simultaneously takes place, e.g., encoding, interpretation and decoding. Semantic noise is a concept introduced here that occurs when sender and receiver apply different meanings to the same message. It happens mostly because of words and phrases, e.g., technical language, certain words and phrases will cause you to deviate from the actual meaning of the communication.

2. Westley and MacLean's Model of Communication

In 1957 Westley and MacLean's model of communication was proposed by Bruce Westley (1915–1990) and Malcolm S. MacLean Jr (1913–2001). Being one of the creators of journalism studies, Westley served as a teacher at the University of Wisconsin, Madison, between 1946 and 1968.

Malcolm was director of University of Journalism School (1967–74) and co founder of the University College at University of Minnesota.

This model can be seen with two contexts—interpersonal and mass communication. The point of difference between interpersonal and mass communication is the feedback. In interpersonal communication, the feedback is direct and fast. In the mass communication, the feedback is indirect and slow.

Explanation

Westely and Maclean realized that communication does not begin when one person starts to talk, but rather when a person responds selectively to his/her physical surroundings. This model considers a strong relation between responses from surroundings and the process of communication. Communication begins only when a person receives message from surroundings. Each receiver responds to the message they received based on their object of orientation.

Components of the Westley and MacLean Model of Communication

Westley and MacLean Model of Communication consists of multiple components, which may sometimes cause confusion (Figure 12.10). However, the model is fairly easy to understand, as is explained per element below. Moreover, the elements are explained in the order in which they appear in contemporary communication.

Source (A): The source is the person who creates and sends a message.

Environment (X): The environment is the physical and psychological state in which the communication process is studied. This doesn't necessarily have to be the same room. Modern communication is a global process, after all.

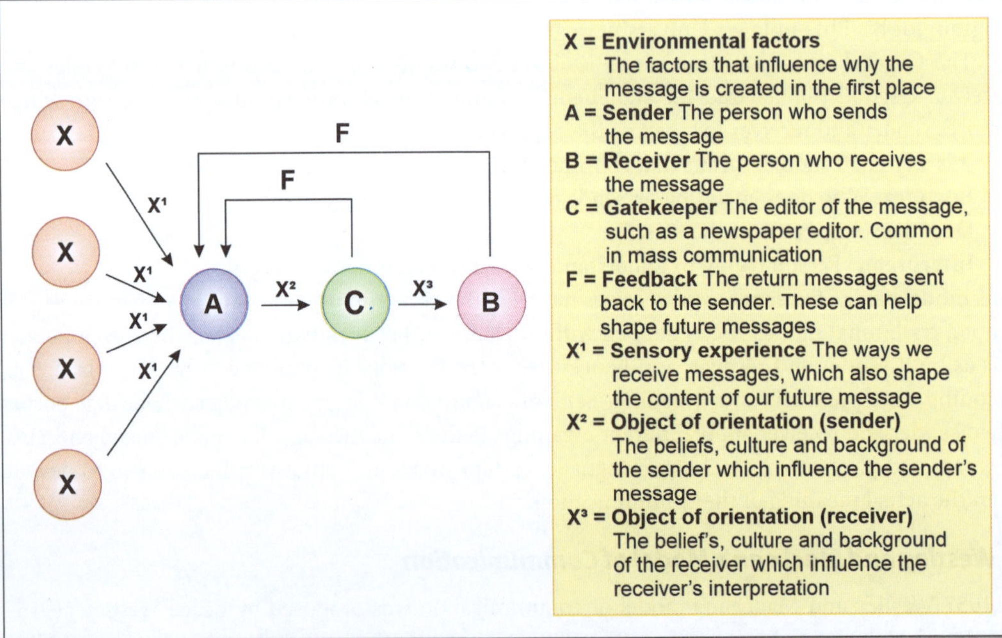

Figure 12.10: The Westley and MacLean's model of communication

Sensory Experience (X1): The sensory experience is the first thing the source sees that gives him/her the idea to write a message or comment.

Object of Orientation (X1, X2, …): Objects of orientation can be many different things. They are what the source is exposed to, both in a social and cultural context. In practice, this may be newsletters or a religious book. The objects of orientation make a person the person they are.

Coding of Interpretation (X'): The information is interpreted by the receiver. In other communication models, such as the Aristotle and Shannon and Weaver model, this component is referred to as decoding.

Receiver (B): Within the Westley and MacLean Model of Communication, the receiver is the person who receives the message from the source, and is the person who interprets the message through the various objects of orientation.

Object of Orientation Receiver (X,b): The beliefs and viewpoints of the receiver are also based on his or her past and objects of orientation. The way in which the information is interpreted is highly dependent on this.

Feedback (F): Once the initial message has been received, the receiver sends a message back to the source. This message is also known as feedback which is very. Crucial part of (interpersonal) communication.

Gatekeepers (C): Gatekeepers are present in mass communication. The gatekeeper is the person who ensures the message is filtered and tailored to the wishes of the public and media companies.

TYPES OF COMMUNICATION

Various types of communications are as follows:

- Nonverbal communication
- Verbal communication
- Written communication
- Symbolic communication
- Metacommunication

Nonverbal Communication

Nonverbal communication deals with the facial expressions and body motions. Nonverbal communication includes facial expression, body movements and gestures and is commonly referred to as body language.

It is considered more reliable because it conveys the emotional part of the message. Nonverbal communication occurs every time. Nonverbal communication includes all of the five senses.

Types of Nonverbal Communications

There are many kinds of nonverbal communication as given in (Fig. 12.11).

Verbal Communication

Verbal communication is when we communicate our messages verbally to the receiver. Verbal communication implies the use of words to convey ideas of the sender. The success of verbal communication is affected by a number of variables. The aim of verbal communication is to promote productive relationship between individuals or group of people.

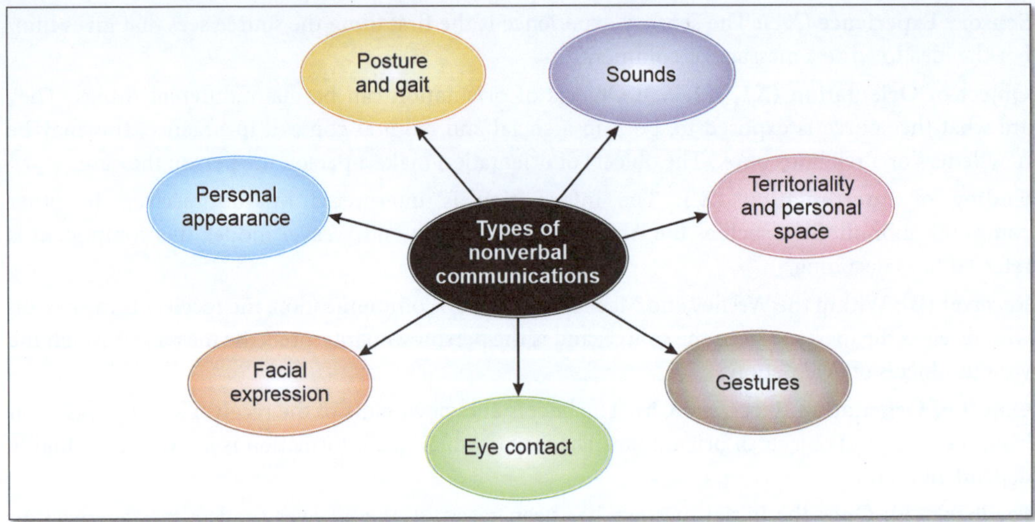

Figure 12.11: Types of nonverbal communications

Written Communication

Written communication is used most often. Many types of written communication are used in the organizations. Organization policy, procedures, events and changes may be announced in writing. Written communication is better for complex and difficult subjects, facts and opinions. Written communication provides opportunity to refer back. It can be circulated.

Symbolic Communication

Symbolic communication is the communication process in which people use symbols like words, gestures and images. Good communication requires awareness of symbolic communication, for example, art and music are forms of symbolic communication.

Metacommunication

Metacommunication is the process of communicating about communication. Metacommunication can be used as a tool for making sense or for understanding events, place, people, etc. Metacommu-nication is important for effective interpersonal interaction messages within a message. Metacommunication can help people understand better what they have communicated.

ORGANIZATIONAL COMMUNICATION

Basically, the two most important medias of communication in an organization are: (i) Formal communication and (ii) Informal communication.

Formal Communication

Formal communication is the easiest way to communicate in the workplace. The organizational chart lays out the reporting structure, lines of authority and channels of communication.

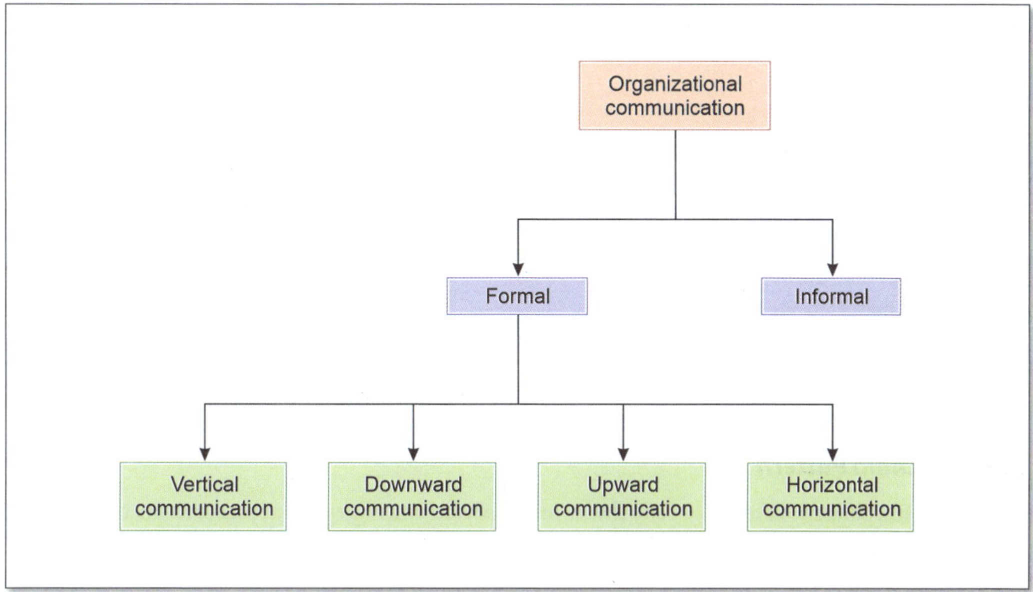

Figure 12.12: Organizational communication

The typical organizational structure looks like a pyramid, within the framework of the organizational structure, the formal channels of communication includes downward, upward, horizontal and matrix communication. Formal communications are those that are official, that are a part of the recognized communication system which is involved in the operation of the organization. A formal communication can be from a superior to a subordinate, from a subordinate to a superior, intra-administrative or external (Fig. 12.12).

Vertical Communication

Vertical communication is also known as upward and downward or interscalar communication. It is the one in which communication flows from top to bottom as well as from the rank-and-file workers toward the management.

Downward Communication

Downward communication is the transmission of ideas or information from nurse leaders to the subordinates. It is generally directive in the sense that it causes action to be initiated by the subordinates.

Upward Communication

Upward communication is getting messages from employees to management. It is difficult to achieve, especially in larger organizations.

Horizontal, Interscalar or Lateral Communication

Horizontal, interscalar or lateral communication is the communication from persons at one level in an organization to others at the same level. It is frequently between the line and staff units (Fig. 12.13).

Informal Communication

Informal communication grows out of the social interactions among people who work together. These are not found by any chart on the wall but are bound by customs and cultures. Such communication provides useful information for events to come in the format grapevine. Informal messages are generally transmitted in a variety of ways such as gestures, silence, written or oral messages. They are often transmitted by unofficial means.

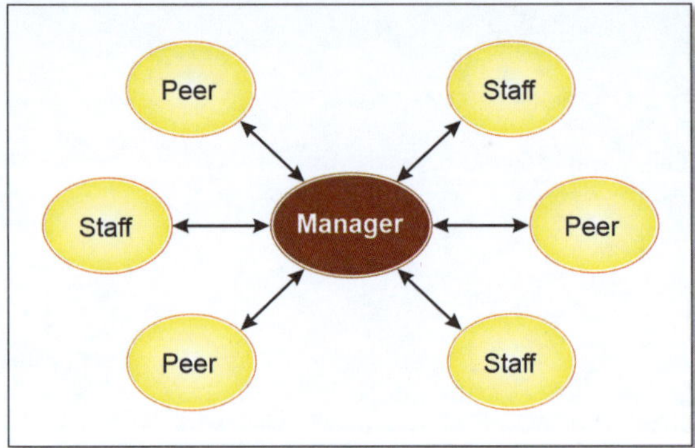

Figure 12.13: Horizontal communication

Straight Chain Pattern

Straight chain pattern develops when the communicated messages are top secret. In this pattern, rumors pass from A to B, B to C and so on (Fig. 12.14).

Star Pattern

Where rumor is disclosed by one person to many others who come in contact with him (Fig. 12.15).

Probability Patterns

Wholesome messages may be accidentally communicated to B and C who in turn communicates it to others, while some members of the group may be left out either because of their absence or lack of opportunity (Fig. 12.16).

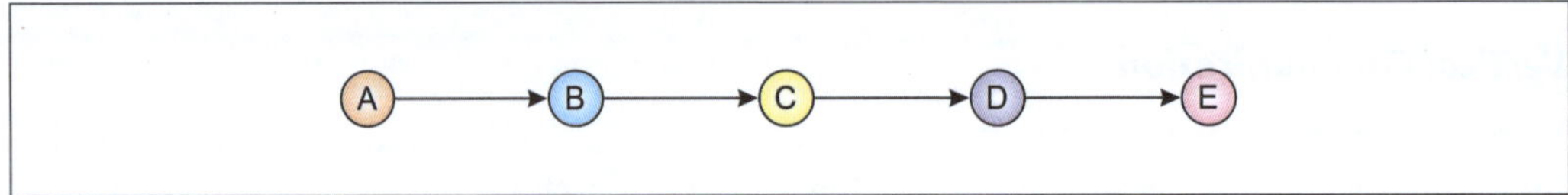

Figure 12.14: Straight chain pattern

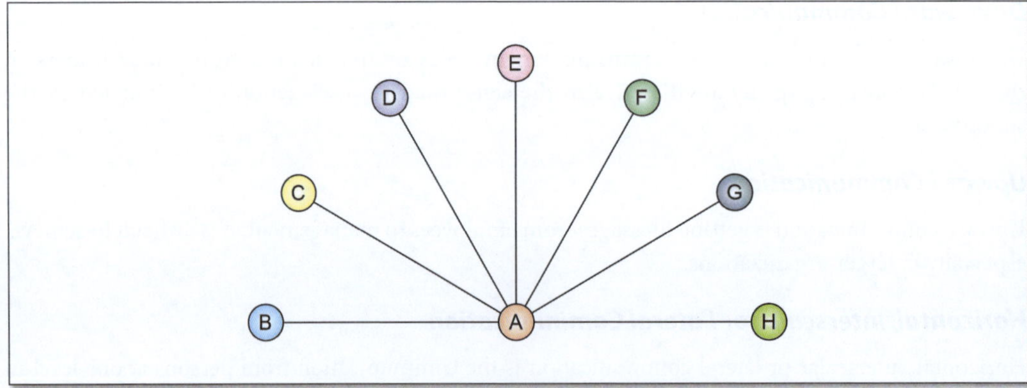

Figure 12.15: Star pattern of communication

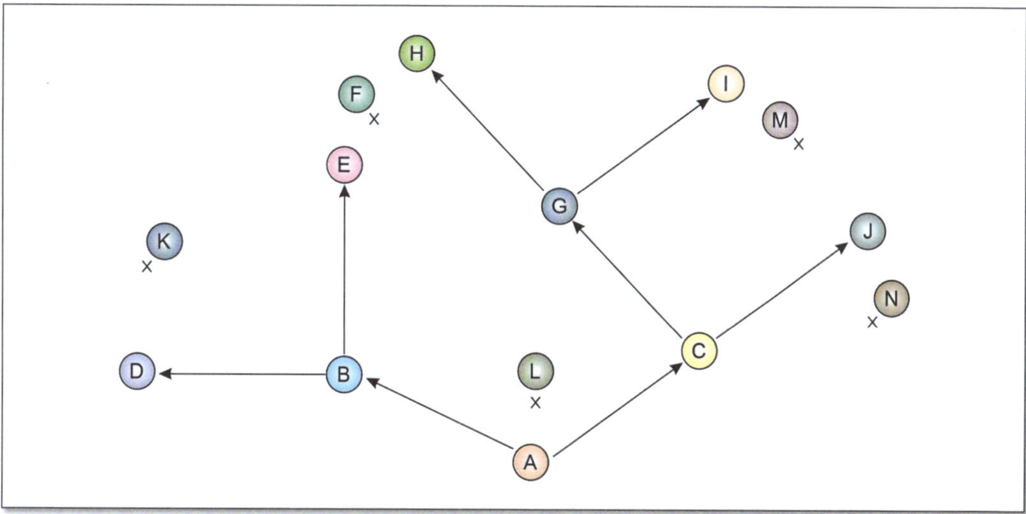

Figure 12.16: Probability pattern of communication

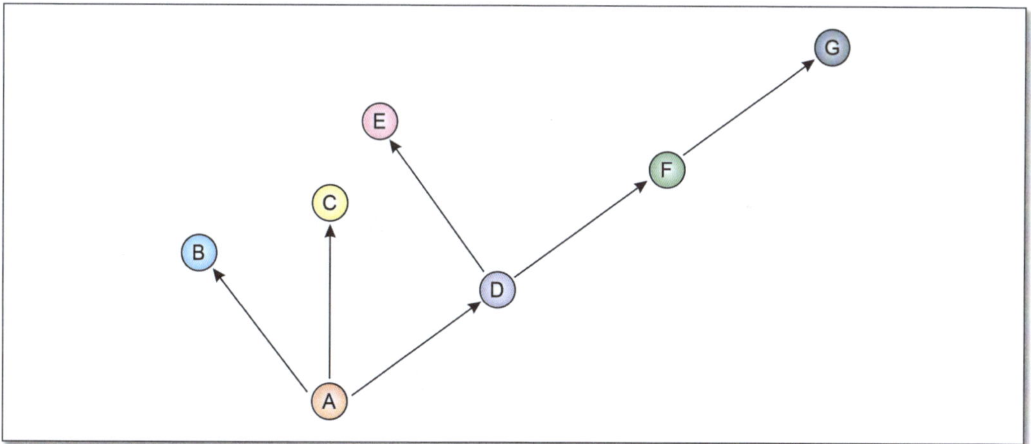

Figure 12.17: Luster net pattern of communication

Luster Net

Where A says something to his three close friends and one of these passes the information to another while a fourth one tells two more either in a straight chain pattern or in an informal star pattern (Fig. 12.17).

COMMUNICATION NETWORK PATTERN

Type I: All the four persons can communicate with one person 'A' but cannot have communication among themselves (Fig. 12.18).

Type II: A is the boss, B and C are his senior assistants and D and E are their junior subordinates. A can directly communicate with B and C but not with D and E (Fig. 12.19).

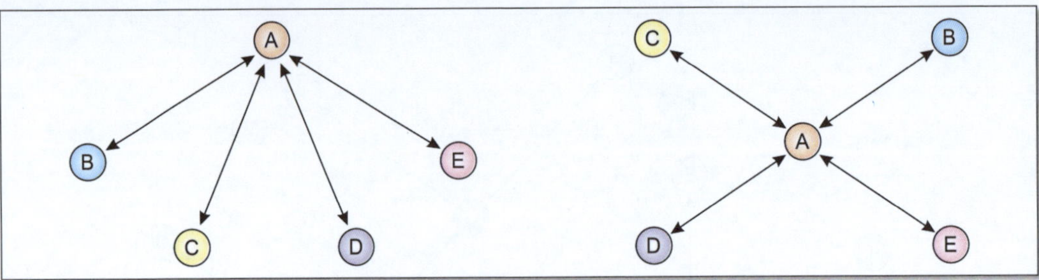

Figure 12.18: Type I communication network

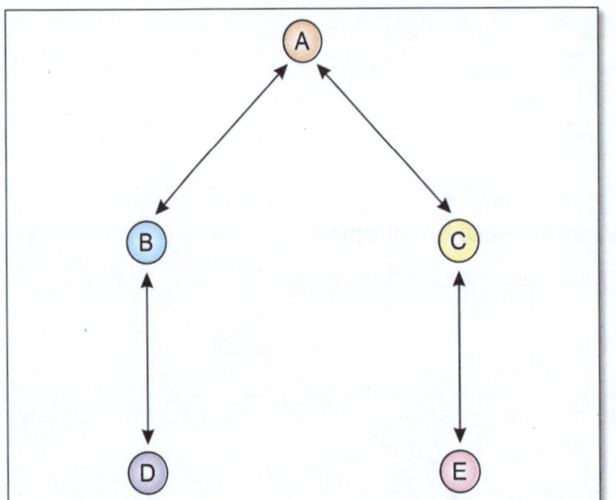

Figure 12.19: Type II communication network

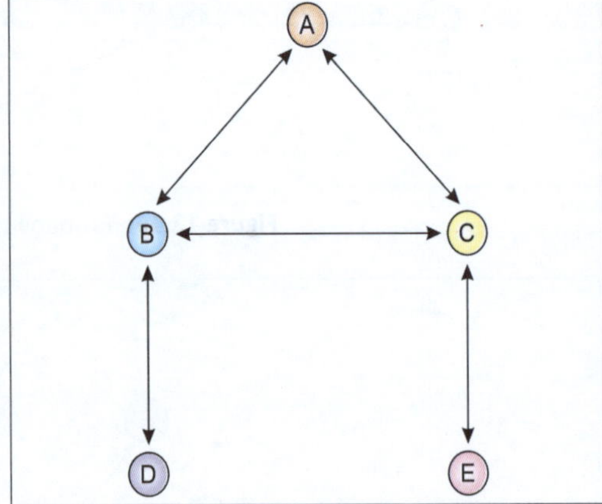

Figure 12.20: Type III communication network

Type III: By allowing direct communication between two seniors members B and C. A, B and C are reduced to a group of equal, in so far as the level of communication is concerned (Fig. 12.20).

Type IV: A can communicate with B but B has the facility to communicate wish C, D and E (Fig. 12.21).

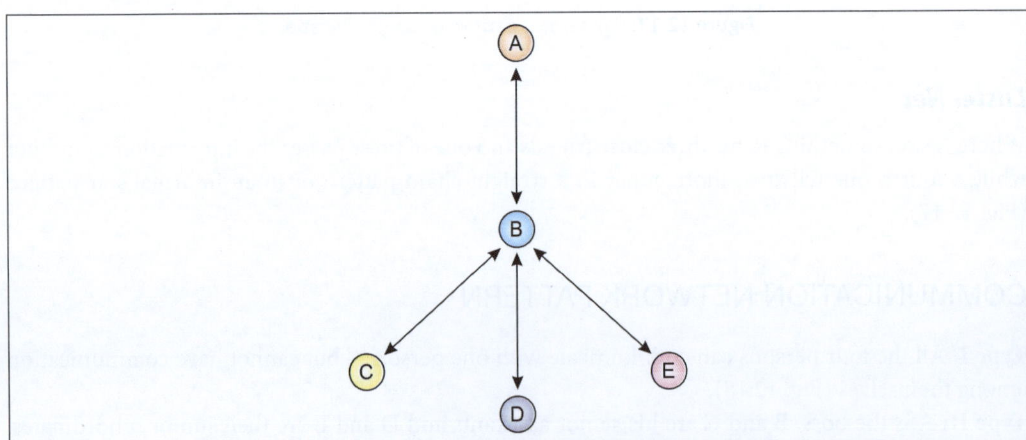

Figure 12.21: Type IV communication network

TABLE 12.1: Various barriers to communications

Human/personal barriers	Semantic barriers	Technical barriers	Physiological barriers	Environmental barriers
Personal emotions	Word interpretation	Mechanical failures	Deaf and dumb	Noise
Perceptual variations	Gesture decoding	Geographical distance	Other disabilities	Cloud
Competencies	Language transactions	Time lags		Rain
Sensual abilities	Signs and symbols	Physical obstruction		Crowd
Mental faults	Cue meaning	Space		

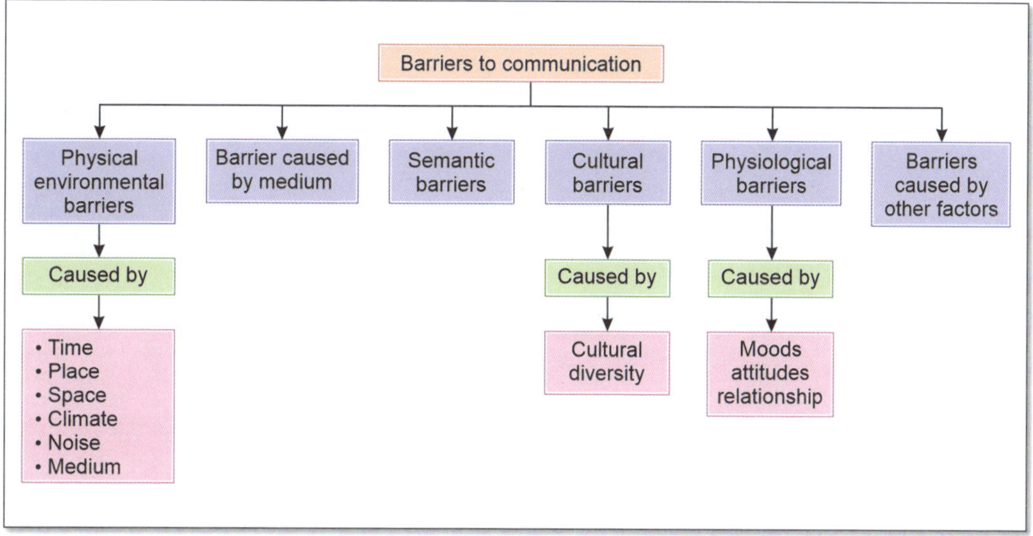

Figure 12.22: Causes of barriers to communication

BARRIERS TO COMMUNICATION

The barriers of communication are summarized in Table 12.1. These barriers to communication are caused by some factors as shown in Figure 12.22.

PRECAUTIONS WHILE COMMUNICATING

The precautions required while communicating are as follows:

- A communication should not disclose sensitive personal facts about an individual.
- A communication should not be threatening or managing.
- A communication should not make a false allegation.
- Systematic analysis of the message is necessary for communication.
- Select and determine appropriate language and medium of communication according to its purpose.

- Avoid being too formal or aloof.
- Avoid distraction.
- Avoid personal biases.

FURTHER READINGS

- Kourkouta L, Papathanasiou IV. Communication in nursing practice. Mater Sociomed. 2014;26(1):65-7.
- University of St. Augustine for Health Sciences. (2023). The importance of effective communication in nursing. [online] Available from https://www.usa.edu/blog/communication-in-nursing/ [Last accessed August, 2023].

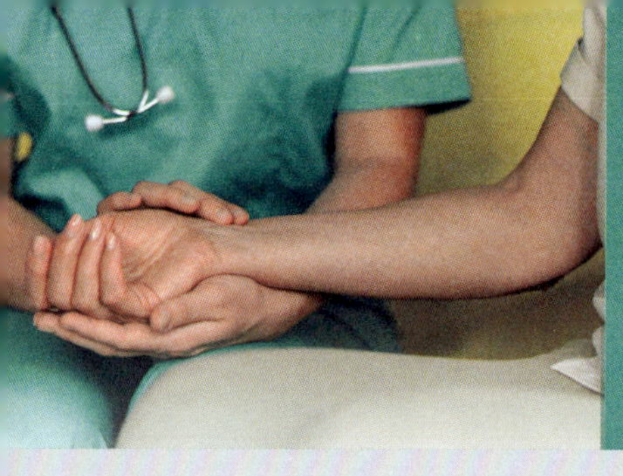

STUDENT ASSIGNMENT

LONG ANSWER QUESTIONS

1. What is communication? What are the types of communication?
2. What are the principles of communication?

SHORT ANSWER QUESTIONS

1. What are barriers of communication?
2. What is the process of communication?
3. What are the precautions while communicating?
4. Write a note on SMCR Model.

MULTIPLE CHOICE QUESTIONS

1. **Communication is a non-stop________.**
   a. Paper
   b. Process
   c. Program
   d. Plan
2. **The __________ is the person who transmits the message.**
   a. Receiver
   b. Driver
   c. Sender
   d. Cleaner
3. **____________ is the person who notices and decodes and attaches some meaning to message.**
   a. Receiver
   b. Driver
   c. Sender
   d. Cleaner
4. **Message is any signal that triggers the response of a __________.**
   a. Receiver
   b. Driver
   c. Sender
   d. Cleaner
5. **The response to a sender's message is called__________.**
   a. Food bank
   b. Feedback
   c. Food
   d. Back
6. **Environmental barriers are the same as_____ noise.**
   a. Physiological
   b. Psychological
   c. Physical
   d. Sociological

ANSWER KEY

1. b   **2.** c   **3.** a   **4.** a   **5.** b   **6.** c

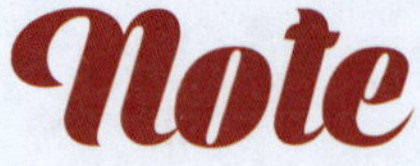

13

Patient Care for Admission, Discharge and Surgery

ADMISSION AND DISCHARGE OF PATIENT

Admission

Admission to the nursing unit prepares the patient for his stay in the healthcare facility.

There are forms of admission a hospital setting. (1) Urgent, (2) Elective.

Goals of Admission Procedure

Various goals of admission procedure are as follows:

- Verify the patient's identity and assess the clinical status.
- Make him as comfortable as possible.
- Obtain critical informations about patient.
- Introduce him to staff and other patients.
- Orient him to the environment and routine.
- Provide supplies and equipment needed for daily care.

Types of Admission

1. Based on patient condition:
    - Emergency
    - Routine/elective
2. Based on the purpose of admission:
    - Therapeutic admission
    - Diagnostic admission
3. Based on length of hospital stay:
    - Long-term duration
    - Short-term duration

Each admission should only occur on the basis of available beds including considerations of the number and experience of nurses in each shift and their current workload.

Procedure of Admission

Assess: At the time of admission, complete assessment of the patient is being done

Following details should be collected at the time of admission:

- Patient name, date and time of admission
- Chief complains
- Medical diagnosis in the admission file or patient file
- Write about the source of information (family, patient, care giver or healthcare person or significant person)
- Check the document if patient has previous hospitalization and past major illness.

Mention type of admission

- Take patient's vital signs (pulse, temperature, respiratory rate, height and weight).
- Document if patient and family have brought valuables to the hospital. If yes, hand it over to the relatives with their signatures.
- At the time of arrival to the unit or ward, patient and family will be given orientation regarding the unit, visiting rooms, patient's rights and responsibilities.

- Position the bed as the patient's condition requires. If the patient is ambulatory, place the bed in low position; if he/she is arriving on a stretcher, place the bed in the high position.
- Fold down the top lines. Prepare any emergency or special equipment, such as oxygen or suction as needed.
- Adjust the room lights, temperature and ventilation.
- Make sure patient is comfortable and safe.

Discharge Planning

Discharge is the termination of care from a healthcare agency or hospital. It means relieving a person from hospital setting, who was admitted as an inpatient in that hospital.

Importance of Discharge Planning

The importance of discharge planning lies in its potential for reducing readmission. Discharge planning must involve the patient, the family and multidisciplinary team of health professionals. The discharge plan may need to be discussed with the patient and his/her family. Discharge planning as a process must begin on admission to hospital and continue throughout the hospital stay.

Steps of Discharge Planning

Determine the appropriate posthospital discharge destination.
- Meet patient's postdischarge needs.
- Follow-up guidance.

Process of Discharge Planning

Discharge planning is a vital aspect of the patient's care. Discharge planning is the process by which the patient is assisted to develop a plan of care for ongoing maintenance and improvement of healthcare even after he/she may be discharged from the acute care hospital.

Discharge planning begins at admission with the initial interview and nursing assessment and continues as an interdisciplinary process throughout hospitalization. The discharge planning is completed as part of initial assessment at admission. Discharge planning is the quality line between hospitals, community-based services, nongovernment organizations and cares. Discharge planning is the critical link between treatment received in a hospital by the patient and postdischarge care provided in the community.

Benefits of Discharge Planning

Various benefits of discharge planning are:
- Improvement in patient health outcomes.
- Reduction in readmission to hospital.
- Reduction in length of stay.
- Reduction in errors

Types of Discharge

Types of discharge are as follows:

- **Planned discharge:** The patient has completed the initial treatment and management procedure in the hospital and no longer requires direct supervision.
- **LAMA:** Leave against medical advice.

- Referral to higher center/lower center.
- DAMA
- Transfer/referral
- Discharge on request
- Abscond
- Death

Features of Discharge Planning

- Discharge planning begins before admission for scheduled admissions and at the time of admission for all other patients.
- Estimated length of stay should be assessed.
- Assessment of patient (beginning on the day of admission and continue assessment during hospitalization).
- Involves the patient's family in the discharge process obtaining discharge orders.
- Check all aspects of discharge and complete discharge check list.
- The family/care giver will be contacted by the nurse to confirm that the patient is being discharged and to ensure that relevant services are activated or reactivated when required.
- Nurse should ensure that the common assessment processes are completed for eligible patients who will require access to long-term residential care.
- The information and education provided to the patient and the family should be provided in the proper language.
- The discharge plan tracks and indicates all stages and progresses in relation to a patient discharge.
- Progress of the discharge plan is discussed with the multidisciplinary team.
- Before discharge the nurse carries out a holistic assessment of the patient.
- Nurse should be familiar with and comply with legislation, regulation and organizational policies concerning patient's discharge.
- Discharge plan should be documented in the healthcare record, reviewed daily and updated.
- Relevant interval referrals should be made to the members of the health team.
- Provide written and verbal instructions to the family according to the patient's level of understanding.
- Nurse should verbally explain instructions to patient/family prior to discharge.
- Ensure that patient has follow-up care arranged at discharge.
- Community resources should be notified.

The discharge planning team is shown in Figure 13.1.

Nursing Considerations

Ideal Discharge Planning
- **Include** the patient and family in planning
- **Discuss** with patient and family to prevent problems at home
- **Educate** the patient and family in simple language
- **Assess** how nurses explain the diagnosis and treatment
- **Listen** to patient and family

PREOPERATIVE CARE

Preoperative care refers to the physical and psychosocial care that prepares a patient to undergo surgery safely. The preoperative period begins when the patient is booked for surgery and ends with

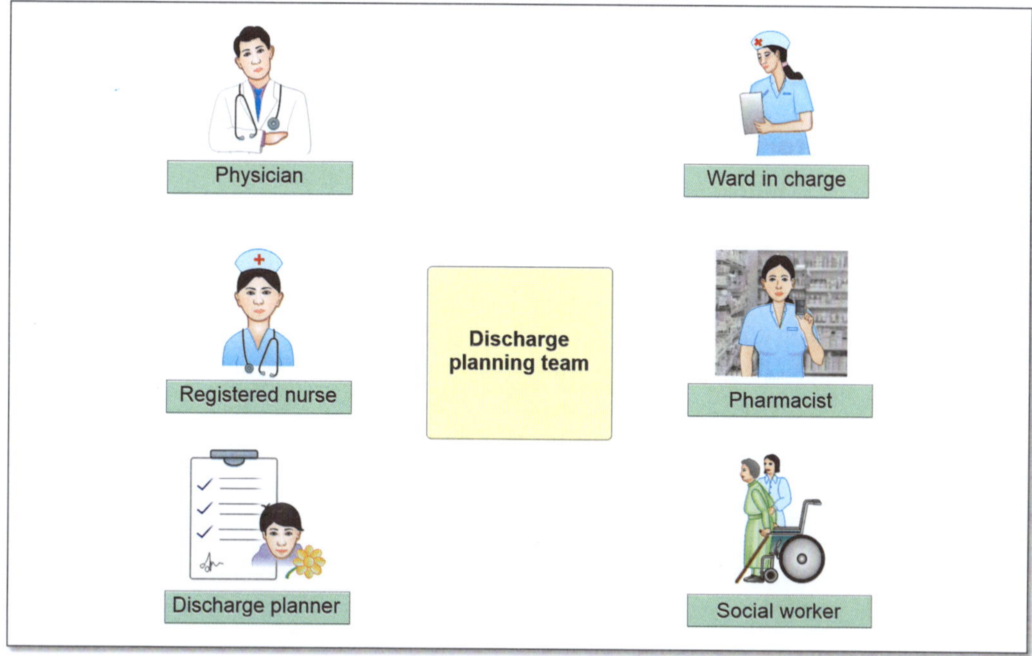

Figure 13.1: Discharge planning team

their transfer to the theater or surgical suite. A careful assessment is necessary, in order to prevent operative complications and alert nurse to postoperative care needs.

Purposes of Preoperative Care

Various purposes of preoperative care are as follows:

- Obtain patient's information.
- Give information.
- Get consent.
- Allow assessment of emotional state and expectations.

Objectives of the Preoperative Care

Various objectives of preoperative care are as follows:

- To meet the patient.
- To identify the present problem requiring surgery.
- To identify any previous ongoing illnesses which may influence the anesthetic or surgery.
- To evaluate any possible concerns about previous anesthetics or any family history of problems with anesthetics.
- To assess any adverse drug reaction and current medications.
- To examine the patient and in particular assess the airway.
- To review any investigations.
- To plan the anesthetic technique.

- To ensure the patient is nothing per oral (NPO) for 6 hours for solids and 4 hours for clear fluids.
- To order any premedication required and all essential routine medications to be given preoperatively.

Preoperative History

A relevant preoperative history includes information as follows:

- Current symptoms suggesting an active cardiopulmonary disorder (e.g., cough, chest pain, dyspnea during exertion, ankle swelling) or infection (e.g., fever, dysuria).
- Risk factors for thromboembolism, excessive bleeding or infection.
- Known disorders that increase risk of complications, particularly hypertension, heart disease, kidney disease, liver disease, diabetes, asthma, chronic obstructive pulmonary disease (COPD) and bleeding disorders.
- Previous surgery, anesthesia or both, particularly their complications.
- Allergies.
- Tobacco and alcohol use.
- Current prescription and nonprescription drug and supplement use.
- If an indwelling catheter may be needed, patients should be asked about prior urinary retention and prostate surgery.

Physical Examination

Physical examination includes:

- When spinal anesthesia is likely, patients should be evaluated for scoliosis and other anatomic abnormalities.
- Any cognitive dysfunction, especially in elderly patients who will be given a general anesthetic, should be noted.

Vital signs:

- Monitor preoperative and baseline vital signs, reports for any changes.
- Past surgical history.

Allergies:

Any allergies to medications, foods, substances. Clearly identify any allergies on the front of the chart.

Nutritional state:

- There is a need to assess nutritional state of the patient.
- Protein is essential for tissue repair. Carbohydrate provides the necessary energy for tissue repair. Vitamins are necessary as vitamin B maintains gastrointestinal (GI) function, vitamin C promotes wound healing and collagen formation and vitamin K promotes clotting.

Body weight:

- Most are weighed before surgery (basis for anesthetic drug dose).
- **Obesity:**
  - More complicated. Increased potential for dehiscence and evisceration, wound infection.
  - Takes more anesthesia and stored in adipose tissue delaying excretion.
  - More postoperative complications—respiratory, ambulation.

- **Underweight:** Lack of protein stores. Diet high in protein, carbohydrate and vitamins is to be recommended in such cases.

Fluid/electrolyte balance: Correction of any imbalance is essential.

Hypervolemia occurs in renal failure, congestive heart failure (CHF), and malnutrition.

Patients prone to hypovolemia have—diarrhea, vomiting, bleeding, insufficient fluid intake, GI bleed. There is a need to assess for dehydration (skin turgor, mucous membranes, intake/output.)

- **Electrolytes:** Na, K, Cl, Ca, Mg. [blood urea nitrogen (BUN), creatinine for kidney function]
- "Routine blood work" concept is giving way to minimal labs based on complexity of procedure and findings in history and physical examination (H & P).

Infections: Unless the surgery is for treating an infection (such as an incision and drainage), it will always be rescheduled if there is any evidence of infection.

Chronic Illness

Chronic illness can complicate the postoperative phase. Few of the chronic illness diseases are as follows:

- **COPD:** Increases pneumonia and decreases the ability to exchange CO_2 and O_2.
- **Asthma:** Intraoperative bronchospasm.
- **Cardiac disease:** Prosthetic valves increase postoperative inflammatory process and potential for infection. Peripheral vascular disease (PVD) impairs tissue and wound healing. Increased risk for thrombophlebitis.
- **Hematologic disorders:** Risk of hemorrhage with clotting disorders. Anemia can compound the surgical loss of blood leading to hypovolemia/shock.
- **Endocrine disorders:** Patient may experience hypo/hyperglycemia during the surgical period. Increased risk of infection, silent myocardial ischemia (MI), peripheral nerve injury, and difficult intubation. Other endocrine disorders can alter the stress response.
- **Neurological disorders:** Neuro assessment provides a baseline for postoperative care. Incorporate chronic neurological disorder care.
- **Gastrointestinal disorders:** Adequate liver function is necessary for the detoxification of drugs.
- **Renal disorders:** Kidneys are responsible for excretion of waste and maintenance of fluid and electrolyte balance. If chronic renal failure (CRF), careful assessment is needed preoperative—intake and output, specific gravity of urine and adequate fluid intake.
- **Musculoskeletal disorders:** Range of motion (ROM).
- **Integumentary status:** Pressure ulcers from immobility.

Drug History

- **Antibiotics:** Combine with cure to prolonged apnea.
  Valvular disease or prosthesis may need antibiotic prophylaxis, anticoagulants—increased bleeding time.
- **Diuretics:** Hypokalemia.
- **Steroids:** Decrease adrenal function.
- **Aspirin:** Decrease platelet aggregation.
- **Tranquilizers:** Hypotension and shock.

> **Note**
>
> Antihypertension medications, usually continue through the aim of surgery. The reason for this is to avoid fearing hypotension, it is done to promote control without as many oscillations.

Laboratory Investigations

These tests vary depending on the patient:

- **Blood counts:** Complete blood counts should be performed on all patients who show signs of anemia or an underlying condition which increases the risk of anemia.
- **Serum electrolytes:** These should be done on all patients over 40 years, those with renal disease, hypertension, diuretic therapy including bowel preparation, diarrhea or vomiting.
- **Liver enzymes:** These are measured if abnormalities are suspected based on the patient's history or examination.
- **Coagulation screening:** It is done if there is a history of bleeding disorder or on anticoagulation therapy.
- **Electrocardiogram:** This should be done on all patients over 40 years, any patient at increased risk of cardiac disease, have symptoms of cardiac disease or show signs of cardiac disease on physical examination.
- **Chest X-ray:** It is required in all patients with symptomatic pulmonary disease or underlying malignancy.
- **Urinalysis:** It is required in all patients.
- **Pulmonary function testing:** This may be done if patients have a known chronic pulmonary disorders or signs and symptoms of pulmonary disease.
  - Patients with symptomatic coronary artery disease need additional tests (e.g., stress testing, coronary angiography) before surgery.
  - All other investigations are ordered if specific problems are identified on history and physical examination.
- **Premedication:** These are given to provide amnesia, anxiolysis, antacid prophylaxis, analgesia, autonomic control, allergy prophylaxis and continuation of specific therapy.

PREOPERATIVE NURSING MANAGEMENT

Preoperative Teaching

Best time to teach is the afternoon or evening before surgery. Challenging when most are same day admits—even carotids or heart surgery. It is important because it decreases anxiety, influences recovery, promotes patient satisfaction.

General Principles of Preoperative Teaching

The general principles of preoperative teaching are as follows:

- Encourages knowledge enhancement.
- Reinforces what the patient has been told about surgery. Finds out that patient understands the procedure, first. Know enough basic information about common procedures to anticipate and answer the common questions.

- Avoids anxiety producing words—"pain" (discomfort).
- Includes family members, if possible.
- Let the patient explain and give return demonstrations.
- Prepares for the situations (cold, bright light and never left alone).

Preoperative Legal Preparation—Informed Consent

It is the surgeon's responsibility to explain the surgical procedure, alternatives, risks and benefits. Purpose is to ensure the patient is not undergoing a procedure without informed consent. Helps protect from liability. Adults must be oriented and not under sedation in order to sign. May take a telephone consent. Consent is witnessed—that is a witness to the signature.

Preparation on the Day of Surgery

Various preparations are done before operation which are as follows:

Physical Preparation

- **Nursing responsibilities:** Orders carried out, final preparations done, records complete and accompany patient to operating room. Patients are might be admitted the evening before, but most tend to be admitted on the same day.
- **Diet:** Regular light diet. Full liquids in some instances. Nothing by mouth (NPO) after midnight (allow time for the stomach to empty, decrease aspiration) or at least 4–8 hours.
- **Skin preparation:** Decrease bacteria to a minimum with mild antiseptic soap and water, the night or day before. Shaving can increase skin bacteria.
- **Bowel preparation:** Type of surgery determines the need for a bowel preparation. Enema or laxative may be administered to permit visualization of the colon and decreases the chance of infection when bowel is resected.

Medications

Sedative to ensure adequate rest and to decrease anxiety.

Preanesthetic agent may be given 30 minutes to 1 hour before surgery to promote sleep and relaxation. No consent if sedated—get it signed before giving. Also, void before giving.

- **Sedatives:** Decreases the anxiety, i.e., benzodiazepines, barbiturates.
- **Narcotic analgesic:** Reduces the amount of anesthetic needed. Given 30 minutes to 1 hour before surgery, often intramuscular.
- **Anticholinergic:** Reduces secretions. Also causes dry mouth and dilatation of the pupils (atropine).
- **Tranquilizer:** May be given instead of a narcotic, especially to the elderly.

Preoperative Checklist/Transportation to the Operating Room

It is nursing responsibility to see that the checklist is completed—important, shows that the patient is ready for transfer to the operating room. Unusual observations and abnormal lab reports are reported to the physician.

Nursing Consideration

"If you want to take care of the patient, take care of the paperwork"

- Nothing by mouth for 6 hours for adults and less for the children. Explain reasons for restriction and importance and inform other caretakers.

NPO before all types of anesthesia.

- Signed operating room consent.
- Current history and physical assessment.
- Completion of physical preparation.
- Prostheses, contacts, dental work, etc.
- Records of preoperative medication.
- Identification band in proper order.
- Do not remove makeup or nail polish. The text says "Take them off"—but they can be kept.
- Jewelry should not be worn—for electrical safety hazard in addition to risk of loss.

Preprocedural Checklist

In the operating room, before the procedure begins, a time-out is held during which the team confirms several important factors:

- Correct procedure and operative site (if applicable).
- Availability of all needed equipment.
- Completion of indicated prophylaxis (e.g., antibiotics, anticoagulants).

Functions of Perioperative Nurse

The following are the major responsibilities and accountabilities (Fig. 13.2) of a perioperative nurse:

- Assessing psychological and physiological conditions, before, during and after the operation of patient.

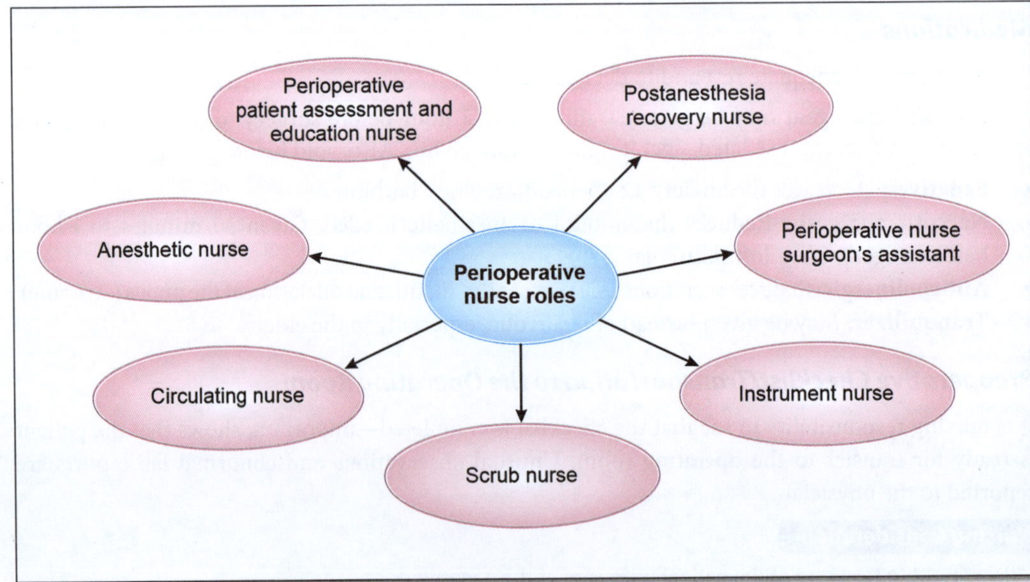

Figure 13.2: Role of perioperative nurse

- Classifying the primary care and priorities to be given to patient based on good nursing decision.
- Giving directions on proper handling of materials, apparatus and equipment for the patient.
- Functioning as a circulating nurse or scrub nurse on a particular procedure.
- Joining ongoing and continuing training programs.

A perioperative nurse:

- Uses the nursing process, designs, coordinates, and delivers care to meet the identified needs of clients.
- Understands the:
  - History and physical assessment, pathophysiology, and lab tests.
  - Nature of the planned procedure.
  - Individual patient's likely responses to stress.
  - Potential risks and complications of the surgical procedure.

POSTOPERATIVE CARE

The postoperative phase of a patient's journey starts when the patient is transferred from the theater to the recovery room. However, preparation for each individual patient commences well before the patient arrives.

All equipment such as resuscitation, oxygen and monitoring are checked and additional resources are acquired if the surgery or anesthesia indicates that this may be so, e.g., patient warming apparatus if the surgery has been long, provision of analgesic pumps or pillows for the patient who needs to be nursed sitting up due to surgery on the neck. The patient's age will also influence the size of the equipment needed, particularly for children.

The transfer cannot occur until the anesthetist is satisfied that the patient's condition is stable, the recovery nurse assesses the patient immediately on arrival, with focus on airway, breathing and circulation.

Airway

Airway includes:

- Observe the movements of the chest to ensure bilateral even movement and feel the air flowing in and out of the mouth. Noisy breathing is obstructed breathing and action must be taken to relieve the obstruction. The nurse may support the patient's airway.

> **Must Know**
>
> Obstructed breathing is not always noisy, as complete obstruction is characterized by silence.

- Skin color (lips, nailbeds) may indicate cyanosis.
- Respiratory rate is taken to include depth. The respiratory pattern changes could be an early indication of future respiratory or cardiac arrest.

Circulation

Circulation includes:

- Once the airway has been established, blood pressure and pulse can be monitored.
- Assessment of perfusion status includes conscious state, skin temperature, pulse and blood pressure as an indication of perfusion to all vital organs.
- Inspecting sounds and drains for signs of hemorrhage is essential. However, it's important to remember that while monitors alert staff to changes in condition, continuous physical assessment and observation are crucial for detecting subtle changes without solely relying on monitors. The patient may be hypoxic despite a 98% reading on the pulse oximeter. The nurse can then carry out a more thorough assessment.

Patient Assessment

Patient is assessed for various signs as follows:

- Checking of consciousness levels and signs of protective reflexes returning.
- **Intravenous infusions:** Type, rate and patency of site.
- **Drains:** Types, amount draining and rate.
- **Urinary catheters:** Patency, color of drainage and amount.

Monitoring

Monitoring includes:

- Temperature, pulse and sensation following arterial or limb surgery
- Wound site
- Plaster of Paris casts
- Pressure areas

Documentation: All postoperative assessment and observations must be recorded in the patient's documentation.

Constant Communication with the Patient

The immediate postoperative period is fraught with potential complications for each patient, and the recovery room nurse plays a vital role in detecting, preventing and managing dangerous life-threatening conditions by continuous, ongoing assessment of the patient visually and with the aid of monitors. Waking up from an anesthetic can be a frightening experience for the patient. The bright lights, uncharacteristic noises, lack of familiarity with the surroundings and pain may disorientate and confuse the patient.

Constant communication with the patient during this phase and throughout their recovery is vital to reduce the patient's anxiety. The nurse should communicate any procedure being undertaken even before the patient regains consciousness, as hearing is the first sense to return.

Managing Patient's Pain

Understanding patient's pain: In the postoperative period, this can be difficult if the patient is drowsy, confused or crying. The recovery nurse can observe nonverbal clues such as restlessness, grimacing and, hyperventilation. Hypoxia, hypothermia, anxiety, nausea, fatigue and pain are all symptoms of the body's stress response to surgery.

Pain postoperatively can magnify these responses and delay a return to normal function, as well as impair wound healing and predispose the patient to infection. Planning an analgesics regime postoperatively can start at the preoperative assessment clinic, where staff can discuss the amount of pain to be expected, how long it will last and the options available for managing this after surgery.

The patient's perception of the pain can be reduced if they are prepared for and expecting it. The administration of early effective analgesics will optimize the recovery outcome.

The patient in pain is anxious, distressed and agitated, yet explanations, reassurance and support can be equally as effective as pharmacological methods.

Analgesics can be administered through a variety of techniques and routes, i.e., intramuscular injection, intravenous bolus, intravenous patient-controlled analgesia (PCA), epidural or rectally.

Recovery nurses must have the knowledge and skills to understand and administer the different methods and analgesics as available, and monitor the incidence and severity of side effects.

The PCA is popular with both patients and clinicians, as it avoids the use of injections, eliminates the delay to the patient in receiving analgesia and allows the patient to feel more in control of their own pain and its management.

Assessment of the patient is ongoing, in order to monitor the efficacy of the pain relief, if the pain is controlled, then the patient should be able to move easily on the trolley/bed.

Taking deep breaths helps in overall feeling of more comfort and less anxiety.

Documentation: Documentation of the assessment and actions taken must be made in the patient's care plan.

Nursing Considerations

Ideal way to give analgesia postoperatively is to:

- Give a small intravenous bolus of about a quarter or a third of the maximum dose.
- Wait for 5–10 minutes to observe the effect—the desired effect is analgesia, but retained consciousness.
- Estimate the correct total dose and give the remaining intramuscularly.

With this method, the patient receives analgesia quickly and the correct dose is given.

General Postoperative Care in the Ward

Regular recording of vital signs and systemic observation can reveal early indicators of postoperative complications. Close monitoring of the patient will allow immediate action to be taken in the event of a complication. Observations should be recorded initially every 30 minutes and compared to baseline assessment by the anesthetist and preassessment clinic, and observations in recovery, to provide an overall view of the patient's condition. Observations and their frequency can be reduced as the patient's condition improves.

Mental Status

All patients are briefly confused when they come out of anesthesia. If delirium occurs, oxygenation should be assessed, and all nonessential drugs should be stopped. Patients should be mobilized as they are able, and any electrolyte or fluid imbalance, should be corrected.

Wound Care

The surgeon must individualize care of each wound, but the sterile dressing placed in the operating room is generally left intact, for 24 hours unless signs of infection (e.g., increasing pain, erythema, drainage) develops.

After 24 hours, the site should be checked twice/day, if possible, for signs of infection. If there are signs of infection, wound exploration and drainage of abscesses, systemic antibiotics or both may be required. Topical antibiotics are usually not helpful.

A drain tube, if present, must be monitored for quantity and quality of the fluid collected. Sutures, skin staples, and other closures are usually left in place 7 days or longer depending on the site and the patient. Face and neck wounds may be superficially healed in 3 days; wounds on the lower extremities may take weeks to heal to a similar degree.

Surgical Wound Care

Surgical dressings should be assessed frequently for drainage, with documentation of the amount, color, and consistency. The Centers for Disease Control and Prevention (CDC) recommend that a surgical incision be covered with a sterile dressing for 24–48 hours. After the surgical dressing is removed, incisions should be left open to air unless drainage is noted. Incisions are monitored for signs of infection, wound approximation, active bleeding, and drainage. Surgical drains may be placed during the procedure to monitor for bleeding.

Postoperative Assessment

Checklist for the postoperative instructions:

- Past medical history
- Medications
- Allergies
- Intraoperative complications
- Postoperative instructions
- Recommended treatment and prophylaxis

Assessment of Respiratory, Circulatory and Mental Status

The assessment of respiratory, circulatory and mental status is completed by a nurse, postoperatively as shown in Figure 13.3.

In addition to the physical assessment, record:

- Any significant symptoms, such as chest pain or breathlessness.
- Pain and adequacy of pain control.

Treatment and Prophylaxis

Following postoperative treatment and prophylaxis options should be discussed preoperatively with the appropriate members of the clinical team:

- Adequate pain control
- Venous thromboembolism prophylaxis

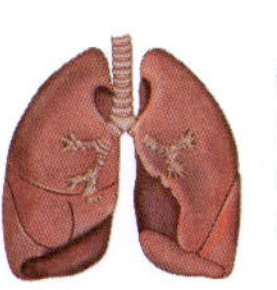
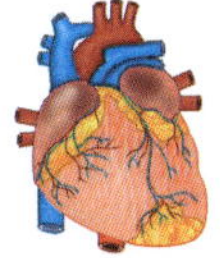
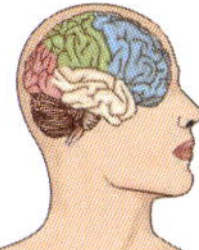

Figure 13.3: Assessment of respiratory, circulatory and mental status

- Antibiotic prophylaxis
- Continuation of current medications (these and in particular cardiorespiratory treatments, should be continued wherever possible).
- Substitution of current medication (e.g., diabetic control, steroid therapy)
- Prophylaxis for postoperative nausea and vomiting
- Ability of patients to take drugs by mouth
- Pressure area management

Postoperatively, consider the need for:

- Physiotherapy
- Nutrition team consultation
- Oral hygiene

Patient Teaching about Postoperative Care

Patients are taught in postoperative care as follows:

- **Therapeutic devices:** Indwelling catheter, nasogastric tube, chest tube.
- **Medications for pain:** Assured that medication will be available.
- **Postoperative self-care procedures:** Splinting, leg exercises, turning.
- **Ambulation:** Do not bound, do not do a sit up, wait for a moment to check dizziness.

ROUTINE MONITORING

Monitoring allows collection of routine data so that trends may be established, assisting in the detection of deterioration or improvement. This is vital for an objective assessment of a patient's response to treatment. In general, the anesthetist will recommend monitoring regimen for the first few hours after surgery, which could normally include:

- Temperature
- Pulse rate
- Blood pressure
- Respiratory rate
- Pain assessment (resting and moving)
- Urine output (postoperative voiding)
- Peripheral oxygen saturation

FURTHER READINGS

- Johnstone J. How to Provide Preoperative Care to Patients. Nurs Stand. 2020;35(12):72-6.
- Soni S. Sam's Operation Theater Techniques, 1st edition. Meerut, India: Amit Publications; 2010.

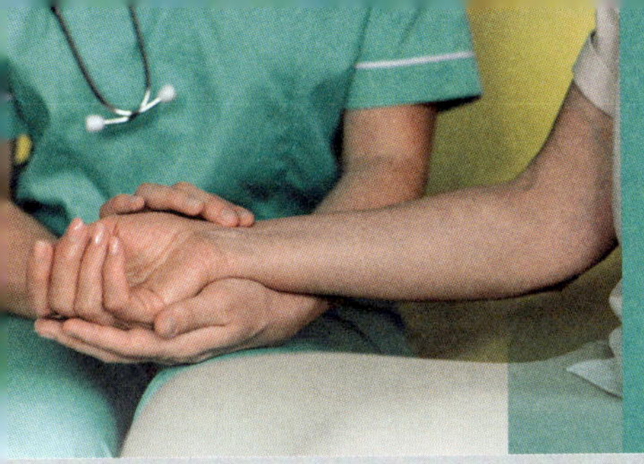

LONG ANSWER QUESTIONS

1. Discuss the admission and discharge of patient.
2. Describe preoperative nursing management.

SHORT ANSWER QUESTIONS

1. Write about the role of a nurse in perioperative nursing.
2. Write a note on postoperative nursing.

MULTIPLE CHOICE QUESTIONS

1. **Common reactions to hospitalization. Select all that apply:**
   a. Fear of the unknown
   b. Disorientation
   c. Separation anxiety
   d. Loss of identity
   e. Excitement

2. **Important procedures for admission. Select all that apply:**
   a. Make a room ready
   b. Greet patient by name using his/her surname if the patient is an adult
   c. Explain hospital routine
   d. Provide directions to closest shopping malls and restaurants
   e. Explain when meals are served and when friends are allowed to visit

3. **Which of the following is not a part of initial assessment?**
   a. Vital signs
   b. Vision and hearing
   c. Height and weight
   d. Culture and sensitivity test

4. **Which is not the nursing assistant's role in the discharge of the resident?**
   a. Giving the resident prescriptions written by the doctor
   b. Helping the resident pack
   c. Helping the resident dress
   d. Making sure all items are collected from drawers and closets

5. **Which of the following is not a valid reason to transfer a person to another unit?**
   a. The person's condition changes
   b. There is a need for closer supervision
   c. Roommates do not get along
   d. The staff do not get along with the resident

ANSWER KEY

1. a to d   **2.** a, b, c, e   **3.** d   **4.** a   **5.** d

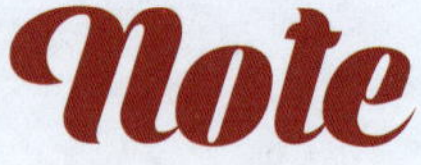

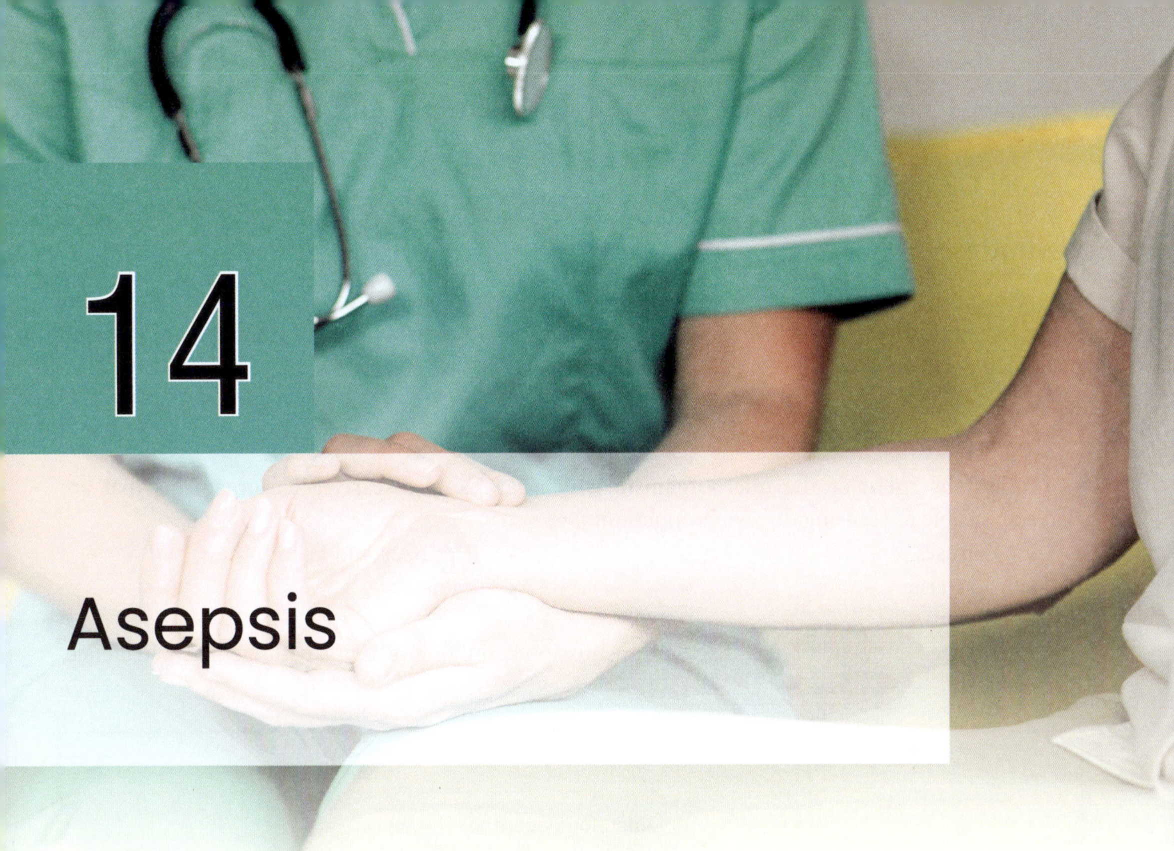

14

Asepsis

After the completion of the chapter, the readers will be able to:
- Discuss asepsis—medical and surgical asepsis.
- Discuss importance of sterile field in a hospital.

CHAPTER OUTLINE

- Chain of Infection
- Asepsis

KEY TERMS

Asepsis: It is a condition in which no living disease-causing microorganisms are present.

Drape: To cover somebody/something.

Medical asepsis: A set of practices that aim to prevent the spread of infection by reducing the number of microorganisms in an environment or on an object.

Surgical asepsis: Also known as sterile technique, is a set of practices and techniques that aims to create and maintain a sterile environment during invasive medical procedures.

CHAIN OF INFECTION

Definition

The "Chain of Infection" describes the process of infection that begins when an infectious agent leaves its reservoir through a portal of exit, and is transmitted by a mode of transmission entering through a portal of entry to infect a susceptible host (Fig. 14.1).

Causes of Infection

- **Infectious agent** or the microorganism which can cause disease. Microorganisms that are responsible for causing disease production:
  - Viruses
  - Bacteria
  - Fungi
  - Protozoa and Helminthes
  - Parasites

Agents are factors that affect disease transmission through infectivity, pathogenicity, virulence, invasiveness.

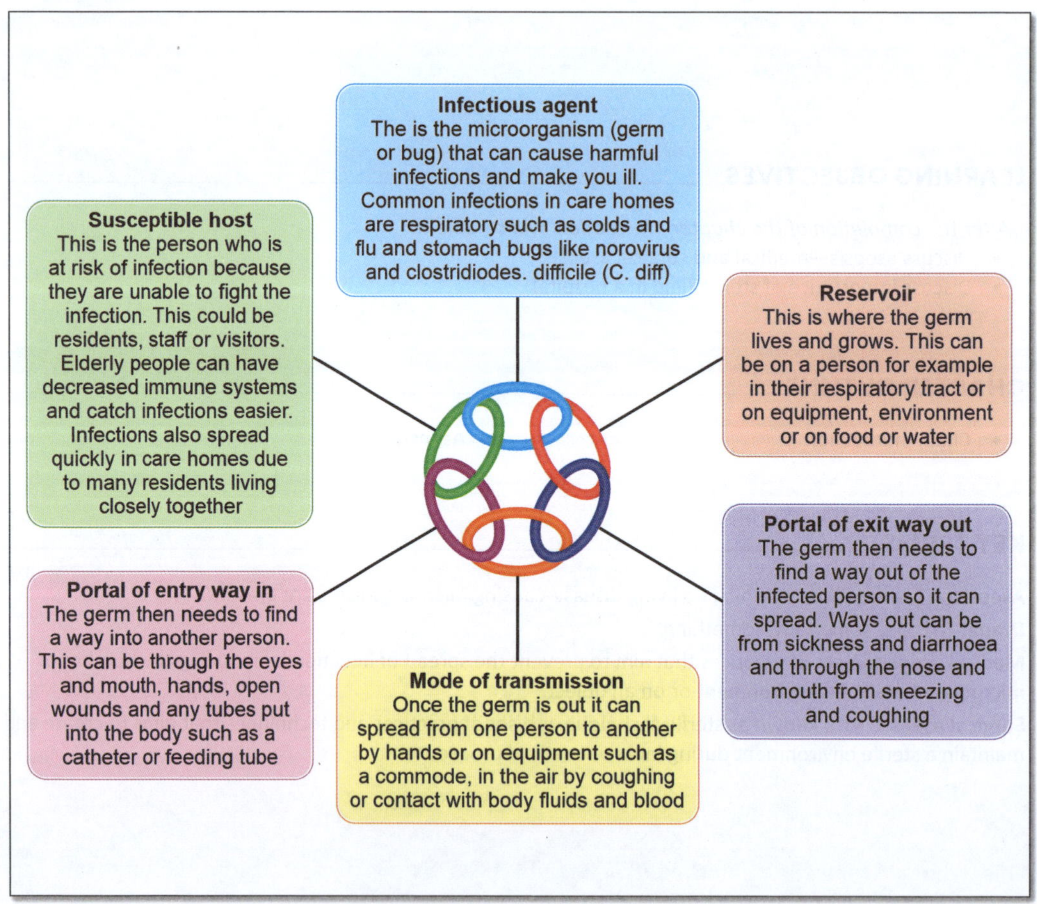

Figure 14.1: Chain of Infection

Reservoir or Source of Infection

Reservoir or source of infection where the microorganism can live and thrive. A reservoir is any person, animal, arthropod, plant, soil or substance (or combination of these) in which an infectious agent normally lives and multiplies. The infectious agent depends on the reservoir for survival, where it can reproduce itself in such manner that it can be transmitted to a susceptible host.

- Animate reservoirs include people, insects, birds, and other animals.
- Inanimate reservoirs include soil, water, food, feces, intravenous fluid, and equipment.

Portal of Exit

Portal of exit from the reservoir. This describes the way the microorganism leaves the reservoir. It is the means by which a pathogen exits from a reservoir. For a human reservoir, the portal of exit can include blood, respiratory secretions, and anything exiting from the gastrointestinal or urinary tracts. Once a pathogen has exited the reservoir, it needs a mode of transmission to transfer itself into a host. This is accomplished by entering the host through a receptive portal of entry. Transmission can be by direct contact, indirect contact, or through the air.

Mode of Transmission

This describes how microorganisms are transmitted from one person or place to another. This could be *via* someone's hands, on an object, through the air or bodily fluid contact.

- **Direct contact**
  - Skin-to-skin contact, kissing, and sexual intercourse.
  - Direct contact refers also to contact with soil, vegetation or water that is contaminated with the infectious agent.
- **Droplet spread**
  - Transmission by direct spray of relatively large, short-range aerosols over a few feet, before the droplets fall to the ground.
  - These aerosols may be produced by sneezing, coughing, or talking.
- **Indirect contact**
  - Indirect transmission of an agent from a reservoir to a susceptible host through suspended particles, vehicles or vectors.
  - **Air particles:** Dust may contain agents, e.g., fungal spores. Droplet nuclei residues (dried droplet spread) coughed or sneezed into the air usually less than 5 µ (microns) in size.
  - **Vehicles:** Infectious agent is carried from a reservoir to a susceptible host by a non-living intermediary, e.g., contaminated food, water, biologics (blood products), and fomites (inanimate objects such as medical equipment, surfaces, bedding).
  - **Vectors:** Infectious agent is carried from a reservoir to a susceptible host by a living intermediary, e.g., insects such as mosquitoes, fleas, and ticks (mechanical or biological)

Portals of Entry

This is how the infection enters another individual. Infectious agents get into the body through various portals of entry, including the mucous membranes, non-intact skin, and the respiratory, gastrointestinal, and genitourinary tracts. Pathogens often enter the body of the host through the same route they exited the reservoir, e.g., airborne pathogens from one person's sneeze can enter through the nose of another person.

Susceptible Host

This describes the person who is vulnerable to infection. Infection does not occur automatically when the pathogen enters the body of a person whose immune system is functioning normally. When a virulent pathogen enters an immune-compromised person, however, infection generally follows.

ASEPSIS

Asepsis is a condition in which no living disease-causing microorganisms are present. Asepsis covers all those procedures designed to reduce the risk of bacterial, fungal or viral contamination, using sterile instruments, sterile draping and the gloved 'no touch' technique. It means absence of disease producing microorganisms.

Definitions of Asepsis

- Asepsis is the state of being free from disease causing contaminants or preventing contact with microorganisms.
- Asepsis is the process of removing pathogenic microorganisms or protecting against infection by such organisms.
- Asepsis is the practice to reduce or eliminate contaminants from entering the operative field in surgery or medicine to prevent infection.

Types of Asepsis

There are two types of asepsis: Medical and surgical.

Medical Asepsis–Clean Technique

All practices that reduce the number, growth, transfer and spread of pathogenic microorganisms. These include hand washing, bathing, cleaning environment, gloving, gowning, wearing mask, hair and shoe covers, disinfecting articles and use of antiseptics. Medical asepsis can be followed by sanitization, antisepsis and disinfection.

- **Sanitization:** Sanitization refers to cleaning practices and techniques that physically remove microorganisms. These include hand washing and cleaning of clients' personal equipment, clothing and linens.
- **Antisepsis:** Antisepsis is the process of killing microorganisms or limiting their growth on the skin and nonliving objects. Chemicals used in antisepsis are called *antiseptics* and the most common ones include rubbing alcohol and iodine. Antiseptics can be used for hand scrubbing, treating cuts, wounds and burns and preoperative skin cleaning.
- **Disinfection:** Disinfection refers to the process of killing microorganisms on objects that are commonly in contact with your clients, such as overbed tables, wheelchairs, stretchers, urinals, bedpans and blood pressure cuffs. It is important to note that disinfection cannot destroy

spores, which are highly resistant forms of microorganisms that develop in conditions that are inconvenient for their growth.

Essential Components of Medical Asepsis

Essential components of maintaining medical asepsis in a hospital/institution include:

- Hand washing
- Utilizing gloves, gown and mask
- Using clean equipment
- Handling linens in ways that prevent germs from spreading. Medical asepsis protects both residents and care givers from becoming ill.

Medical aseptic practices are involved in all nursing activities because microorganisms are always present in the environment.

Methods of Medical Asepsis

Various methods involved in medical asepsis are as follows:

- Isolation precautions
- Hand washing
- Use of disposables, clean surfaces
- Use of gown, mask, gloves and glasses
- Concurrent and terminal disinfection
- Control of visitors/relatives
- Teaching of visitors/relatives
- Developing staff health, hygiene and education
- Preventive vaccination, inoculation and medicines
- Use of efficient devices for aseptic practices

Surgical Asepsis–Sterile Technique

Surgical asepsis is a practice that keeps an area or an object free from all microorganisms including spores. It is the exclusion of all microorganisms before they can enter an open surgical wound or contaminate a sterile field during surgery to break the chain of infection. Surgical asepsis is practiced in operating rooms and special diagnostic areas. It may be practiced in general care areas too (Fig. 14.2).

Principles of Surgical Asepsis

The principles of surgical asepsis are as follows:

- Surgical asepsis starts with sterile equipment and setting up the sterile field.
- All objects used in a sterile field must be sterile.
- Confirm sterility of the package. Check expiration date and ensure package is clean and dry. Only sterile items are used within the sterile field. If in doubt about the sterility of the packaged item, it is not considered sterile.

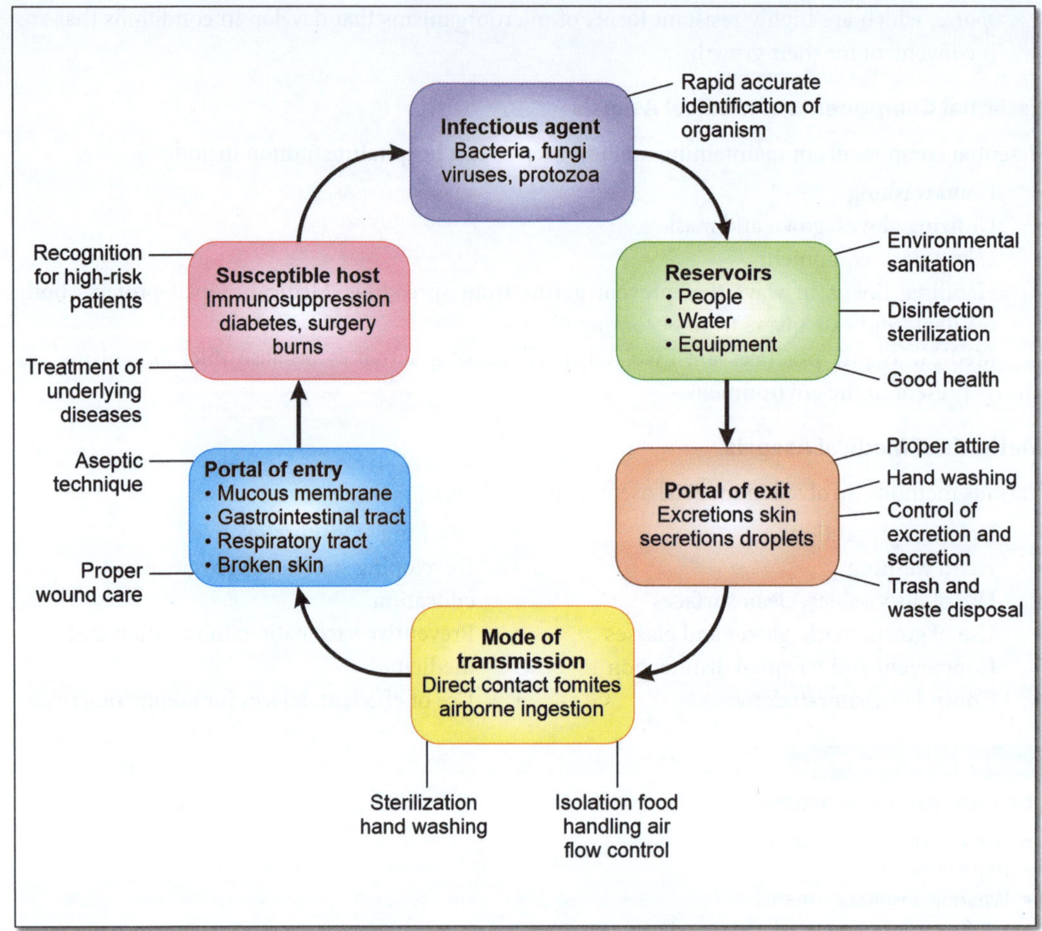

Figure 14.2: Breaking chain of infection

- Whenever a sterile item has been compromised, the package contents, gown or the sterile field involved must be considered contaminated.
- Single use medical devices shall only be used on an individual client for a single procedure and then must be discarded.
- Reusable medical devices shall be reprocessed according to the manufacturer's directions for use.

Must Know

Four Rules of Surgical Asepsis

1. Know what is sterile.
2. Know what is not sterile.
3. Separate sterile from non-sterile.
4. Remove contamination immediately.

Comparison of medical and surgical asepsis is given in Table 14.1.

TABLE 14.1: Comparison of medical and surgical asepsis	
Medical asepsis	**Surgical asepsis**

• Reduces number of pathogens
• Referred to as clean techniques
• Used in administration of:
  ▪ Medicine
  ▪ Enema
  ▪ Tube feeding
  ▪ Hygiene
  ▪ Hand washing
	• Eliminates all pathogens
	• Referred to as sterile techniques
	• Used in:
	  ▪ Dressing·changes
	  ▪ Surgical procedure
	  ▪ Catheterization
	  ▪ Scrubbing

Sterile Field

Sterile field is a microorganism-free area, including free of spores. To maintain an area free of microorganisms, sterile gloves, gowns and drapes are used to create a barrier between the environment and the client.

Establishing a Sterile Field

Sterile drapes used to cover surfaces or operative fields shall provide a barrier against microorganisms, liquids and particulate matter. Drapes are only sterile at table level. The drapes below the working surface are not under direct vision of the surgical team and is not considered sterile. If the drape does not cover the entire surface, a 1 inch margin around the edge of the drapes is not considered sterile.

Sterile and Unsterile Area

- The edges of the tabletop serve as a demarcation line between sterile and nonsterile.
- Any item that falls below the table level is considered unsterile.
- The edges of packages are not considered sterile. When opening packages for a sterile procedure, the packaging must be managed in a manner that prevents the wrapper from touching the sterile field or packaged contents.
- All flat surfaces shall be dry and dust free before placing a sterile bundle or drape on them.
- The skin cannot be sterilized and is unsterile. Sterile persons and items contact only sterile areas, unsterile persons and items contact only unsterile areas. Sterile object become unsterile when touched by unsterile objects.
- Sterile objects become unsterile by prolonged exposure to airborne microorganisms.

Precautions Observed in a Sterile Field

- Do not cough, sneeze or talk excessively over a sterile field. Always maintain some space with the sterile field.
- Movement within and around a sterile field must be such as not to cause contamination of that sterile field.
- Sterile gowns are considered sterile in front, shoulder to table level. The sleeves are also sterile.

Note: Conscientiousness, alertness and honesty are essential qualities in maintaining surgical asepsis.

Principles for Maintaining a Sterile Field

- The circulatory nurse shall not touch or reach over sterile items or areas.
- The scrubbed assistant shall not touch or reach over unsterile items or areas.
- When a scrubbed assistant opens a sterile table cover or drape, it is opened first toward the sterile individual.
- If the circulating assistant opens a sterile pack, the wrap is opened first away from the circulating assistant to prevent contamination of the pack.
- Movement within the sterile field must not contaminate the field.
- Sterile personnel stay close to the sterile field.
- Sterile personnel must never turn their back on the sterile field.
- Open sterile supplies shall not be left unattended and continuously monitored for possible contamination.
- The sterile set up shall not be covered.

Sterile Supplies

Supplies shall be opened as close as possible to the surgical start time. Sterile supplies shall be handled as little as possible. All articles added to sterile field shall be assessed prior to opening for sterility by checking package integrity and that chemical indicators should show, a "pass" result. Large bundles or packages shall be opened on a flat surface. Items introduced on to a sterile field should be opened, dispensed and transferred by methods that maintain sterility and integrity.

Sterile solution must be paused into a sterile receptacle. Once the sterile solution of the bottle has been dispensed into the sterile receptacle, discard the remaining solution (if any).

Once a patient has entered the operation theater where sterile supplies have been opened, those supplies shall be discarded in the event the procedure is canceled or if they are not used.

Surgical Hand Scrubbing

- Surgical hand scrubbing is a process of removing as many microorganisms as possible from the hands and forearms by mechanical washing and chemical antisepsis before surgery.
- It should be performed prior to donning sterile gloves or sterile gowns for surgical or other procedure.
- If hands are visibly soiled, they must be washed and dried prior to surgical hand scrub.
- All rings, wrist watch, bracelets and bangles must be removed before starting surgical scrub.
- Haircap, eye wear and surgical mask must be donned prior to initiating the surgical hand scrub.
- Hands should be held above the level of the elbow both during the scrub and rinsing. Contact with the faucet must be avoided.
- Wash hands with plain soap and water, warm water, cleanse nails with disposable nail cleaning device.

- Rinse hands and forearms under running water.
- Don sterile surgical gown and gloves.
- Nails must be natural, clean, short and healthy.
- Do not wear artificial nails.
- Remove all hands and arm jewelry.

Gloving and Gowning

- Gowns are only considered sterile in the front from the axilla to the level of the sterile field and sleeves from 5 cm above the elbow to cuff.
- The neckline shoulders, under arms, gloves cuff and the back are considered unsterile.
- Gowns are donned before gloves.
- The sterile gown is lifted out of its sterile wrapper without contamination.
- The gown is held away from the body and unfolded so that the inside is toward the wearer.
- The hands are slipped into the gown while keeping them away from the body and at shoulder level.
- The hands are advanced up the sleeves of the gown to the proximal end of the cuffs.
- Gloving is performed by the closed and open method.

Hand Washing

- After touching an animal, animal feed, or animal waste
- After handing pet food or pet treats
- After touching garbage

To maintain optimum hand hygiene, it is recommended that nothing is worn below the elbows (except for a plain bands), and that the fingernails are clean and trimmed. The use of soap and water is specifically indicated when the hands are visibly soiled or when they have come into contact with spore-forming pathogens, such as clostridium difficile.

Procedure

- Wet hands with water, and apply soap to cover hand surfaces
- Rub hands palm to palm
- Right palm over left dorsum with interlaced fingers and vice versa
- Palm to palm with fingers interlaced
- Rotational rubbing, backwards and forwards with clasped fingers of the right hand, and vice versa
- Rinse hands with water and dry with a single use towel
- Use the towel to turn off the tap

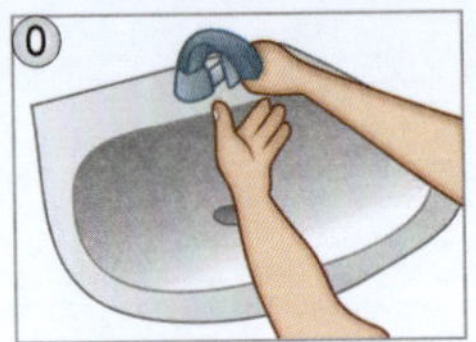

Wet hands with water

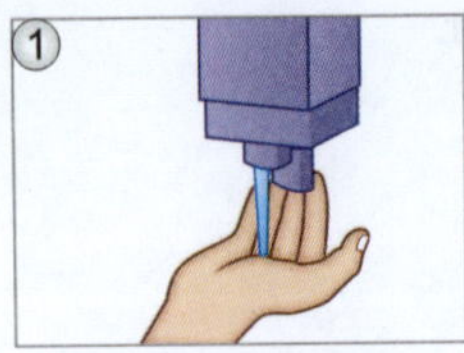

Apply enough soap to cover all hand surfaces

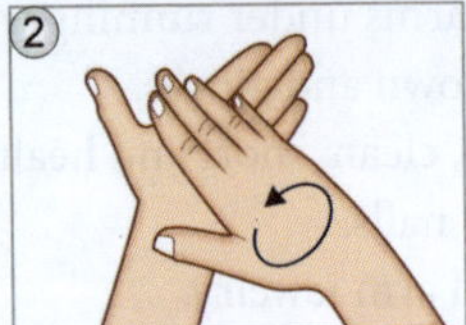

Rub hands palm to palm

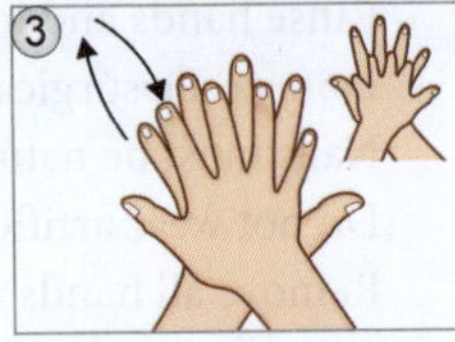

Right palm over left dorsum with interlaced fingers and vice versa

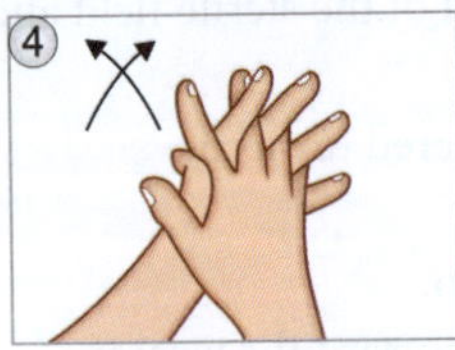

Palm to palm with fingers interlaced

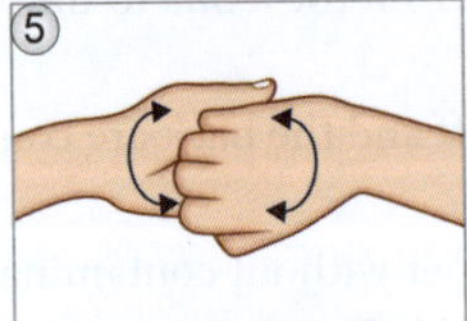

Backs of fingers to opposing palms with fingers interlocked

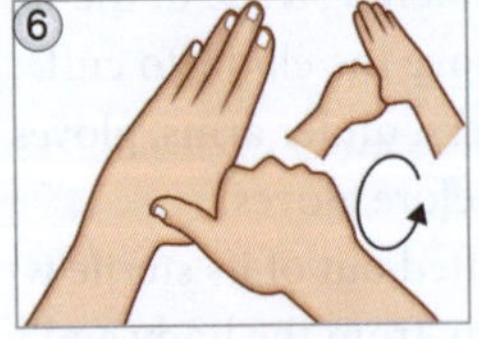

Rotational rubbing of left thumb clasped in right palm and vice versa

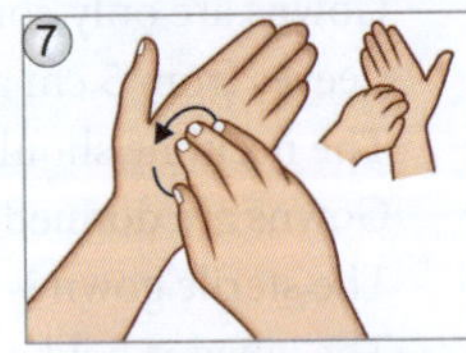

Rotational rubbing backwards and forwards with clasped fingers of right hand in left palm and vice versa

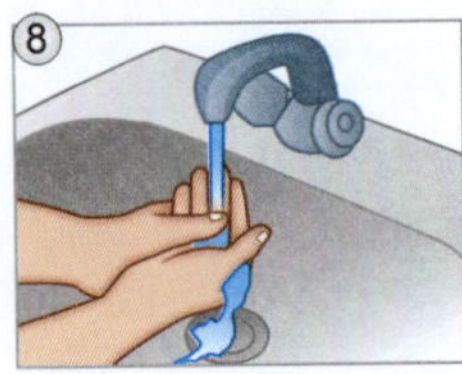

Rinse hands with water

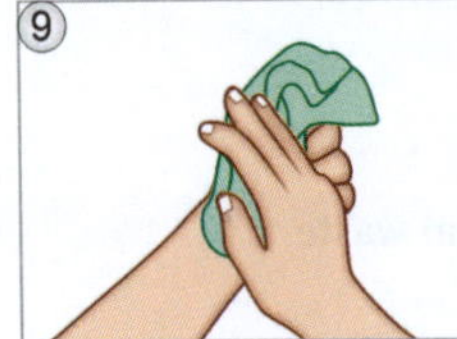

Dry hands thoroughly with a single use towel

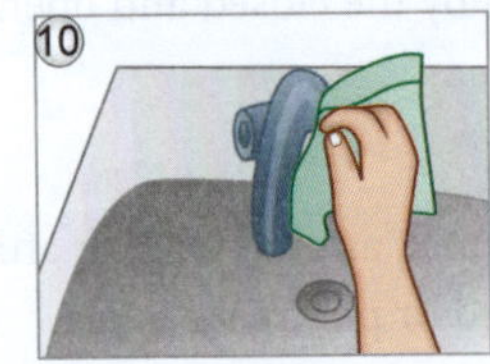

Use towel to turn off faucet

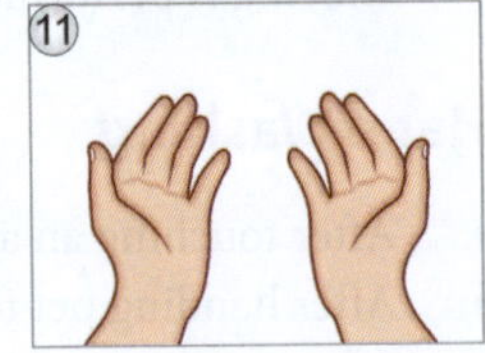

Your hands are now safe

FURTHER READINGS

- Asepsis. [online] Available from https://www.sciencedirect.com/topics/immunology-and-microbiology/asepsis [Last accessed August, 2023].
- Osmosis (Elsevier). Medical and surgical asepsis: Clinical skills notes. [online] Available from https://www.osmosis.org/learn/Medical_and_surgical_asepsis:_Clinical_skills_notes [Last accessed August, 2023].

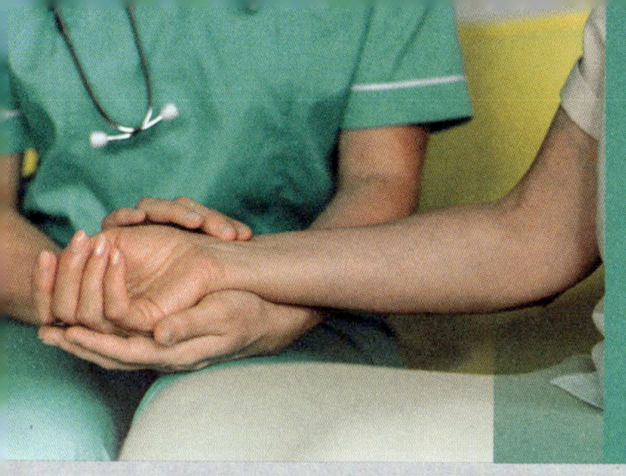

LONG ANSWER QUESTIONS

1. What do you know about asepsis?
2. What are the precautions required to maintain the sterile field?

SHORT ANSWER QUESTIONS

1. Write notes on:
   a. Medical asepsis
   b. Surgical asepsis
   c. Differences between medical and surgical asepsis
2. Write in brief about surgical hand scrubbing.

MULTIPLE CHOICE QUESTIONS

1. **Hand washing is an example of:**
   a. Surgical asepsis
   b. Safety
   c. Medical asepsis
   d. Sterility
2. **All are ways to break the chain of infection; except:**
   a. Hand washing
   b. Disinfection
   c. Sterilization
   d. Reusing gloves
3. **What is the single most effective way to break the chain of infection?**
   a. Hand washing
   b. Cleaning surfaces
   c. Sterilization
   d. Nutrition
4. **The process that eliminates most but not necessarily all microorganisms on nonliving surfaces is called:**
   a. Fumigation
   b. Disinfection
   c. Extermination
   d. Sterilization
5. **______________ is the absence of all microorganisms within any type of invasive procedure.**
   a. Asepsis
   b. Surgical asepsis
   c. Sterile technique
   d. Clean
6. **What is infection prevention?**
   a. An object has been prevented from being contaminated with pathogens
   b. The way in which infections occur
   c. An infection that is prevented from traveling from one part of the body to another
   d. A set of methods used to prevent the spread of disease

ANSWER KEY

1. c   **2.** d   **3.** a   **4.** b   **5.** b   **6.** d

Note

Most Probable Questions Asked in University

LONG ANSWER QUESTIONS

1. Describe nursing as a profession.
2. Describe the expanded role of graduate nurse.
3. What are the components of nursing process? Discuss
4. Describe the steps in nursing process with examples.
5. Write in detail about team nursing.
6. Explain ethical principles or nursing.
7. Define health. Explain self care theory in detail.
8. Define stress. What are the stages of stress? Describe any two models of stress and adaptation.
9. Describe the ICN's code of conduct.

SHORT ANSWER QUESTIONS/SHORT NOTES

1. Define nursing process.
2. List out the functions of Indian nursing council.
3. Expanded roles or nurses.
4. Write in brief about Nightingale's theory.
5. Legal issues in nursing.
6. Purpose and methods of physical examination.

7. Characteristics of nursing process.
8. Problem oriented nursing.
9. Nursing standards.
10. Nursing audit and professional conducts for nurses.
11. Qualities and functions of a nurse.
12. Orlando's nursing process theory.
13. Four types of nursing documentation.

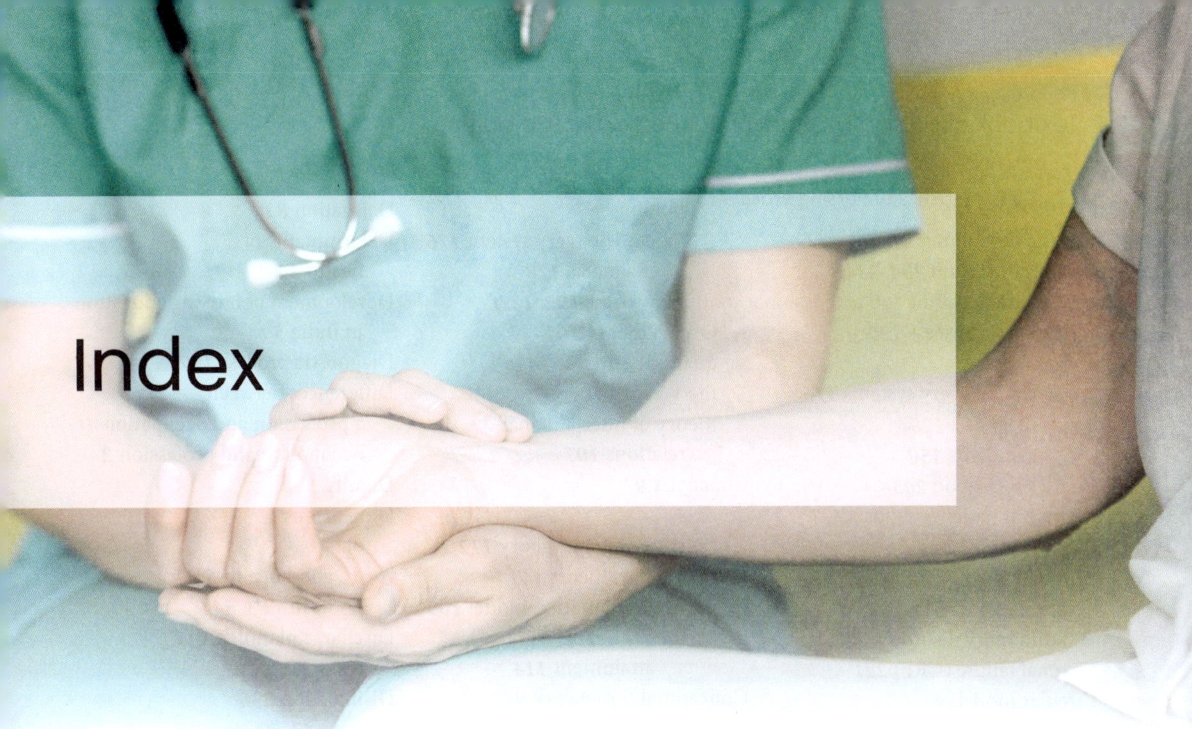

Index

Refer 'f' for figure and 't' for table, respectively